Hospital Management

AF654054

Hospital Management

Text and Cases

K.V. Ramani

Professor

Centre for Management of Health Services

Indian Institute of Management, Ahmedabad

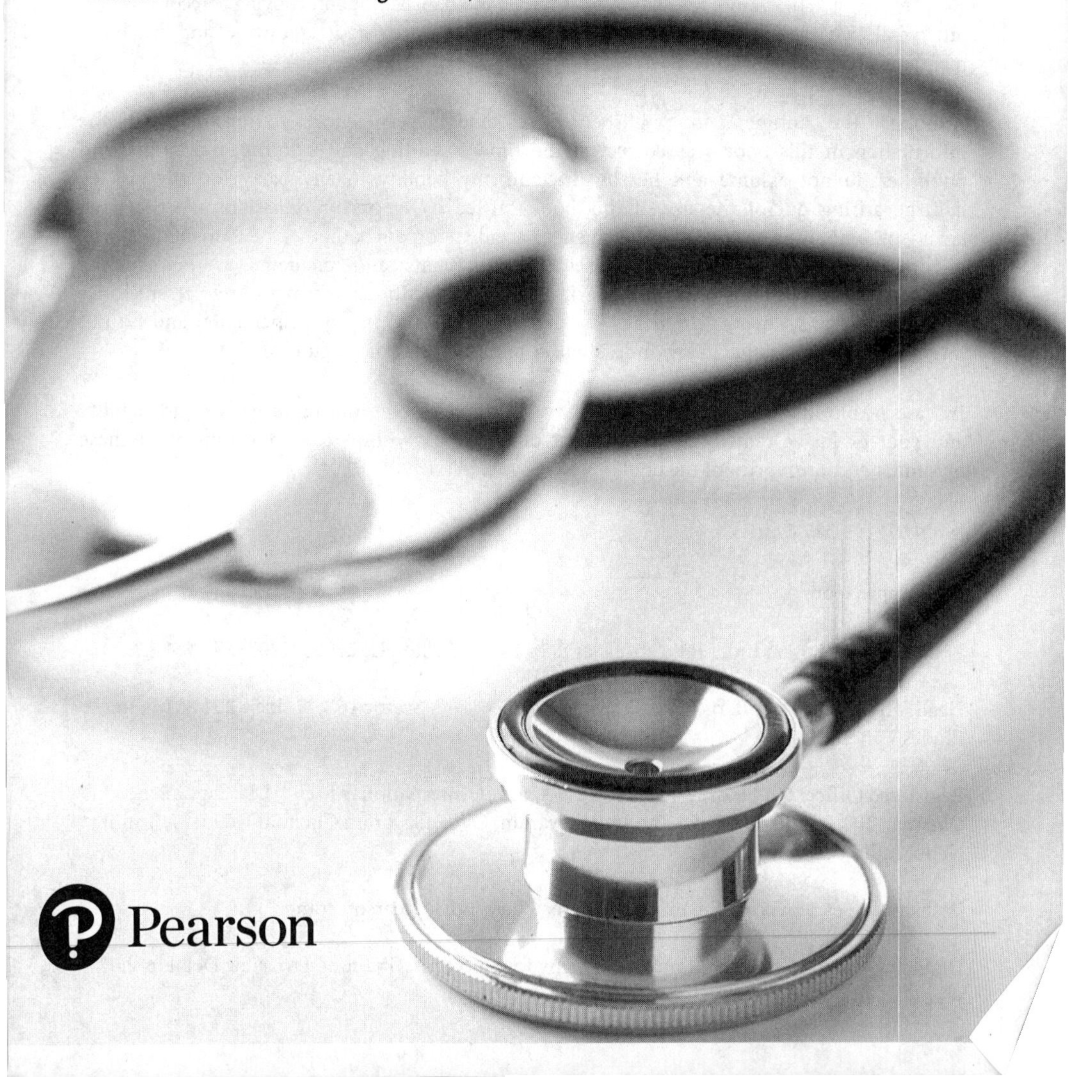

Pearson

Associate Editor–Acquisitions: Neeraj Bhalla *Associate Editor–Production*: Amrita Naskar

Copyright © 2013 Dorling Kindersley (India) Pvt. Ltd

This book is sold subject to the condition that it shall not, by way of trade or otherwise, be lent, resold, hired out, or otherwise circulated without the publisher's prior written consent in any form of binding or cover other than that in which it is published and without a similar condition including this condition being imposed on the subsequent purchaser and without limiting the rights under copyright reserved above, no part of this publication may be reproduced, stored in or introduced into a retrieval system, or trans-mitted in any form or by any means (electronic, mechanical, photocopying, recording or otherwise), without the prior written permission of both the copyright owner and the above-mentioned publisher of this book.

Although the author and publisher have made every effort to ensure that the information in this book was correct at the time of editing and printing, the author and publisher do not assume and hereby disclaim any liability to any party for any loss or damage arising out of the use of this book caused by errors or omissions, whether such errors or omissions result from negligence, accident or any other cause. Further, names, pictures, images, characters, businesses, places, events and incidents are either the products of the author's imagination or used in a fictitious manner. Any resemblance to actual persons, living or dead or actual events is purely coincidental and do not intend to hurt sentiments of any individual, community, sect or religion.

In case of binding mistake, misprints or missing pages etc., the publisher's entire liability and your exclusive remedy is replacement of this book within reasonable time of purchase by similar edition/reprint of the book.

ISBN 978-81-317-9401-2

First Impression

Published by Pearson India Education Services Pvt. Ltd, CIN: U72200TN2005PTC057128.

Head Office: 1st Floor, Berger Tower, Plot No. C-001A/2, Sector 16B, Noida - 201 301, Uttar Pradesh, India.

Registered Office: 6th Floor, Tower A, Unit A and B, International Tech Park, CapitaLand Chennai, 200 Feet Radial Road,Zamin Pallavaram, Old Pallavaram Chennai – 600117, Tamil Nadu, India

Website: in.pearson.com; Email: companysecretary.india@pearson.com

Digitally printed in India by Trinity Academy for Corporate Training Ltd, New Delhi in the year of 2026

Contents

List of Tables

List of Figures

Preface

If there's a book that you want to read but it hasn't been written yet, then you must write it.

—Toni Morrison

This book on 'Hospital Management: Text and Cases' is based on my experience in teaching this subject at the Indian Institute of Management, Ahmedabad (IIMA), over the last 12 years.

At IIMA, we have been offering a one-week Executive Development Programme on Hospital Management since 2001, which is attended by senior managers and administrators from medium to large hospitals, both from India and abroad. All the case studies included in this book are based on my research and consulting to the hospitals who have sponsored their managers to the above programme. Following the success of our one-week Executive Development Programme, we introduced an elective course on Hospital Management to our MBA students in 2005 and to our Faculty Development Programme for the university teachers in 2007. The feedback from teaching in the above programmes have helped me to properly organize the materials in this book to address the issues and challenges in hospital management.

Hospitals have become complex organizations as they consume vast amount of resources in delivering a wide range of healthcare services. The increased cost for medical care, ageing population, and the potentially declining levels of service threaten the quality of service delivered. The poor quality of services not only wastes resources but is positively dangerous to the health and welfare of the patients and the community at large. Hospital managers, current and future aspirants, therefore, need a certain amount of professional management inputs so as to manage the hospitals effectively and efficiently.

Chapters 1 and 2 provide a profile of the Indian healthcare industry within the overall global market, and, thereby, bring out the importance of hospital management in the Indian health sector.

Chapters 3, 4, and 5 explain the hospital management concepts, starting with a focus on the issues and challenges in delivering good quality hospital services. An introduction to queuing systems in Chapter 3 prepares the hospital managers to satisfactorily address the concerns on customer satisfaction. Hospital management functions, namely, operations management, finance and cost management, human resource management, and materials management are explained in detail in Chapter 4. Chapter 5 discusses the important role of hospital support systems, namely, clinical support, information support and administrative support systems in the delivery of hospital services.

Besides conceptual clarity, hospital managers need to develop problem-solving skills to diagnose the issues and address the challenges effectively and efficiently. Towards this, we discuss several real-life case studies from medium to large hospitals in chapters 6–10, which highlight the magnitude, complexity and nature of managerial challenges in delivering hospital services. These case studies focus on the management of outpatient services, inpatient discharge, cathlab scheduling, analysis of financial statements, cost management, impact of organizational changes on service quality, reengineering the purchase process, monitor and control of clinical lab errors, and so on.

A framework for analysing hospital management case studies is discussed in the last chapter along with an application of this framework in analysing a sample case—CMC Hospital, Vellore (A). The readers are expected to use this framework for solving other case studies presented in this book.

The organization of materials in this book is as shown below:

	Importance of Hospital Management	Objective
PART 1	Chapter 1 Healthcare Industry	Highlight the importance of hospital management in the Indian health sector.
	Chapter 2 Health Sector in India	

	Hospital Management Challenges	Objective
PART 2	Chapter 3 Hospital Management: Service Quality	Provide a working knowledge on concepts in hospital management.
	Chapter 4 Hospital Management Functions	
	Chapter 5 Hospital Management Support Systems	

	Hospital Management Case Studies	Objective
PART 3	Chapter 6 Hospital Operations Management	Develop skills in applying the concepts to address real-life issues in hospital management.
	Chapter 7 Hospital Finance and Cost Management	
	Chapter 8 Hospital Human Resource Management	
	Chapter 9 Hospital Materials Management	
	Chapter 10 Hospital MIS	

	A Framework for Case Analysis	Objective
PART 4	Chapter 11 Hospital Management Cases: A Framework for Analysis	Build a logical sequence of steps for case analysis.

I hope this book would serve as a textbook for a second year elective course on Hospital Management in the MBA programme on General Management, and as a textbook for a first year compulsory course in the MBA programme on Healthcare Management, as well as serve the needs of practicing hospital managers to augment their management capacity.

K.V. Ramani

Acknowledgements

I would like to express my sincere thanks to:

The Indian Institute of Management, Ahmedabad (IIMA), for supporting my research and teaching interests in the areas on hospital and healthcare management.

The co-authors of case studies, both from IIMA and the hospitals, for all their contributions in case development.

All the hospitals for their excellent support in developing the case studies. Special thanks to Apollo Hospitals for allowing me to reproduce certain financial statements from the Annual Report 2010–11.

The Ministry of Health and Family Welfare, Government of India for granting permission to use data from government publications.

The MBA students at IIMA, who have taken my elective course on Hospital Management, for their active class participation in case analysis and discussions.

The participants of our Executive Development Programme on Hospital Management for sharing with me their valuable insights into hospital management practices.

Reshmi at IIMA for her excellent secretarial assistance in preparing the manuscript.

The reviewers of this book whose suggestions helped me to improve the quality of the materials presented.

Neeraj, Shadan and Amrita at Pearson Education—Neeraj for his wholehearted support throughout this project and useful suggestions in the preparation of the manuscript; Shadan and Amrita for their painstaking efforts in coordinating the editing and layout of the material.

My family, Hema, Abhinay and Akshay, for their constant encouragement to write this book.

K.V. Ramani

About the Author

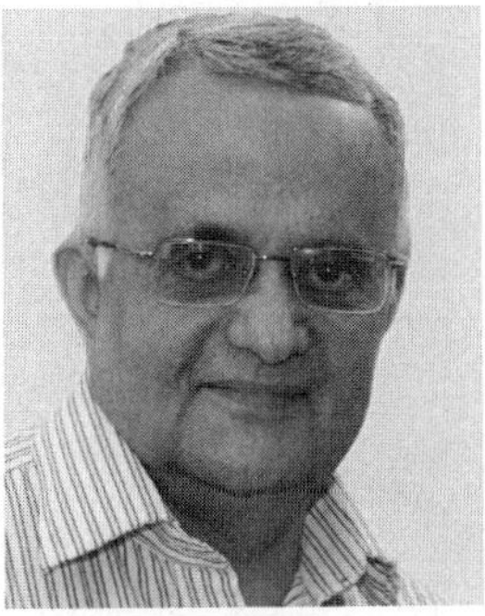

Prof. K.V. Ramani obtained his Ph.D. in Operations Research from Cornell University, USA in 1977. He is currently a Professor at the Centre for Management of Health Services at the Indian Institute of Management, Ahmedabad. He has also taught at Cornell University and Florida International University in USA, as well as the National University of Singapore. He has been a visiting research scholar at the University of Texas, Austin, USA; University of Leeds, UK; University of Warwick, UK; University of Western Sydney, Australia and the Helsinki School of Economics and Business Administration, Finland.

His current teaching and research interests are in the areas of Hospital Management, Governance and Management of Health Sector, HMIS, Maternal Health, Child Health, Urban Health, HIV/AIDS and so on. Dr Ramani has published extensively in international referred journals such as *Journal of Health Policy, Health Policy and Planning, Journal of Health Organization and Management, Interfaces, Naval Research Logistics, Journal of Strategic Information Systems, Simulation*, and so on. He has been a consultant to the World Bank, European Commission, UNOPS, USAID, Sida, Ministry of Health and Family Welfare, and a number of hospitals in India and abroad.

Prof. Ramani has served as a member on the Governing Board of IIM, Ahmedabad, Gujarat State Health Society, Gujarat Cancer Society and a few public sector units.

part 1

Importance of Hospital Management

CHAPTERS

OBJECTIVE

The main objective of this part is to highlight the importance of hospital management in the Indian health sector.

The Indian health sector faces a unique '1-2-3 challenge':

We need

1 million doctors
2 million nurses
3 million hospital beds,

so as to achieve the world average of the above indicators per 1,000 population.

chapter 1

Healthcare Industry

CHAPTER OUTLINE

CHAPTER OBJECTIVE

The main objective of this introductory chapter is to profile India's healthcare industry in the overall global context, and the challenges it faces for improving the health system performance to help hospital managers understand the overall context in which they work.

1.1 AN INTRODUCTION

The global healthcare industry, estimated at \$5[i] trillion, is one of the world's largest and fastest-growing industries consuming over 10 per cent of the Gross Domestic Product (GDP) of most developed nations. Health plays an important role in the national economic development of any country. Improvement in the GDP depends on the country's ability to increase productivity, which is possible only if the country's workforce is healthy.

> Health is a state of complete physical, mental and social well-being and not merely the absence of disease or infirmity (WHO).

Ancillary sectors of the healthcare industry include pharmaceuticals, medical equipments and devices, biotechnology, IT in healthcare, medical insurance, medical tourism, and so on.

Healthcare industry in India has grown from \$4 billion in 1990–91 to almost \$40 billion by 2011–12. Unfortunately, the Government of India's contribution to healthcare expenditure is only one per cent of the GDP, which accounts for less than 25 per cent of the total expenditure, while 'out-of-pocket' expenditure accounts for almost two-thirds of the private sector expenditure. India is ranked 171 out of 191 WHO member countries for public health spending and ranked 118 in health system performance.

> Healthcare services include inpatient care, outpatient care and non-medical health services such as nursing, midwifery, physiotherapy and so on (UN classification).

As India is on a path of economic development, we have to address several challenges to improve our health system performance.

1.2 A GLOBAL VIEW

The World Health Organization (WHO) defines health as a state of complete physical, mental and social well-being and not merely the absence of disease or infirmity.

Health services are the most visible part of any health system, both to the users and the general public. Good health services are those which deliver effective, safe and good quality services. Availability, access, affordability and equity are important determinants of health service delivery. Improving access, coverage and quality of health services depends on the ways services are organized and managed, and on the incentives influencing providers and users.[1]

According to the United Nations International Standard Industrial Classification,[2] healthcare industry consists of three categories, namely:

---

[i] \$ indicates USD.

- Hospital activities
- Medical and dental practice activities
- Other human health activities

Hospital activities are mostly inpatient services. Medical and dental practice activities are mostly outpatient services in hospitals, outpatient clinics, home, and so on. Other human health activities are mostly non-medical healthcare services, such as nursing, midwifery, physiotherapy, and so on.

Ancillary sectors of the healthcare industry include pharmaceuticals, medical equipment and devices, biotechnology, information technology (IT), medical insurance, medical tourism, and so on.

Healthcare Industry	Hospital services Outpatient services All other health services	Medical Medical Non-medical
Ancillary Sectors	Pharmaceuticals Medical equipment and devices Biotechnology Information technology Medical insurance Medical tourism	

1.2.1 Healthcare Industry

Healthcare industry is one of the world's largest and fastest growing industries consuming over 10 per cent of the GDP of most developed nations. In the year 2009, a group of 34 countries, called the Organization of Economic Cooperation and Development (OECD), accounted for about 75 per cent of the total expenditure. Emerging economies, namely, Brazil, Russia, India, China and South Africa (BRICS), accounted for 10–12 per cent of the global health spending, and the remaining expenditure was accounted by the rest of the world. The industry is expected to cross $5 trillion by the end of 2012.

The WHO, in its report on World Health Statistics 2011,[3] estimated 35.3 million healthcare workforce in the year 2009, consisting of 9.2 million physicians, 19.4 million nurses and midwives, 1.9 million dentists and other dentistry personnel, 2.6 million pharmacists and other pharmaceutical personnel, and over 1.3 million community health workers worldwide, making the healthcare industry one of the largest segments of the workforce.

1.2.2 Pharmaceuticals

The global market share of pharmaceutical industry was 800 billion in 2009 and is expected to cross $1 trillion by 2015.[4] The pharmaceutical industry is involved in research and development, production, marketing and distribution of drugs and medicines for prevention, cure and diagnostic needs. The R&D segment of this industry alone contributes to almost $200 billion, as it costs almost $1 billion for developing a safe drug. The GAVI alliance (Global Alliance for Vaccines and Immunization), a public–private partnership founded in 2000 by the UN, WHO and Gates Foundation is very actively engaged in vaccine research and distribution.

1.2.3 Medical Equipments

The global medical equipment and devices industry was valued at $300 billion in 2009 and is expected to cross the $500 billion by 2015.[5] This industry includes surgical and medical instruments, dental equipments and supplies, clinical laboratory and radiology/imaging diagnostic equipment, orthopedic devices, and so on. Home healthcare products are expected to become one of the fastest growing segments of the medical device industry as a result of the influence of the aging population. Developments in medical technology allow for earlier detection of diseases and more effective treatment options. For example, Picture Archiving and Communications Systems (PACS) which integrate radiology with information system for diagnostic imaging are expected to transform the healthcare delivery system. The OECD countries have a very large share of the medical equipment market at present, while emerging economies like China and India are expected to play a significant role in the next five years.

1.2.4 Biotechnology

Biotechnology, a major research area in the healthcare industry, is a $50 billion industry. It uses living organisms and bioprocesses in making a wide variety of biotech products. Biotechnology led to the development of antibiotics which led to the discovery of Penicillium by Alexander Fleming in 1928. Biotechnology is being applied to develop products for preventing, diagnosing and care for many chronic diseases. Though biotechnology is primarily used by the pharmaceutical industry, it has applications in agriculture, mining, waste treatment industries, and so on. China, United States, India, Australia and France are the market leaders of biotech products in the world.[6]

1.2.5 Information Technology

IT applications in healthcare industry is gaining wider acceptance now. The world healthcare IT market is expected to grow from $100 billion in 2009 to over $160 billion by 2015.[7] Increasing cost of healthcare service delivery is forcing many healthcare providers to use IT to enhance clinical/administrative workflow of hospitals. Systems such as Computerized Physician Order Entry Systems (CPOE), PACS, Electronic Medical Records (EMR), and so on help in reducing medical errors, and, thereby, improve the management of healthcare.

1.2.6 Medical Tourism

'Medical tourism' is a term coined by the travel industry to promote tourism combined with less expensive healthcare services across international borders. Over 50 countries have identified medical tourism as a national industry. However, accreditation and other measures of quality vary widely across the globe, and some destinations may become hazardous or even dangerous for medical tourists.[8] Thailand has taken the lead in medical tourism. Bumrungrad International is an internationally accredited, multi-specialty hospital located in the heart of Bangkok, Thailand. Founded in 1980, today it is the largest private hospital in Southeast Asia, with 554 beds and serves over a million patients (40 per cent are internationals) annually over 30 specialty centres.[9]

1.3 THE INDIA SCENARIO

1.3.1 Healthcare Industry

Healthcare industry in India has grown from $4 billion industry in 1990–91 to $20 billion by 2000–01 and is expected to grow to almost $40 billion by 2011–12.[10] The healthcare industry in India, thus, registered a compounded annual growth rate of almost 17 per cent during the period 1990–91 to 2000–01 and seven per cent during the period 2000–01 to 2011–12. The overall annual compounded growth rate over the period 1990–91 to 2011–12 has been around 11 per cent.

While the growth of the Indian healthcare industry has been good, India's current share of $40 billion is less than one per cent of the global healthcare industry estimated at $5 trillion. Our per capita expenditure on health estimated at $33 is very low. The WHO estimates that a minimum of $35–50 per person per year is needed to provide basic healthcare services. India, therefore, faces tremendous challenges to improve the health status of its citizens.

1.3.2 Pharmaceuticals

The Indian pharmaceutical industry, estimated at $18 billion in 2008–09,[11] is the world's fourth largest by volume and is likely to lead the manufacturing sector of India. It accounts for about 1.8 per cent of the global pharmaceutical industry. This industry is expected to grow by 12 per cent annually. About 10,000 units operate in this sector with almost two-thirds of them in the five states of Maharashtra, Gujarat, West Bengal, Andhra Pradesh and Tamil Nadu, and the top ten companies account for almost one-third of the total market.[12] This industry is different from many others; competition among the drug manufacturers has not brought down the prices. There is an urgent need to revise and strengthen the archaic drug regulatory system in India.

1.3.3 Medical Equipments

The medical equipment industry in India is very small. Its market in India was around $5 billion in 2010 and is likely to be a $7 billion by the end of 2012.[13] The report of the National Commission on Macroeconomics on Health[14] highlighted the poor investment in capital expenditure by the healthcare sector and argued for scaling it up to improve the quality of service delivery. India continues to import most of the equipments from the United States and other developed nations, which enjoy almost 70 per cent of this market share. Many large hospitals, pathological laboratories and imaging centres in the private sector have started making huge investments in medical technology, and project their investments in medical technology as a marketing tool to attract specialist doctors and patients.

1.3.4 Biotechnology

The Indian biotech industry accounts for almost two per cent of the global biotech market of $50 billion. Biopharmaceuticals account for almost 70 per cent of this market, with vaccines playing the leading role. India could play a very active role in biogenerics as an estimated $103 billion of patented products would lose their patents by 2012.[15] Since the establishment of the Department of Biotechnology by the Government of India in 1986 under the Ministry of Science and Technology, many small start-up companies have entered this market. The government is also encouraging foreign investment in biotech sector. This sector is likely to be a leader in the employment of skilled human resources like the IT sector.

1.3.5 Medical Insurance

Medical insurance started in India in 1987 when mediclaim policy was announced by the government-owned insurance companies.[16] This market is dominated by the government-run General Insurance Company (GIC) with its four subsidiaries. The Government of India opened this sector for private companies in 2000, but successful private sector participation has been minimal, may be due to lack of quality healthcare service delivery. Total premiums under voluntary health insurance account for barely three per cent of the total health spending in India.[17]

The Employees State Insurance Scheme (ESIS) launched in 1952[18] by the Ministry of Labour, Government of India, offers a comprehensive social and medical insurance cover for low-paid workers in small-scale units.

Rashtriya Swasthya Bima Yojana (RSBY) was launched on 1 April 2008 by the Ministry of Labour and Employment, Government of India, to provide health insurance coverage for below poverty line (BPL) families. This scheme jointly funded by the central government (75 per cent) and state government (25 per cent) provides cashless insurance for hospitalization in public as well private hospitals, up to ₹30,000 (approx. $670 as of March 2011) per family per year. More than 27.3 million families are currently enrolled in RSBY, it has been implemented in 24 states and 396 districts, 3.1 million hospitalization cases have been benefited since the inception of the scheme in 2008.[19]

Having provided an overview of the healthcare industry, we highlight in the next section, the role of healthcare in the national economic development.

1.4 HEALTH AND NATIONAL ECONOMY

Healthcare industry plays an important role in the national economic development of any country. The ultimate goal of the national economic policy of any country is to improve the living standards of its individuals and the community. A common measure of the standard of living is the GDP per capita. Improvement in the GDP depends on the country's ability to increase productivity. Increased productivity is possible only if the country's workforce is healthy. While good health leads to increased productivity, poor health status reduces productivity and leads to higher consumption. The positive correlation between good health and economic performance has been well established.[20]

We first define certain indicators of economic development and healthcare expenditure.

GDP (Nominal): The market value of all final goods and services from a nation in a given year, usually expressed in USD using the government official exchange rate.

GDP (PPP): The market value of all final goods and services from a nation in a given year derived from purchasing power parity (PPP) calculations. This is expressed in equivalent international dollars.[ii]

[ii] Unless otherwise mentioned, we use international dollar (PPP) for all economic indicators.

GDP per Capita (PPP): GDP (PPP) divided by the average or mid-year population for the same year.

Total Health Expenditure per Capita (PPP): Total expenditure on health measures the final consumption of health goods and services (current health expenditure) plus capital investment infrastructure. This includes both public and private sources on medical services and goods, public health and prevention programmes and administration.

Total Health Expenditure as a Percentage of GDP: Total health expenditure divided by GDP for same year.

To compare countries across the world on their expenditure on health, it would be useful to classify all the countries in the world into three groups, namely, OECD, BRICS and others. The OECD and BRICS groups of countries account for almost 55 per cent and 20 per cent of the world GDP, respectively.

In tables 1.1 and 1.2, we give the International Monitory Fund (IMF) estimates[iii] of the above indicators (accessed through Wikipedia web site) for the OECD group of developed countries and the BRICS group of developing countries, respectively.

These tables give the estimates of a number of important indicators to relate health expenditure with the national economy of the OECD and BRICS countries.

Tables 1.1 and 1.2 have the OECD and BRICS countries ranked on GDP (PPP).

Figure 1.1 has the OECD and BRICS countries sorted on GDP per capita.

Figure 1.2 has the OECD and BRICS countries sorted on health expenditure per capita.

> About 70 per cent of the global healthcare expenditure is spent by the OECD countries which account for 18 per cent of the world population.

It can be seen from tables 1.1 and 1.2 that India with a GDP (PPP) of four trillion international dollars is the fourth largest economy in the world after the United States ($14.5 trillion), China ($10 trillion) and Japan ($4.3 trillion).

An analysis of healthcare spending in relation to a nation's GDP reveals some very interesting facts. The OECD countries spend an average of nine per cent of their GDP on health. India, the fourth largest economy in the world, spends only 4.2 per cent of its GDP on health.

[iii] While estimates from other sources may differ from IMF estimates, the overall picture would be more or less the same.

Table 1.1 Indicators of Economic Development and Health Expenditure: OECD Countries

Sr. No.	OECD Countries	GDP (PPP) Intl $ Million 2010	GDP (PPP) per Capita Intl $ 2010	Total Health Exp per Capita PPP Intl $ 2009	Total Health Exp as % GDP 2009
1	The United States	14,526,550	46,860	7,960	17.4
2	Japan	4,323,504	33,885	2,878	8.5
3	Germany	2,944,352	36,081	4,218	11.6
4	The United Kingdom	2,181,456	35,059	3,487	9.8
5	France	2,134,941	33,910	3,978	11.8
6	Italy	1,778,832	29,480	3,137	9.5
7	Mexico	1,564,872	14,406	918	6.4
8	S Korea	1,466,125	29,997	1,879	6.9
9	Spain	1,372,720	29,830	3,067	9.5
10	Canada	1,334,143	39,171	4,363	11.4
11	Turkey	968,604	13,577	902	6.1
12	Australia	883,807	39,764	3,445	8.7
13	Poland	723,032	18,981	1,394	7.4
14	Netherlands	680,772	40,973	4,914	12.0
15	Belgium	396,035	36,274	3,946	10.9
16	Sweden	356,321	38,204	3,722	10.0
17	Austria	333,537	39,761	3,445	8.7
18	Switzerland	326,741	41,950	5,144	11.4
19	Greece	318,670	28,496	2,724	9.6
20	Czech Rep	262,144	24,950	2,108	6.8
21	Chile	258,536	15,040	1,186	8.4
22	Norway	255,022	51,959	5,352	9.6
23	Portugal	247,458	23,262	2,508	10.1
24	Israel	219,954	29,602	2,104	7.9
25	Denmark	201,702	36,443	4,348	11.5
26	Hungary	188,677	22,195	1,511	7.4
27	Finland	187,696	34,918	3,226	9.2
28	Ireland	176,555	39,492	3,781	9.5
29	Slovakia	120,524	18,841	2,084	9.1
30	New Zealand	118,522	27,130	2,983	10.3
31	Slovenia	56,663	28,073	2,579	9.3
32	Luxemburg	41,271	81,466	4,808	7.8
33	Estonia	24,762	18,527	1,393	7.0
34	Iceland	11,853	36,730	3,538	9.7

Sources: Wikipedia and World Bank web sites

List of countries by GDP (PPP). Available at http://en.wikipedia.org/wiki/List_of_countries_by_GDP_PPP. Last accessed on 31 Dec 2011.

List of countries by GDP (PPP) per capita. Available at http://en.wikipedia.org/wiki/List_of_countries_by_GDP_PPP_per_capita. Last accessed on 31 Dec 2011.

List of countries by total health expenditure (PPP) per capita: http://en.wikipedia.org/wiki/List_of_countries_by_total_health_expenditure_PPP_per_capita, accessed on 31 Dec 2011.

Health expenditure, total (% of GDP). Available at http://data.worldbank.org/indicator/SH.XPD.TOTL.ZS. Last accessed on 31 Dec 2011.

Table 1.2 Indicators of Economic Development and Health Expenditure: BRICS Countries

Sr. No.	BRICS Countries	GDP (PPP) Intl $ Million 2010	GDP (PPP) per Capita Intl $ 2010	Total Health Exp per Capita PPP Intl $ 2009	Total Health Exp as % GDP 2009
1	China	10,119,896	7,544	345	4.6
2	India	4,000,002	3,408	142	4.2
3	Russia	2,230,954	15,612	842	5.4
4	Brazil	2,178,529	11,273	1,025	9.1
5	South Africa	525,806	10,518	890	8.5

Sources: Wikipedia and World Bank web sites

List of countries by GDP (PPP). Available at http://en.wikipedia.org/wiki/List_of_countries_by_GDP_PPP. Last accessed on 31 Dec 2011.

List of countries by GDP (PPP) per capita. Available at http://en.wikipedia.org/wiki/List_of_countries_by_GDP_PPP_per_capita. Last accessed on 31 Dec 2011.

List of countries by total health expenditure (PPP) per capita: http://en.wikipedia.org/wiki/List_of_countries_by_total_health_expenditure_PPP_per_capita, accessed on 31 Dec 2011.

Health expenditure, total (% of GDP). Available at http://data.worldbank.org/indicator/SH.XPD.TOTL.ZS. Last accessed on 31 Dec 2011.

While countries with higher GDP tend to spend more on healthcare, there are wide variations. The United States is the highest spender on health services; it spends $7,960 per capita, 2.5 times the OECD average spending of $3,200 (PPP) per capita. Norway and Switzerland spend two-thirds of the per capita level of the United States. Most of the northern and western European countries spend between $3,200 and 4,400 (110 per cent to 150 per cent OECD average). The OECD countries spending below the OECD average are Mexico, Turkey, and many in southern and eastern Europe. About 75 per cent of the healthcare expenditure is spent by OECD countries which account for 18 per cent of the world population.

The GDP is not the sole factor influencing health expenditure levels. For example, Germany and Finland have similar GDP per capita, but their health spending per capita differs considerably with Germany spending 11.6 per cent, and Finland only 9.2 per cent. In other words, Germany spent 25 per cent more than Finland on health per capita even though they are at similar levels of GDP per capita. Figure 1.1 shows the GDP per capita and health expenditure per capita for the top 10 countries in the world and India.

Next, we examine the source of health spending by the developed and developing countries. Tables 1.3 and 1.4 give the total spending and the government share of health spending by OECD and BRICS countries, respectively.

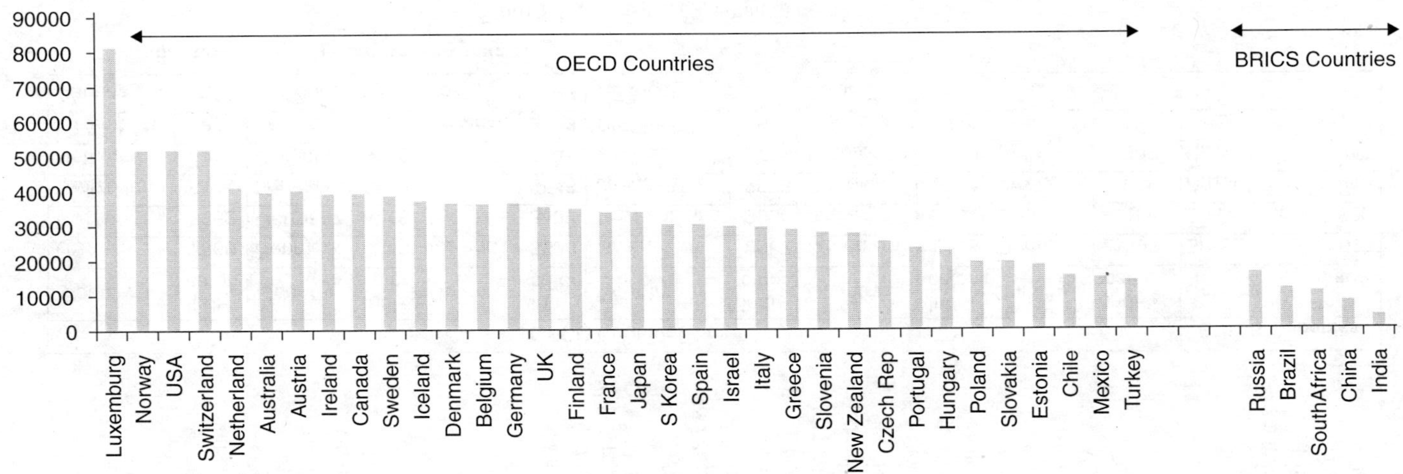

OECD Countries												BRICS Countries	
Country	Indi-cator	Country	Indi-cator	Country	Indi-cator	Country	Indi-cator	Country	Indi-cator	Country	Indi-cator	Country	Indi-cator
Luxemburg	81466	Austria	39761	Belgium	36274	S Korea	29997	New Zealand	27130	Estonia	18527	Russia	15612
Norway	51959	Ireland	39492	Germany	36081	Spain	29830	Czech Rep	24950	Chile	15040	Brazil	11273
USA	46860	Canada	39171	UK	35059	Israel	29602	Portugal	23262	Mexico	14406	South Africa	10518
Switzerland	41950	Sweden	38204	Finland	34918	Italy	29480	Hungary	22195	Turkey	13577	China	7544
Netherlands	40973	Iceland	36730	France	33910	Greece	28496	Poland	18981			India	3408
Australia	39764	Denmark	36443	Japan	33885	Slovenia	28073	Slovakia	18841				

Indicator: GDP per capita

Figure 1.1 GDP Per Capita (PPP)

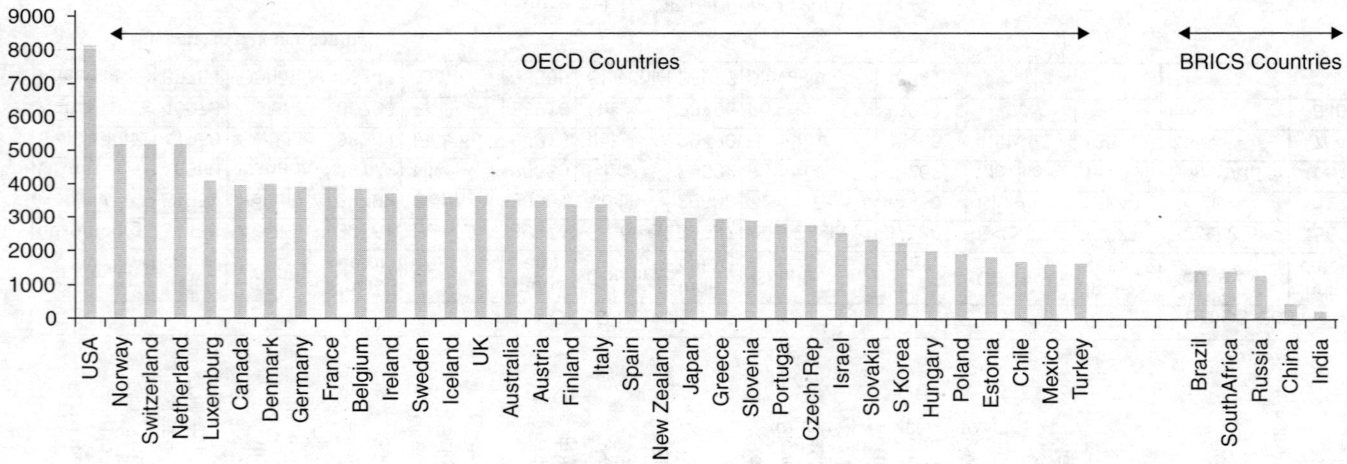

OECD Countries												BRICS Countries	
Country	Indi-cator	Country	Indi-cator	Country	Indi-cator	Country	Indi-cator	Country	Indi-cator	Country	Indi-cator	Country	Indi-cator
USA	7960	Denmark	4348	Iceland	3538	Spain	3067	Czech Rep	2108	Estonia	1393	Brazil	1025
Norway	5352	Germany	4218	UK	3487	New Zealand	2983	Israel	2104	Chile	1186	South Africa	890
Switzerland	5144	France	3978	Australia	3445	Japan	2878	Slovakia	2084	Mexico	918	Russia	842
Netherlands	4914	Belgium	3946	Austria	3445	Greece	2724	S Korea	1879	Turkey	902	China	345
Luxemburg	4808	Ireland	3781	Finland	3226	Slovenia	2579	Hungary	1511			India	142
Canada	4363	Sweden	3722	Italy	3137	Portugal	2508	Poland	1394				

Indicator: Health expenditure per capita

Figure 1.2 Health Expenditure Per Capita (PPP)

Table 1.3 Public Health Expenditure as Percentage Total Health Expenditure: OECD Countries

Sr. No.	OECD Countries	Total Health Exp as % GDP 2009	Public Health Exp as % of Total Health Expenditure 2009
1	The United Kingdom	9.8	83.6
2	Iceland	9.7	82.3
3	Czech Rep	6.8	80.2
4	New Zealand	10.3	80.2
5	Denmark	11.5	80.1
6	Japan	8.5	80.0
7	Ireland	9.5	79.6
8	Sweden	10.0	78.6
9	Norway	9.6	78.6
10	Italy	9.5	77.3
11	Netherlands	12.0	77.3
12	France	11.8	76.6
13	Germany	11.6	75.7
14	Estonia	7.0	75.5
15	Turkey	6.1	75.2
16	Austria	8.7	74.5
17	Luxemburg	7.8	74.2
18	Finland	9.2	72.1
19	Spain	9.5	72.1
20	Slovenia	9.3	70.2
21	Portugal	10.1	69.9
22	Hungary	7.4	69.6
23	Canada	11.4	68.7
24	Belgium	10.9	68.4
25	Poland	7.4	68.2
26	Slovakia	9.1	67.3
27	Australia	8.7	65.4
28	Greece	9.6	62.6
29	Switzerland	11.4	59.6
30	Israel	7.9	58.9
31	S Korea	6.9	54.1
32	The United States	17.4	48.6
33	Mexico	6.4	48.3
34	Chile	8.4	46.8

Sources: World Bank web site

Health expenditure, total (% of GDP). Available at http://data.worldbank.org/indicator/SH.XPD.TOTL.ZS. Last accessed on 31 Dec 2011.

Health expenditure, total (% of GDP). Available at http://data.worldbank.org/indicator/SH.XPD.TOTL.ZS. Last accessed on 31 Dec 2011.

Table 1.4 Public Health Expenditure as Percentage Total Health Expenditure: BRICS Countries

Sr. No.	BRICS Countries	Total Health Exp as % GDP 2009	Public Health Exp as % of Total Health Expenditure 2009
1	Russia	5.4	64.4
2	China	4.6	50.1
3	Brazil	9.1	45.7
4	South Africa	8.5	40.1
5	India	4.2	32.8

Sources: World Bank web site

Health expenditure, total (% of GDP). Available at http://data.worldbank.org/indicator/SH.XPD.TOTL.ZS. Last accessed on 31 Dec 2011.

Health expenditure, total (% of GDP). Available at http://data.worldbank.org/indicator/SH.XPD.TOTL.ZS. Last accessed on 31 Dec 2011.

Figures 1.3 and 1.4 rank these countries on health expenditure (as a percentage of GDP) and public health expenditure (as a percentage of total health expenditure).

It can be seen from tables 1.3 and 1.4 that the United States (ranked first among the 34 OECD countries on healthcare expenditure per capita) is ranked 32 among the 34 OECD countries on public health expenditure as a percentage of total health expenditure.

Most of the developed nations spend around 10–12 per cent of their GDP on healthcare. Public health spending as a percentage of total health spending is very high in developed OECD countries than in the developing BRICS countries. Japan, which is ranked third on GDP (PPP), has 80 per cent of its health expenditure contributed by the public sector, while India ranked fourth on GDP (PPP) has its public sector contributing to less than 25 per cent of the total health expenditure.

Global inequality in healthcare spending is large as is evident from Table 1.5. Countries in the highest five percentile spend $2,337 per capita on healthcare, which is almost 45 times the per capita spending on healthcare by the countries in the lowest 20th percentile, and almost 14 times the per capita spending on healthcare by the countries in the lower 40th percentile which includes India.

In spite of large inequity in health spending, higher spending on healthcare need not necessarily lead to better health indicators. We discuss this issue in the next section, by bringing out some very interesting observations on the relationship between health expenditure and health outcomes.

In the next section, we provide a comparison between healthcare expenditure and the health system performance in the OECD, BRICS and a few other countries.

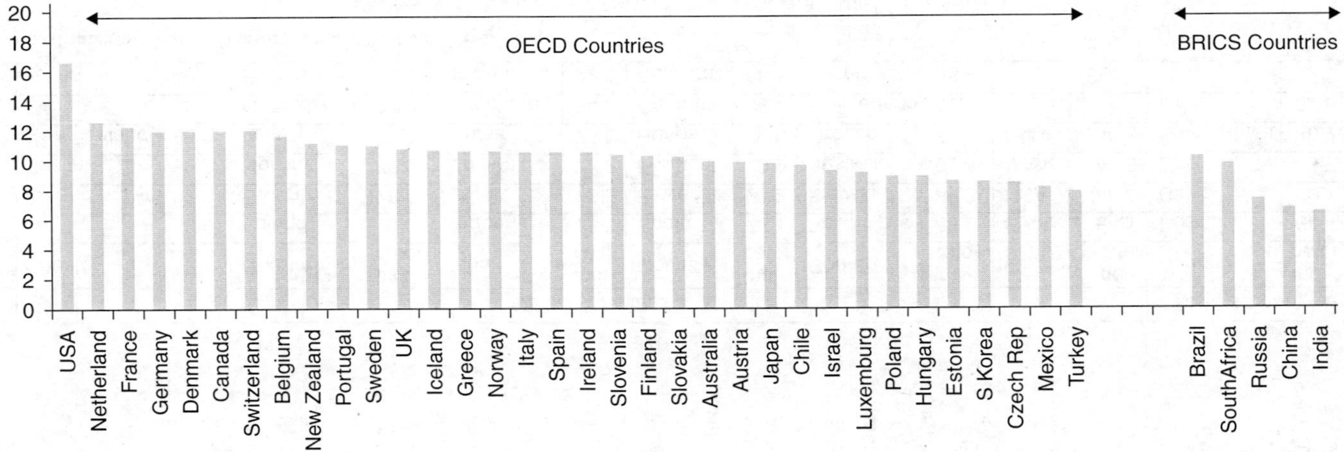

OECD Countries												BRICS Countries	
Country	Indi-cator	Country	Indi-cator	Country	Indi-cator	Country	Indi-cator	Country	Indi-cator	Country	Indi-cator	Country	Indi-cator
USA	17.4	Switzerland	11.4	Iceland	9.7	Slovenia	9.3	Chile	8.4	S Korea	6.9	Brazil	9.1
Netherlands	12.0	Belgium	10.9	Greece	9.6	Finland	9.2	Israel	7.9	Czech Rep	6.8	South Africa	8.5
France	11.8	New Zealand	10.3	Norway	9.6	Slovakia	9.1	Luxemburg	7.8	Mexico	6.4	Russia	5.4
Germany	11.6	Portugal	10.1	Italy	9.5	Australia	8.7	Poland	7.4	Turkey	6.1	China	4.6
Denmark	11.5	Sweden	10.0	Spain	9.5	Austria	8.7	Hungary	7.4			India	4.2
Canada	11.4	UK	9.8	Ireland	9.5	Japan	8.5	Estonia	7.0				

Indicator: Health expenditure as a % GDP

Figure 1.3 Health Expenditure as % GDP

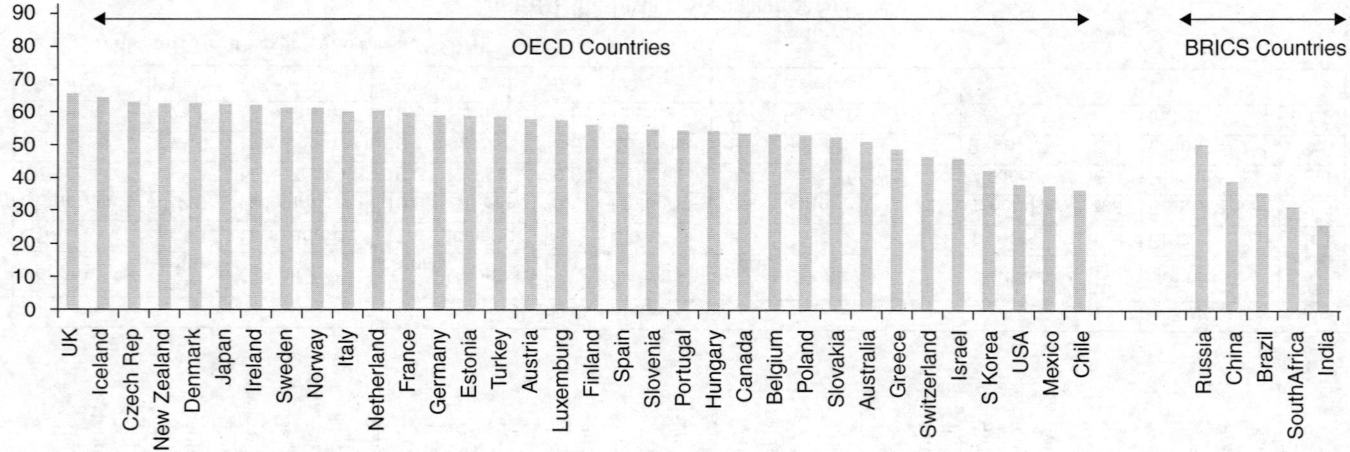

OECD Countries												BRICS Countries	
Country	Indi-cator	Country	Indi-cator	Country	Indi-cator	Country	Indi-cator	Country	Indi-cator	Country	Indi-cator	Country	Indi-cator
UK	83.6	Ireland	79.6	Germany	75.7	Spain	72.1	Poland	68.2	S Korea	54.1	Russia	64.4
Iceland	82.3	Sweden	78.6	Estonia	75.5	Slovenia	70.2	Slovakia	67.3	USA	48.6	China	50.1
Czech Rep	80.2	Norway	78.6	Turkey	75.2	Portugal	69.9	Australia	65.4	Mexico	48.3	Brazil	45.7
New Zealand	80.2	Italy	77.3	Austria	74.5	Hungary	69.6	Greece	62.6	Chile	46.8	South Africa	40.1
Denmark	80.1	Netherlands	77.3	Luxemburg	74.2	Canada	68.7	Switzerland	59.6			India	32.8
Japan	80.0	France	76.6	Finland	72.1	Belgium	68.4	Israel	58.9				

Indicator: Public Health Exp as a % Total Health Exp

Figure 1.4 Public Health Expenditure as % Total Health Expenditure

Table 1.5 Inequity in Healthcare Spending

Per Capita Spending (International Dollars) PPP	Percentile
2,337	95
849	80
369	60
171	40
52	20

Source: Healthcare Spending, UC Atlas of global inequality.
Available at http://ucatlas.ucsc.edu/spemd.php. Last accessed 31 Dec 2011.

1.5 HEALTH SYSTEM PERFORMANCE

The WHO defines health systems as comprising all the organizations, institutions and resources that are devoted to producing health actions.[21] A health action is defined as any effort, whether in personal healthcare, public health services or through intersectoral initiatives, whose primary purpose is to improve health.

As per the WHO, health systems started evolving soon after the First World War with a few European countries adopting the 1883 German model of state-funded social insurance for low-wage workers. After the Second World War, many more countries introduced social insurance. By the early 1970s, the social insurance models became very costly and, hence, inequitable. This led to the birth of primary healthcare as an approach to address affordability and equity in heathcare provision. Unfortunately, primary healthcare services in many developing and poor countries did not satisfactorily meet the community needs, due to resource constraints, lack of good governance and poor management practices.

Investments in financial resources, human resources and infrastructure are essential for any health system to deliver. We reproduce in Table 1.6 (OECD countries) and Table 1.7 (BRICS countries) the estimates of three important indicators of health system, namely:

- Number of hospital beds per 1,000 people
- Number of physicians per 1,000 people
- Number of nurses per 1,000 people

> The United States with the highest per capita spending on health was ranked 32 out of 34 OECD countries on public health spending and 37 among 191 member countries on health system performance by the WHO.

Table 1.6 Health System in the OECD Countries

Rank by Number of Beds per 1,000 People	Country	Hospital Beds per 1,000 People	Physicians per 1,000 People	Nurses per 1,000 People
1	Japan	14.3	2.0	9.0
2	Germany	9.0	3.4	10.1
3	Czech Republic	8.8	3.5	10.2
4	Austria	8.3	3.4	6.2
5	Hungary	7.9	3.2	8.8
6	Iceland	7.6	3.62	9.9
7	France	7.7	3.4	7.3
8	Australia	7.5	2.5	9.2
9	Slovakia	7.2	3.1	7.0
10	Finland	7.2	2.6	22.2
11	South Korea	7.1	1.6	4.0
12	Belgium	7.0	3.9	11.8
13	New Zealand	6.2	2.2	9.0
14	Switzerland	6.1	3.6	9.0
15	Israel	6.1	3.9	6.2
16	Estonia	6.1	3.1	6.7
17	Luxemburg	6	2.7	9.5
18	Poland	5.7	2.5	5.4
19	Slovenia	5.0	2.3	7.2
20	Netherlands	5.0	3.1	13.8
21	Greece	4.8	4.4	3.6
22	Italy	4.5	4.2	4.8
23	Ireland	4.3	2.8	18.5
24	The United Kingdom	4.2	2.2	5.4
25	Denmark	4.0	2.9	7.5
26	Norway	4.0	3.1	15.2
27	Spain	3.8	3.2	4.0
28	Canada	3.8	2.1	7.5
29	Sweden	3.8	3.3	10.9
30	Portugal	3.7	3.3	4.0
31	The United States	3.3	2.3	10.0
32	Chile	2.6	1.1	0.7
33	Turkey	2.5	1.3	3.0
34	Mexico	1.0	1.5	3.1
World Average *		**3.6**	**1.7**	**3.3**

Source: World Health Statistics 2011 – Table 6: Health workforce, infrastructure and essential medicines.

Table 1.7 Health System in BRICS Countries

Rank	Country	Beds/1000	Physicians per 1,000 People	Nurses per 1,000 People
1	Russia	10.5	4.25	8.5
2	Brazil	2.8	2.2	0.7
3	China	2.4	1.5	1.1
4	India	1	0.6	1.0
5	South Africa	2.84	0.77	4.08
World Average		**3.6**	**1.7**	**3.3**

Source: World Health Statistics 2011 – Table 6: Health workforce, infrastructure and essential medicines.

Health system performance is judged by availability, access, affordability and equity in healthcare provision. The world health report[22] showed that beyond a point, increase in healthcare expenditure need not necessarily result in improved health system performance. The United States, which has the highest per capita expenditure on health, was ranked 37 on overall health system performance by the WHO among 191 member countries.[iv] Of the 36 countries ranked by the WHO better than the United States on overall health system performance, 22 countries are from OECD and 14 are non-OECD non-BRICS countries. Table 1.8 lists these countries by rank, ahead of the United States on overall health system performance.

It can be seen from Table 1.8 that Morocco ranked 99th and Dominica ranked 70th on health expenditure per capita in international dollars are ranked 29th and 36th, respectively, on overall health system performance ahead of the United States.

There may be many answers to the intriguing question as to why the nation which tops the list of health spending does not top the list of health system performance. One such answer (author's hypothesis based on the information given in Table 1.8) could be that public health spending in the United States is very low; the United States is ranked 32 among the 34 OECD countries on public health spending. It is difficult to provide a comprehensive answer due to paucity of reliable data from all countries.

It may be that public health spending is more critical than total health spending in explaining the health system performance in any country. If the above hypothesis is true, it could explain why India's health indicators are bad (ranked 117 by

---

[iv] These rankings reflect the ranking as per the WHO study World Health Report, 2000. No recent data on health system performance is available on all WHO countries since then. It is possible that the rankings have changed; but the United States still continues to top the list of countries on health spending, but not on health system performance.

Table 1.8 Countries Better Than the United States on Overall Health System Performance

Rank Health System Performance	Country	OECD Country Yes/No	Ranking on Health Expenditure per Capita (PPP)
1	France	Yes	4
2	Italy	Yes	11
3	San Marino	No	21
4	Andorra	No	23
5	Malta	No	37
6	Singapore	No	38
7	Spain	Yes	24
8	Oman	No	62
9	Austria	Yes	6
10	Japan	Yes	13
11	Norway	Yes	16
12	Portugal	Yes	28
13	Monaco	No	12
14	Greece	Yes	30
15	Iceland	Yes	14
16	Luxemburg	Yes	5
17	Netherlands	Yes	9
18	The United Kingdom	Yes	26
19	Ireland	Yes	25
20	Switzerland	Yes	2
21	Belgium	Yes	15
22	Columbia	No	49
23	Sweden	Yes	7
24	Cyprus	No	39
25	Germany	Yes	3
26	Saudi Arabia	No	63
27	UAE	No	35
28	Israel	Yes	19
29	Morocco	No	99
30	Canada	Yes	10
31	Finland	Yes	18
32	Australia	Yes	17
33	Chile	Yes	44
34	Denmark	Yes	8
35	Dominica	No	70
36	Costa Rica	No	50
37	The United States	Yes	1

Source: The World Health Report, 2000, Health Systems: Improving Performance, WHO.

the WHO on overall health performance), while Cuba is doing better than the United States on many health indicators except maternal mortality rate, as can be seen in Table 1.9. South Africa's problems lie in its high rate of HIV/AIDS infection among the most vulnerable age group of 15–49 years.

The Indian health system has shown some improvements;[23] life expectancy at birth has gone up from 30 years in 1950 to 63.5 years by 2006; maternal mortality has come down from 460 deaths from 100,000 live births in 1984 to 254 by

Table 1.9 Comparison of Health Statistics: The United States, Cuba, India and South Africa

Statistics	The United States	Cuba	India	S Africa
Health expenditure per capita current $ (2004)	6096.2	229.8	31.4	390.2
Total health expenditure as a % of GDP (2004)	15.4	6.3	5.0	8.6
Public health spending as a % of total health spending (*)	43.7 (2000)	90.9 (2000)	21.8 (2000)	42.4 (2000)
Life expectancy at birth (2005)	77.71 years	77.25 years	63.5 years	47.66 years
Maternal mortality per 100,000 live births)	8 per 100,000	33 per 100,000	540 per 100,000	150 per 100,000 live births
Infant mortality per 1,000 live births	6.81	5.12	52.91	54.81
Prevalence of HIV as a % of population 15–49 years (2005)	0.6%	0.09%	0.92%	18.78%
Physicians per 1,000 people (2002)	2.3	5.91	0.55	0.77
No. of beds per 1,000 people (2003)	3.3	4.9	0.9	2.84

Sources: Health Stats: Cuba Vs United States. Available at www.nationmaster.com/compare/Cuba/United-States/Health. Last accessed on 21 Mar 2012.

Health Stats: India Vs United States. Available at www.nationmaster.com/cpmpare/India/Unired-States/Health. Last accessed on 21 Mar 2012.

Health Stats: India Vs South Africa. Available at www.nationmaster.com/cpmpare/India/South-Africa/Health. Last accessed on 21 Mar 2012.

List of countries by Infant Mortality Rate. Available at http://en.wikipedia.org/wiki/List_of_countries_by_infant_mortality_rate. Last accessed on 30 Mar 2012.

Government of India (Sep 2010); Annual Report, Ministry of Health and Family Welfare, Government of India; New Delhi: Government of India.

2006; infant mortality rate has come down from 129 deaths per 1,000 live births in 1971 to 53 by 2006. Small pox is eradicated, and the WHO has taken India off the polio list.[24] India achieved a major milestone on 13 January 2012, following a 12-month period without any case of polio, considering that in 2009, India had more polio cases than any other country in the world (741). Complete immunization against vaccine preventable diseases is only 49 per cent,[25] child malnutrition rate is twice as high as some sub-Saharan countries. Managerial challenges to improve the India health system performance should address the problems facing India's inter-sectoral health system:[26] which collaborates with several sectors such as nutrition, education, women and child welfare, and youth and culture sectors in delivering a wide range of health services.

The Indian rural health system got considerably strengthened when the Government of India launched the National Rural Health Mission in April 2005 to carry out the necessary architectural corrections in the basic healthcare delivery system. As per the NRHM Mission Document,[27]

> The goal of NRHM is to improve the availability of and access to quality healthcare services. The mission adopts a synergistic approach by relating health to determinants of good health, such as nutrition, sanitation, hygiene and safe drinking water. It also aims at mainstreaming the Indian system of medicine to facilitate healthcare. The mission is an articulation of the Government of India's commitment to increase public health spending from the current levels of one percentage of GDP to 2–3 percentage of GDP. It seeks decentralization of programmes for district management of health and to address inter-state and inter-district disparities.

There is a proposal to launch a National Urban Health Mission (NUHM) to provide an integrated and sustainable system for primary healthcare services. As per the NUHM document of the Government of India,[28]

> The goal of NUHM is to improve the health status of the urban poor and particularly the slum dwellers and other disadvantaged sections, by facilitating equitable access to quality healthcare through a revamped public health system and partnerships. NUHM would provide flexibility to the states to choose which model suits the needs and capacities of the states to best address the healthcare needs of the urban poor. The states will be free to choose from non-governmental partnership for public health goals, PPP, extending the extant primary public health system, an optimal mix of these or to propose other innovative models best suitable to their state needs.

Unfortunately, India has very high maternal and infant mortality rates in the world.[29] The maternal mortality rate in India translates into one mother dying every 6–7 minutes; it is possible to save at least 70 per cent of maternal deaths through appropriate and timely medical interventions. For every maternal death, about 15 women who survived complicated childbirth develop some form of disability. What is worst is that about 5,000 children under the age of five die in India every day,[30] while 60 per cent of these deaths could be prevented with minimal medical interventions and more community awareness. India is unlikely to achieve Millenium Development Goals (MDG) on maternal and infant mortality.

1.6 SUMMARY

India faces several challenges in improving its health system performance. While many developed countries spend about 9–10 per cent of their GDP on healthcare, India's healthcare expenditure is only about 4.5 per cent of its GDP, with the government share at only one per cent. The per capita expenditure on health by developed nations ranges between $3,000 and $4,000 (the United States tops this list with more than $7,000), while India's per capita expenditure on health at $33 is less than $50, the minimum level as per WHO norms for basic healthcare services. Contribution from the government of India (central and states combined) is only about one per cent of GDP, or equivalently less than 25 per cent of the total health expenditure as against 50–80 per cent public health spending by developed nations. Leaving the healthcare delivery mostly in the hands of the private sector has led to 'out-of-pocket' expenditure accounting for almost three-fourths of the private sector health spending. The Government of India has committed to increase its spending on healthcare to 2–3 per cent of GDP by the end of the 12th Five Year Plan, 2012–17. Political priority for additional government expenditure for socio-economic developments is essential to sustain our economic developments. Health has also been identified as an integral component of sustainable development.[31]

The Indian health sector faces many challenges. The government has to increase its share of the total health expenditure to provide healthcare services which are available, accessible, affordable and equitable to all. In the next chapter, we discuss these and other issues by reviewing the status of the health sector in India across three important determinants, namely, health financing, health infrastructure and health HR.

QUESTIONS

1. If you were a consultant to the Ministry of Health and Family Welfare,
   (a) What steps would you recommend for the Indian healthcare industry to achieve the projected growth of 10–12 per cent for the next 5–10 years?
   (b) What should be the increase in public health spending and private health spending to achieve the projected growth?

(c) Do you think the government's commitment to increase public health spending from the current level of one per cent to three per cent by the end of 12th Five Year Plan would help the health sector to achieve its projected growth? Or would you leave it to the private sector to become even more dominant?

(d) What are the consequences if the private health expenditure grows faster than public health expenditure?

2. Who are the major players in the Indian pharmaceutical industry? List the top 10 companies and their share of the industry. What are their market segments? Should the industry focus on communicable or non-communicable diseases?
3. If you are a consultant to a pharmaceutical industry, would you or would you not recommend a revision of the current drug regulatory system in India?
4. In the Indian medical equipment industry, who are the major players and what are their market shares? List the top 10 leaders in this field and their contribution to the industry.
5. What are your views on the growth of biotechnology in India?
6. What steps are required to provide medical insurance coverage to more people?
7. Is public–private partnership a solution to deliver healthcare services better?
8. Comment on the health system performance vs public health expenditure in the OECD and BRICS countries.
9. Comment on the health system performance vs total health expenditure in the OECD and BRICS countries.

REFERENCES

1. World Health Organization. (2011). Health Service Delivery. Available at http://www.who.int/healthsystems/topics/delivery/en/index.html. Last accessed on 27 Dec 2011.
2. International Standards Industrial Classification of Economic Activities. Statistical papers, Series M, No.4, Rev 4. Available at unstats.un.org/unsd/publication/seriesm_4rev4e.pdf. Last accessed on 14 Mar 2012.
3. World Health Statistics 2011—Table 6: Health workforce, infrastructure and essential medicines.
4. Pharmaceutical Market Trends, 2010–2014. Available at http://www.pharmaceutical-market-research.com/publications/general_industry/pharmaceutical_market_trends_2008_2012.html,. Last accessed on 19 Feb 2012.
5. S&N and the global medical device industry—by numbers. Available at http://www.telegraph.co.uk/finance/newsbysector/pharmaceuticalsandchemicals/8257936/SandN-and-the-global-medical-device-industry-by-numbers.html). Last accessed on 12 Feb 2012.
6. Biotechnology. Available at http://en.wikipedia.org/wiki/Biotechnology. Last accessed on 12 Feb 2012.
7. World Healthcare IT Market: Tends and Forecast (2010–2015). Available at http://www.reportlinker.com/p0593564/World-Healthcare-IT-Market-Trends-Forecast. Last accessed on 12 Feb 2012.

8. Medical tourism. Available at http://en.wikipedia.org/wiki/Medical_tourism. Last accessed on 12 Feb 2012.
9. Bumrungrad International Hospital; http://www.bumrungrad.com/en/about-us/overview. Last accessed on 12 Feb 2012.
10. Pricewaterhouse Coopers. (2009). Emerging Market Report: Health in India 2009. Available at http://www.pwc.com/en_GX/gx/healthcare/pdf/emerging-market-report-hc-in-india.pdf. Last accessed on 12 Feb 2012.
11. Mahal, Ajay; Debroy, Bibek; Bhandari, Laveesh (2010); India Health Report 2010; Indicus Analytics: BS Books.
12. Ibid.
13. ASSOCHAM, The Associated Chambers of Commerce and Industry of India. (March 22, 2010). Medical Equipment Industry To Touch US$7 Bln. By 2012: ASSOCHAM Available at http://www.assocham.org/prels/shownews.php?id=2365. Last accessed on 2 Mar 2012.
14. Government of India (Aug 2005); Report of the National Commission on Macroeconomics and Health; Ministry of Health and Family Welfare, Government of India; New Delhi: Government of India.
15. Mahal, et al (2010); India Health Report 2010.
16. Bhat, Ramesh; Jain, Nishant. (July 2006). Factors Affecting the Demand for Health Insurance; IIMA working Paper. No. 2006-07-02.
17. Government of India (2004–05); National Health Accounts India, 2004–05, Ministry of Health and Family Welfare, Government of India; New Delhi: Government of India.
18. Employee State Insurance Corporation, Government of India. Available at http://esic.nic.in/. Last accessed on 14 Mar 2012.
19. Government of India. Rashtriya Swasthya Bima Yojana (RSBY). Available at http://rsby.gov.in/about_rsby.aspx. Last accessed on 14 Mar 2012.
20. Hsiao W & Heller P; (2007); What should macroeconomists know about healthcare Policy? IMF Working paper, n. WP/07/13, IMF Washington DC.
21. The World Health Report, 2000, Health Systems: Improving Performance, WHO.
22. Ibid.
23. Government of India (Sep 2010); Annual Report, Ministry of Health and Family Welfare, Government of India; New Delhi: Government of India.
24. UNICEF. Polio Eradication: India no longer a polio endemic country. Available at http://www.unicef.org/india/health_3729.htm. Last accessed on 10 Mar 2012.
25. NFHS. NFHS-3: Fact Sheets For Key Indicators Based On Final Data. Available at http://www.nfhsindia.org/factsheet.html. Last accessed on 12 Feb 2012.
26. Ramani KV, Dileep Mavalankar. (2006 a). Health System in India: Opportunities and challenges for improvements. Journal of Health Organization and Management 20 (6); p 560–572.
27. Government of India. National Rural Health Mission (2005–12): Mission Document; Government of India. Available at www.mofhw.nic.in. Last accessed on 3 Mar 2012.

28. Ministry of Health and Family Welfare, Government of India. (June 2010). National Urban Health Mission; Framework for Implementation (Draft for Discussion) Available at www.mohfw.nic.in. Last accessed on 12 Feb 2012.
29. Black, ER; Morris, SS; Bryce, J (2003). Where and Why are 10 Million Children Dying Every Year? Lancet; 361(9376), p2226–2234.
30. Ramani KV et al. (April–June 2010). 'Why should 5000 children die in India every day: Major Causes of Death and Managerial Challenges' Vikalpa. 35 (2).
31. (Sep 2002,). The World summit on sustainable development. Available at http://www.un.org/events/wssd/. Last accessed on 10 Feb 2012.

chapter 2

Health Sector in India

CHAPTER OUTLINE

CHAPTER OBJECTIVE

The main objective of this chapter is to provide an overview of the health sector in India and to bring out the critical role of hospitals in the delivery of health services. India needs to add 1 million physicians, 2 million nurses and 3 million hospital beds to achieve the world average of 1.7 physicians, 3.3 nurses and 3.6 beds per 1,000 people.

2.1 AN INTRODUCTION

Our National Population Policy 2000[1] and the National Health Policy 2002[2] are the two important policy documents of the Indian health sector.

As per the WHO, the goals of a nation's health sector are good health, responsiveness to the expectations of the population, and fair financial contribution.

The Indian health sector is at a crossroads today. The health sector has achieved some noteworthy successes such as increased life expectancy, reduced maternal and infant mortality rates, eradication of small pox, and getting off the WHO list of polio-endemic countries. Yet, our health system performances are very poor; 200 mothers and 5,000 children die every day; 75 per cent of maternal and child deaths can be prevented if health services can be delivered on time. Child malnutrition, which is twice as bad as some sub-Saharan countries, is a major cause for 50 per cent of childhood illness-related morbidity.

The WHO Report on Macroeconomics and Health,[3] followed by the Report of the National Commission on Macroeconomics and Health (NCMH)[4] provide strategic directions to improve our heath sector performance. Effective and efficient management of health services calls for a significant scaling up of resources currently spent in the health sector and tackling the non-financial obstacles that have limited the capacity to deliver health services. Building health systems that are responsive to client needs requires politically difficult and administratively demanding choices.

This chapter is divided into four sections:

1. Health financing
2. Health infrastructure
3. Health human resources
4. Role of hospitals in the Indian health sector

2.2 HEALTH FINANCING

In this section, we present an overview of health financing in India, using a detailed classification of health expenditure for 2004–05 (the year for which the latest data is available) published by the National Health Accounts, Government of India.

The National Health Accounts 2004–05[5] provides a very detailed classification of healthcare expenditure, such as:

- Expenditure by source of funding (public, private, external flows)
- Current expenditure vs capital assets
- Expenditure by service providers (public, private, NGOs)
- Public expenditure (Centre, states)
- Private expenditure (out-of-pocket, insurance, firms)
- Expenditure by function (curative, preventive, and so on)

We present these figures and draw important conclusions on health financing, only for the year 2004–05, since a detailed classification of health expenditure is not available for years beyond 2004–05. The scenario has changed slightly during the last five years of National Rural Health Mission (NRHM); 2005–10, but not drastically.

We start our discussion on health financing with an analysis of the sources of funding.

2.2.1 Health Expenditure: Source of Funding

It can be seen from Table 2.1 that India's dependence on external funds is very negligible, that is, 2.3 per cent of the total health spending.

Table 2.1 Health Expenditure: Sources of Funding

Sources of Funding	2004–05 Billion ₹	2005–06 Billion ₹	2006–07 Billion ₹	2007–08 Billion ₹	2008–09 Billion ₹
Public	263.13	344	407	487	587
Private	1,044.14	1,150	1,278	1,427	1,574
External flows	30.49	21	22	26	37
Total	1,337.76	1,515	1,707	1,940	2,198
GDP	31,495	35,800	41,460	47,235	53,220
Health as a % GDP	4.2%	4.2%	4.1%	4.1%	4.1%
Public exp as % GDP	0.83%	0.96%	0.98%	1.03%	1.1%

Source: Government of India (2004–05), National Health Accounts India, 2004–05, Ministry of Health and Family Welfare, Government of India, New Delhi.

2.2.2 Health Expenditure: Service Providers

External flows mentioned in Table 2.1 are mostly routed through the Central government and disbursed by the Centre as grants to the healthcare providers in the public sector, private sector and the NGOs. A reclassification of the total health expenditure by service providers is given in Table 2. 2.

Table 2.2 Health Expenditure: Service Providers 2004–05

Type of Expenditure	Billion ₹	Percentage
Public: Central government	75.31	5.63
State governments	209.23	15.64
Private providers	1,026.57	76.74
NGO providers	11.46	0.86
Others	15.19	1.14
Total spending	1,337.76	100

Source: Government of India (2004–05), National Health Accounts India, 2004–05, Ministry of Health and Family Welfare, Government of India, New Delhi.

2.2.3 Public Health Expenditure

Public health expenditure consists of expenditure by the Central government, state governments, municipals and local government bodies. Expenditure by the municipals and local bodies are not shown separately here, since most of their expenditures are based on government grants. The contribution from the Central government and the state governments towards total public health expenditure are ₹75.31 billion and ₹209.23 billion, respectively.

The share of the Central government is 26.5 per cent and that of the state government is 73.5 per cent in the total public health spending[i]. A large share of the public health spending is in the hands of the states as health is a subject of the state governments in India as per our constitution.

In 2004–05, 95 per cent of public health expenditure constituted current consumption expenditure and only 5 per cent accounted for creation of capital assets in health sector[6] as can be seen from Table 2.3. Neglect of capital investment in health sector has been pointed out by many experts earlier, including the NCMH report on Macroeconomics and Health.[7] This is a very worrying trend in the Indian health sector.

Table 2.3 Current Expenditure vs Capital Assets: Public Sector (2004–05)

Public Health Expenditure	Percentage of Total
Current expenditure	95%
Capital expenditure	5%
Total expenditure	100%

Source: Government of India (2004–05), National Health Accounts India, 2004–05, Ministry of Health and Family Welfare, Government of India, New Delhi.

2.2.4 Private Health Expenditure

Next, we carry out an analysis of the private health sector spending. Private health expenditure includes the following components:

- Out-of-pocket expenditure by households for availing healthcare services
- Healthcare expenditure through insurance mechanism
- Expenditure by corporate bodies on their employees and families

[i]It is true that the government health budget has increased since the announcement of the NRHM in April 2005. The share of Central government in the total public health expenditure has gone up to almost 30 per cent by 2009. The challenge now is to use the additional resources to improve healthcare service delivery, both effectively and efficiently.

Out-of-Pocket Expenditure: An analysis of out-of-pocket expenditure is given in Table 2.4.

The out-of-pocket expenditure at ₹930 billion accounts for almost 90 per cent of the total private healthcare expenditure (₹ 1,026 billion), with a per capita expenditure of ₹854.

The combined expenditure for inpatient and outpatient services account for 90 per cent of the total out-of-pocket expenditure in rural, urban or India as a whole.

Outpatient care accounts for almost two-thirds of the out-of-pocket expenditure in the country as a whole; 69 per cent rural areas and 62 per cent in urban areas.

A break-up of the inpatient care into its components is given in Table 2.5 for the public and private sectors.

Table 2.4 Out-of-Pocket Expenditure: Private Sector (2004–05)

Type of Service	Rural (%)	Urban (%)	Total (%)	Per Cap Exp.
Outpatient care	396.72 (69)	218.06 (62)	614.77 (66)	565
Inpatient care	123.06 (21)	95.28 (27)	218.33 (24)	201
RCH services*	29.02 (5)	21.29 (6)	50.31 (5)	46
Other services†	30.20 (5)	16.37 (5)	46.58 (5)	43
Total	579.00 (100)	351.00 (100)	930.00 (100)	854

Source: Government of India (2004–05), National Health Accounts India, 2004–05, Ministry of Health and Family Welfare, Government of India, New Delhi.

*Anti-natal, intra-natal, post-natal and abortion services.

†Includes immunization, family planning and death-related services.

Table 2.5 Out-of-Pocket Inpatient Care: Public vs Private Sector (2004–05)

Items of Expenditure	Public Sector		Private Sector	
	Per cent Expenditure Rural	Per cent Expenditure Urban	Per cent Expenditure Rural	Per cent Expenditure Urban
Doctor's fee	4.16	4.64	25.84	27.31
Investigations	11.92	15.12	9.37	10.84
Medicines	66.49	62.31	40.43	37.77
Other services*	17.43	17.93	24.36	24.08
Total	100	100	100	100

Source: Government of India (2004–05), National Health Accounts India, 2004–05, Ministry of Health and Family Welfare, Government of India, New Delhi.

*Includes food, bed, blood, and so on.

It can be seen from Table 2.5 that medicines alone account for two-thirds of the total inpatient care expenditure in public sector, while doctor's fee and medicines together account for two-thirds of the total inpatient care expenditure in the private sector, whether in rural or urban areas. Even though doctor's consultation is free in public sector, medicines are expensive.

Expenditure on Insurance: An analysis of expenditure on health insurance is given in Table 2.6. Health insurance is broadly classified into social health insurance (e.g. ESIS) and voluntary health insurance provided by both public and private sector companies.

Table 2.6 Healthcare Insurance (2004–05) Curative, Preventive, Others

Components	Expenditure Billion ₹	Percentage
Employee state insurance scheme	12.58	34.4
Central government health scheme	2.49	6.8
Public insurance companies	19.31	52.7
Private insurance companies	2.23	6.1
Total	36.61	100

Source: Government of India (2004–05), National Health Accounts India, 2004–05, Ministry of Health and Family Welfare, Government of India, New Delhi.

It can be seen that private sector companies account for a mere 6 per cent of the total insurance market in India. Data on another government insurance scheme, namely, RSBY insurance scheme started in 2008, are not available.

2.2.5 Health Expenditure by Function

Next, we show the breakdown of the total expenditure by function in Table 2.7.

Table 2.7 Health Expenditure by Function (2004–05)

Function	Billion ₹	Percentage
Curative care	1,042.87	77.96
RCH an FW	107.97	8.01
Control of communicable diseases	18.01	1.35
Control of non-communicable diseases	2.42	0.18
Other public health activities	6.54	0.49
Medical education and research	30.14	2.25
Health administration and insurance	43.32	3.24
Others	86.49	6.47
Total	1,337.76	100

Source: Government of India (2004–05), National Health Accounts India, 2004–05, Ministry of Health and Family Welfare, Government of India, New Delhi.

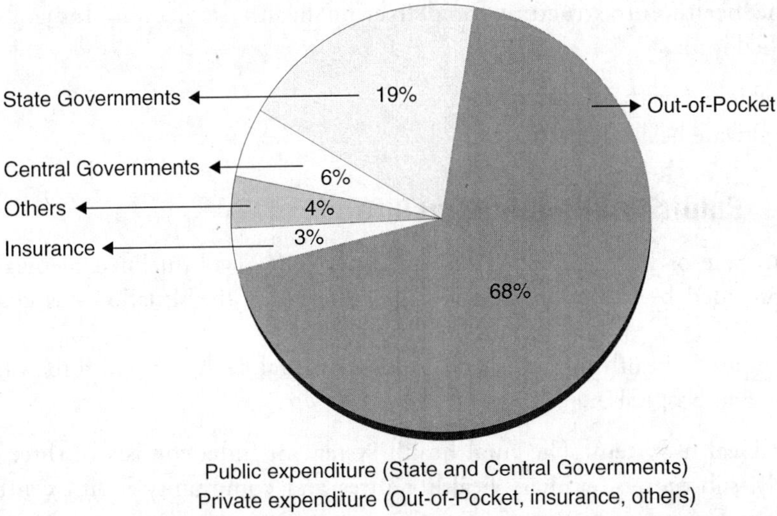

Figure 2.1 Health Expenditure (Public vs Private)

It can be seen that curative care alone accounts for almost 80 per cent of the total health expenditure. Hospitals, therefore, play an important role in health financing.

To summarize health financing, India's dependence on external funds is negligible at 2.3 per cent of the total health expenditure in the country. Public health spending is around 25 per cent with the share of Central and state governments being 25 per cent and 75 per cent, respectively. Within the private sector, out-of-pocket component alone accounts for 90 per cent, and the expenditure on health and social insurance accounts for a mere 4 per cent.

Curative care accounts for almost 80 per cent of the total health spending in India. Hospitals play the most important role in offering curative care services for primary, secondary and tertiary care, and hence their importance in the health financing.

In the next section, we describe the health infrastructure in the public and private sectors which support the delivery of services.

2.3 HEALTH INFRASTRUCTURE

Infrastructure forms a critical part of health service delivery in any country. Availability, access, affordability and equity of quality services highly depend on the distribution, functionality and quality of infrastructure. India's record of investing in infrastructure has not been very satisfactory.

The health infrastructure for delivering health services in India can be classified into:

- Public health infrastructure
- Private health infrastructure

2.3.1 Public Health Infrastructure

At the time of independence, almost 92 per cent of all qualified medical care was provided by the public sector.[8] Over the years, the situation has changed drastically.

The public health infrastructure consists of rural health system, urban health system and hospitals.

Rural Health System: The rural health system in India consists of three tiers, namely, sub-centres, primary health centres and community health centres as shown in Figure 2.2.

- **Health sub-centre:** A health sub-centre, known as a sub-centre (SC) is the most peripheral health facility and is, therefore, the first contact point for the community with the primary healthcare system. SCs provide basic minimum public health services to a population of 5,000 people (3,000 in the case of hard-to-reach areas). Each SC has two (one male and one female) multiple purpose workers (MPH) and one female auxiliary nurse midwife (ANM).
- **Primary health centre:** A primary health centre (PHC) is the first contact point for the community with a medical doctor. PHCs provide integrated preventive, promotive and curative care services, for a population of 30,000 (20,000 in the case of hard-to-reach areas). Each PHC has 4–6 beds and is

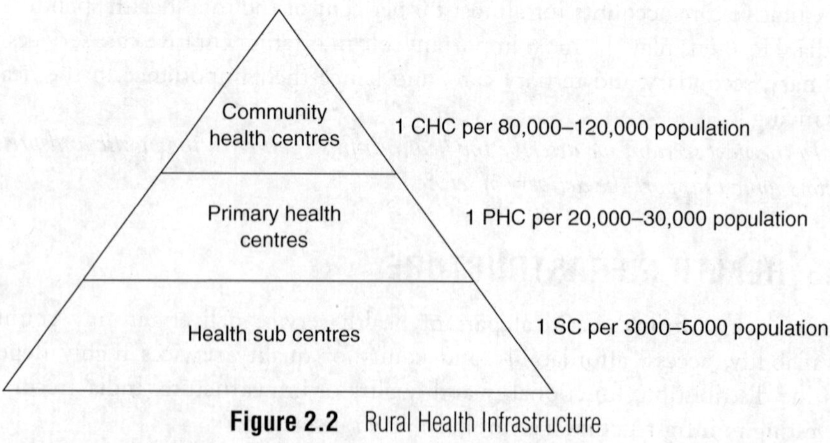

Figure 2.2 Rural Health Infrastructure

under the administrative control of a medical officer, assisted by one nurse and 14 other health workers. PHCs serve as referral centres for a group of 4–6 SCs in its area.

- **Community health centre:** A community health centre (CHC) provides specialized services in gynecology, pediatrics, surgery and medicine to a population of 120,000 (80,000 for hard-to-reach areas). A CHC has 30 beds, four specialists, three medical officers, seven nurses and 16 other health workers. Every CHC has an operating theatre, labour room, and laboratory and X-ray investigation facilities. CHCs are referral centres for PHCs.

SCs, PHCs and CHCs constitute the backbone of our rural public health service delivery system. Many states have upgraded some of their CHCs (and even some PHCs) as first referral units (FRUs). An FRU provides 24×7 emergency obstetric care and newborn care services.

Rural health infrastructure got considerably strengthened when the Government of India launched the NRHM in April 2005 to carry out the necessary architectural corrections in the basic healthcare delivery system.[9] As on March 2010, the rural health infrastructure in India had 147068 Sub Centres, 23673 Primary Health Centres and 4535 Community Health Centers, besides 1579 District and sub-divisional hospitals.[10]

> The real *big* worrying question is *not* the shortfall in health facilities, but 'How many of the existing health facilities are functional?' What is the definition of functionality of a health facility?

> As on 31 March 2010, India had 147,069 SCs, 23,673 PHCs and 4,535 CHCs. Even this seemingly large number of facilities falls short of government norms.

Assuming a rural population of 80 crores in 2010, the number of rural health facilities, namely, 147,069 SCs, 23,673 PHCs and 4,535 CHCs work out to only 1 SC per 5,400 population, 1 PHC per 34,000 population and 1 CHC per 176,000 population, which are below the government norms. Hence, there is still a shortfall of rural health facilities. Shortfall in the availability of health facilities is an indication of poor investment. Recall that as per National Health Accounts 2004–05,[11] the government's expenditure on capital assets was only 5 per cent of the total public health expenditure.

As of 2010, about 45 per cent of existing SCs and 12 per cent of the existing PHCs were operating from rented premises.[12] Mere presence of a facility (either in a government building or rented building) does not necessarily mean the health facility serves its intended purpose of delivering services. For example, when would a PHC be called functional?

A PHC would be functional if it provides consultation, investigation and medication.

- **Consultation:** Consultation would be available only when the medical officer is present. In the absence of the medical officer (who may be away on official work, personal leave, and so on), the PHC is almost non-functional since the PHC nurse is not empowered to prescribe medication or order investigation. Many medical officers in rural PHCs do not stay in the same village and, therefore, their availability in PHC is very limited, even when they are 'at work' in their PHC.

  For consultation, the medical officer needs the assistance of the PHC nurse.

  In short, the medical officer and nurse must be available to claim functionality of consultation service.
- **Investigation:** For investigation, the lab technologist and the materials for investigations must be available. Also, the lab microscope should be in working condition.
- **Medication:** For medication services, the pharmacist and all the essential drugs should be available.

  Hence for a PHC to be functional, all the resources should be available, namely, PHC staff (medical officer, nurse, lab technician and pharmacist), materials (for investigation and all the essential medicines and drugs) and the lab microscope.

  What are the chances that a PHC is functional on any given working day, since the PHCs remain officially closed on Sundays, and on all public holidays?

Referral System: Providing effective referral services (transportation and communication) in case of emergencies is an important part of health service delivery. Unfortunately, referral system in India is not very functional. It is assumed that sub-centres would refer patients to the PHCs, PHCs to CHCs, and CHCs to district hospitals. In practice, any patient is free to go anywhere, and complete records are not maintained on the outcome of referrals.

Urban Health System: Urbanization is an important demographic shift worldwide. Urban population is 50 per cent of the global population now, and is increasing at a rapid rate. The current urban population in India is estimated at 350 million and the UN projections put urban population at 45 per cent of the total population by 2030.

Urban health did not receive any recognition from our national planners till the census of 2001 projected India's urban population at 300 million constituting 28 per cent of our population. Urban health found a mention for the first time in the 10th Five Year Plan 2002–2007 and the National Health Policy 2002. A proposal to set up a National Urban Health Mission (NUHM) is pending with the Government of India.[13]

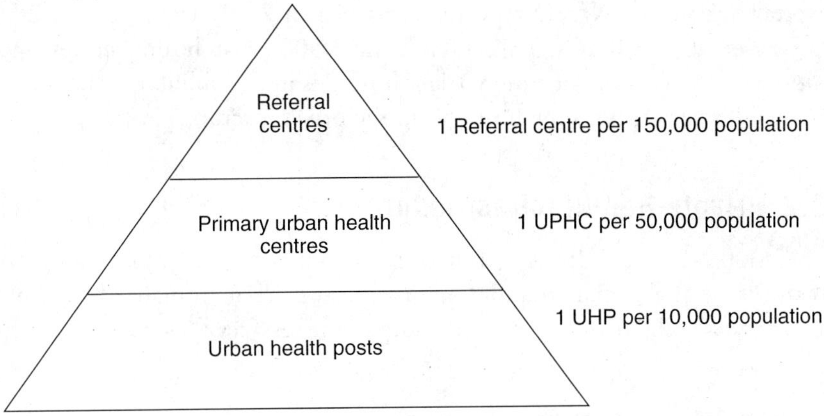

Figure 2.3 Urban Health Infrastructure

The NUHM recommends a three-tier[ii] health infrastructure for urban health system as shown in Figure 2.3:

- **First tier:** Urban health posts (1 UHP per 10,000 population). A Tier-1 urban health centre has been recently established on a public–private partnership (PPP) model.[14] The main objective is to provide outreach, primary healthcare, family welfare, maternal and child health services.
- **Second tier:** One primary urban health centre (PUHC) for a population of 50,000 to offer outpatient services on primary health.
- **Third tier:** A referral centre for a population of 150,000. Referral facility includes maternity homes, 50–100 bed general hospital, and so on. Service delivery would include emergency maternal obstetric care, child care, abortion services, family planning, and so on.

Unfortunately, no recent statistics are available from the government on the number of urban health facilities in India. The poor status of urban health[15] is a reflection of the continued neglect of this sector. There is even a proposal to include NUHM under NRHM, even though the priority areas for urban health are *not* the same as those of rural health. For example, large levels of migration from rural areas into urban cities are raising concerns on the spread of HIV/AIDS. Unplanned and rapid urban developments are threatening the quality of basic public health services such as drinking water, drainage, sanitation, and so on. Non-communicable diseases such as diabetes, cardiovascular diseases and renal failures are on the rise due to the lifestyles of people in cities and towns. Urban health cannot remain neglected any longer. The Government of India must launch NUHM as soon as possible.

[ii] Compare urban health system with the three-tier rural health system.

Hospitals: As per the WHO report,[16] India had in 2001, 137,311 SCs, 28,000 dispensaries, 22,842 PHCs, 3,043 CHCs and 3,500 urban health centres, and an additional 12,000 secondary and tertiary hospitals in the public sector, besides an estimated 68 per cent of total hospitals in the private sector.

2.3.2 Private Health Infrastructure

As per 2004–05 data from our national sample survey (NSS), more than two-thirds of the Indian population, including the marginalized sections of our society, use the private sector for outpatient services,[17] as can be seen from Table 2.8.

Table 2.8 Outpatient Service Providers

Population	Government (%)	Private (%)	Total (%)
Rural areas	24	76	100
Urban areas	20	80	100
SC	27	73	100
ST	37	63	100
Others	21	79	100

The situation is not very different for inpatient services as well. The private sector serves almost two-thirds of the population, rural or urban.[18] The move towards private sector for healthcare needs would be more in the years to come, if the public sector does not perform satisfactorily to meet the community demands. As per the government estimates,[19] more than three-fourths of human resources and advanced medical technology is in the private sector. The dominant position of the private sector in health service delivery is raising serious issues regarding the quality and inequity of service provision.

The private health sector in India is not regulated and so there is no reliable source to provide complete information on private healthcare facilities. Private healthcare facilities include dispensaries, clinics, nursing homes and hospitals, big and small.

> The private sector in India has a dominant presence in all the sub-markets—medical education and training, medical technology and diagnostics, pharmaceutical manufacture and sale, hospital construction and ancillary services, and finally the provisioning of medical care. Over 75 per cent of the human resources and 37 per cent of 623,819 beds in the country are in the private sector. Of these, most are located in the urban areas. Of concern is the abysmally poor quality of services being provided at the rural periphery by the large number of unqualified persons. Its relationship to health

outcomes at the population level has never been established. The private sector's predominance in the health sector has led to inequities in access to healthcare. Hospitalization among the well-off is six times higher than that of the poor.[20]

2.3.3 Public–Private Partnerships

PPP has become a very attractive proposition recently. PPP is, in a way, an acknowledgement of unsatisfactory performance of the public health system. Health is, and will continue to be, an obligation of the government to people. PPPs cannot substitute public health delivery system.

It is important to realize the need for regulating (not control) of the private health sector, if the government's push for PPP in health has to succeed.

How is it possible to sustain a PPP without sharing of information between the public and the private sectors?

An important element for the success of any PPP in healthcare service delivery is to have a legal contract (instead of an MoU) binding the public and the private sectors for resource input and service delivery. This is probably one reason for the success of Vasna Urban Health Centre in Ahmedabad Municipal Corporation.[21] The earlier urban health centre for Vasna ward was getting an OPD load of 4–5 patients per day, but the new centre based on a PPP contract is attracting 60–70 OPD patients every day; and there is demand to add new services.

In the next section, we will discuss the human resources in the Indian health sector. Human resource management in our health sector has been the subject of debate over the last few decades. While staff shortfall at all levels has been a concern in the public sector, the presence of unqualified staff practising in the private sector is a major concern.

2.4 HUMAN RESOURCES IN HEALTH

Health service delivery is highly labour-intensive and, therefore, health workforce is the most critical component of the health sector in any country. Health workforce is not merely the number of doctors and nurses; it includes all health service providers and administrators from remotest sub-centres to large hospitals, both public and private.

2.4.1 Demand for Health Workforce

As per government estimates, more than three-fourths of human resources and advanced medical technology is in the private sector.

One of the most important functions of the HR management is to estimate the requirements of medical, paramedical and administrative staff, and do the necessary follow up for filling up the sanctioned posts, so as to ensure good quality service delivery. Non-availability and uneven distribution of healthcare providers are challenging issues in the Indian health sector, both public and private.

As per the government estimates,[22] more than three-fourths of human resources and advanced medical technology are in the private sector.

Launch of NRHM led to induction of almost 108,000 more staff, both regular and on contract, consisting of 2,460 specialists, 8,600 allopath doctors, 8,000 AYUSH doctors, 27,000 nurses, 47,000 ANMs and 15,000 paramedical workers, in addition to introducing a new cadre of 700,000 ASHAs (accredited social health workers).[23]

As per the Planning Commission of India,[24] the human resource situation is particularly bad in the public health sector, which has witnessed a serious decline during the last two or three decades because of non-availability of medical and paramedical staff, diagnostic services and medicines.

The shortage of doctors in PHCs and CHCs against sanctioned posts is estimated at 13794 in 2010.[25] A break-up of the above shortfall into specialties[26] shows that shortages are as high as 59.4 per cent surgeons, 45 per cent obstetricians and gynecologists, 61 per cent physicians and 53 per cent pediatricians[iii] (see Figure 2.4).

Such a high level of non-availability of highly skilled doctors and other healthcare providers is a basic reason for the poor quality of public health service delivery

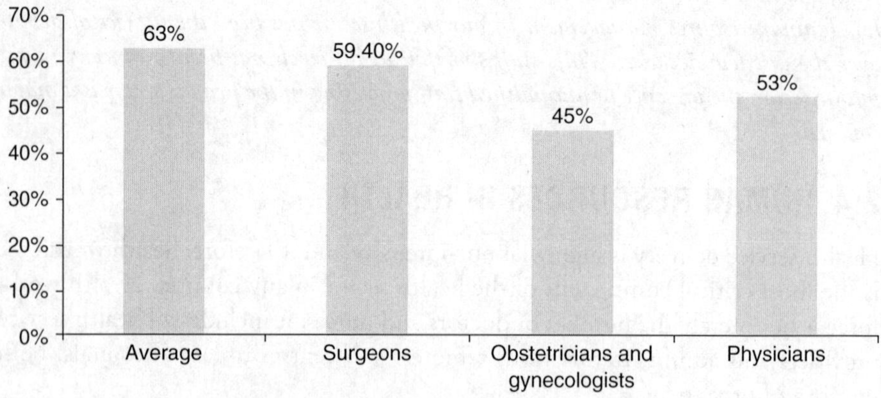

Figure 2.4 Shortfall of Specialists in CHCs

[iii] The government is proposing to establish rural MBBS programmes to overcome the shortages of doctors in rural areas.

in the rural areas of the country. Non-availability of any resource makes the facility less functional.

Uncertainty in the functionality of public health sector facilities is the main reason for the rural and urban population to rely extensively on the private sector for their healthcare needs, even though there are 'non-qualified' doctors and nurses practising in the private sector.

2.4.2 Supply of Health Workforce

As per the Ministry of Health and Family Welfare,[27] India has 335 medical colleges with (154 medical colleges) in the public sector and 181 in the private sector. The public sector has about 45 per cent medical colleges and account for almost 45 per cent of the annual admissions estimated at 41,500.

The southern states of Andhra Pradesh, Karnataka, Kerala and Tamil Nadu have 42 per cent of medical colleges (141 out of 335 medical colleges) and account for 45 per cent of annual admissions (annual intake of 18,040 students out of 40,525 seats all over the country). The two western states of Maharashtra and Gujarat have 60 medical colleges and together offer 7,240 admissions annually. In short, the four southern states of Andhra Pradesh, Karnataka, Kerala and Tamil Nadu and the two western states of Maharashtra and Gujarat have between them 60 per cent of medical colleges (201 out of 335 medical colleges) and an annual intake of 62 per cent of the entire country. Such an uneven distribution in the supply of healthcare providers is one of the reasons for the shortfall and uneven availability of healthcare providers.

> India has a shortfall of 1.2 million doctors and 2 million nurses to achieve the world average of 1.7 physicians and 3.3 nurses per 1,000 population.

India produces around 40,000 medical graduates and 21,000 post graduate students every year. During the year 2011–12, 4442 medical seats and 2398 post graduate seats ware added.[28]

As per the WHO,[29] India stands unfavourably when compared with world levels, even with low-income countries, in the capacity of human resources.

The number of doctors registered by different state councils stood at 696,747 during the year 2007.[30] This number of registered doctors probably includes those who have migrated or retired. Therefore, the doctor to population ratio in India is no more than 60 per 100,000 people. In urban areas, this ratio is probably six times more than that in the rural areas.[31]

Similarly, the number of nursing[iv] institutions in India in 2011 was estimated to be around 6,000 consisting of 935 ANM institutions, 2,351 GNM institutions, 1570 B.Sc. nursing institutions, 500 P.B.B.Sc. institutions and 450 M.Sc. institutions. Assuming an average of 25–35 students per course, the above number of institutions produces around 180,000 nurses every year. India had only 1.1 million nurses in 2007.[32]

> If we want to meet the world average of 3.3 per 1,000 population, we need to add another 2.5 million nurses.

Nurses include midwives, professional nurses, professional midwives, auxiliary nurses, auxiliary midwives, enrolled nurses, enrolled midwives and other associated personnel such as dental nurses and primary care nurses.

The four southern states of Andhra Pradesh, Karnataka, Kerala and Tamil Nadu have more than 50 per cent of GNM training institutions (1,234 GNM institutions out of 2,351) and more than 55 per cent of B.Sc. nursing training institutions (894 out of 1,570). The states of Madhya Pradesh, Punjab, Rajasthan and Uttar Pradesh have between them 625 GNM training institutions and 379 B.Sc. nursing training institutions.

> In short, the four southern states of Andhra Pradesh, Karnataka, Kerala and Tamil Nadu have more than 50 per cent of medical colleges and nursing institutions, and produce more than 50 per cent of MBBS doctors and nurses in the whole country. Such an uneven distribution in the supply of doctors and nurses in the country is one of the reasons for the uneven availability of healthcare providers in India.

2.5 ROLE OF HOSPITALS IN THE HEALTH SECTOR

As per the WHO,[33] India had in 2001, 137,311 SCs, 28,000 dispensaries, 22,842 PHCs, 3,043 CHCs and 3,500 UFWCs and an additional 12,000 secondary and tertiary hospitals in the public sector, besides an estimated 68 per cent of total hospitals in the private sector. Over 75 per cent of the human resources and 37 per cent of beds in the country are in the private sector.

[iv] Nursing courses available include

ANM	Auxiliary Nurse and Midwife
GNM	General Nurse and Midwife
B.Sc.	Bachelor of Science in Nursing
P.B.B.Sc.	Post Basic B.Sc. Nursing
M.Sc.	Master of Science in Nursing

More than two-thirds of the Indian population, including the marginalized sections of the society, use the private sector for outpatient and inpatient services.[34]

There is an acute shortage of doctors, nurses and allied workforce in our hospitals. The Government of India's estimate[35] of 623,819 beds in the country implies a ratio of only 0.6 beds per 1,000 people. The world average of 3.6 beds per 1,000 people[36] means a requirement of at least 4,000,000 beds (4 million beds) for our population of 1.2 billion, and thereby a shortfall of about 3.4 million beds. This is a huge shortfall even to meet the world average of 3.6 beds per 1,000 people.

India needs to add 1.2 million doctors, 2.5 million nurses and 3 million hospital beds to achieve the world average of 1.7 physicians, 3.3 nurses and 3.6 beds per 1,000 population.

The above observations on the Indian health sector along with the fact that curative care accounts for 80 per cent of the total health expenditure highlights the important role of hospitals in the Indian health sector.

The biggest challenge is not just the additional requirement of financial resources, but to utilize the financial resources effectively and efficiently in delivering health services. Optimal utilization of resources for service delivery is the managerial challenge facing the Indian health sector, especially the hospital sector.

India needs to add 1.2 million doctors, 2.5 million nurses and 3 million hospital beds to achieve the world average of 1.7 physicians, 3.3 nurses and 3.6 beds per 1,000 population.

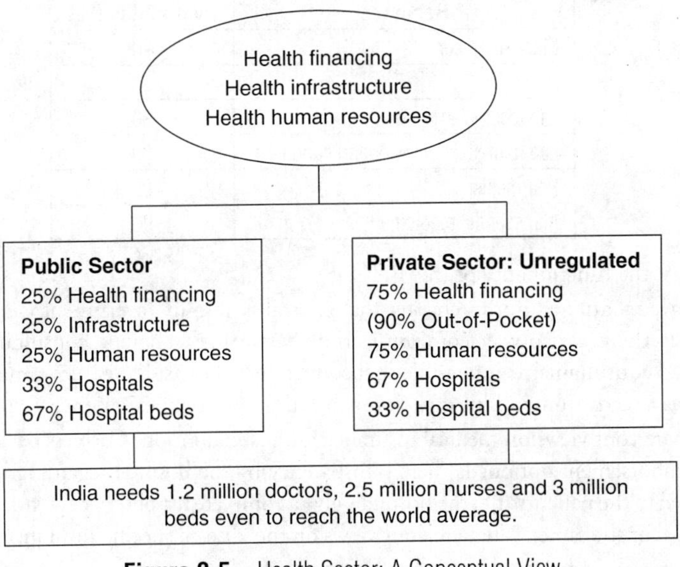

Figure 2.5 Health Sector: A Conceptual View

2.6 SUMMARY

In this chapter, we have described the health sector in India across three important dimensions, namely, health financing, health infrastructure and health human resources.

The Government of India's poor investments in the health sector (only 1 per cent of total health expenditure) has led to an unregulated growth of the private health sector, raising concerns on the equity of health service delivery.

In the next three chapters (chapters 3, 4 and 5), we will discuss the basic concepts in hospital management, challenges in service delivery and the managerial response to these challenges.

QUESTIONS

1. Collect the data on India's health expenditure, health infrastructure and HR in health sector for a period of 10 years from 2001 to 2010. You may use the data from the web site of the Ministry of Health and Family Welfare for the above period, which captures the pre-NRHM (2005) and post-NRHM periods.
   (a) Compare the health expenditure: public vs private during the pre- and post-NRHM period.
   (b) Compare health infrastructure: public vs private during the pre- and post-NRHM period.
   (c) Compare HR profile: public vs private during the pre- and post-NRHM period.
2. Assume that the resource availability in a PHC is as in the table below:

Resource	Availability (%)
Medical officer	90
Nurse	90
Lab technician	90
Lab microscope in working condition	90
Pharmacist	90
All essential medicine	90

   What is the functionality of this PHC?
3. We have mentioned in this chapter that referral system in government is not working well. Is there a two-way communication between the parent consultant and the referred consultants? Is it possible that some referred consultants recommend investigations already done? (This question is based on personal experience.)
4. What are your views on medical insurance for hospitalization? Cashless package service vs reimbursement option? Is there transparency by the hospital regarding the amount charged to the patients? Do the hospitals give a complete list of services rendered and the charges for the same? What are your views on the 'disease specific insurance package'?
5. What are the advantages and disadvantages of allowing government doctors to do private practice?

6. The private health sector is not regulated. As a result, we see many maternity nursing homes and orthopedic hospitals in residential complexes and shopping centres. What are its implications on the community? How do these 'hospitals' manage bio-medical wastes and x-ray emissions?
7. Do you or do you not recommend regulation (not control) of the Indian private health sector? Explain your choice rationally.
8. The Government of India is promoting PPP for delivery of health services. Given the fact that the private sector is not regulated, what are the consequences of PPPs?
9. What steps are required to get the Indian health sector perform better?

REFERENCES

1. Government of India (2000), National Population Policy 2000, New Delhi, Government of India. Available at www.mohfw.nic.in/npp2000. Last accessed on Nov 2004.
2. Government of India (2002), National Health Policy 2002, New Delhi, Government of India. Available at www.mohfw.nic.in//nhp2002. Last accessed on Nov 2004.
3. Sachs, Jeffery and Singh, Manmohan et al (Dec 2001), *Macroeconomics and Health: Investing in Health for Economic Development*, WHO.
4. Government of India (Aug 2005), Report of the National Commission on Macroeconomics and Health, Ministry of Health and Family Welfare, Government of India, New Delhi.
5. Government of India (2004–05), National Health Accounts India, 2004–05, Ministry of Health and Family Welfare, Government of India, New Delhi.
6. Ibid.
7. Rao, K. Sujatha; V. Selvaraju; S. Nagpal; S. Sakhivel (2005), *Financing and Delivery of Healthcare Services in India*, New Delhi.
8. Government of India (Sep 2010), Annual Report, Ministry of Health and Family Welfare, Government of India, New Delhi.
9. Government of India. National Rural Health Mission (2005–12): Mission Document, Government of India. Available at www.mofhw.nic.in. Last accessed on 3 Mar 2012.
10. Annual Report, Government of India, Ministry of Health and Family Welfare, December 2011.
11. Government of India (2004–05), National Health Accounts India, 2004–05, Ministry of Health and Family Welfare, Government of India, New Delhi.
12. Government of India (2010), Rural Healthcare System in India, Ministry of Health and Family Welfare, Government of India. Available at http://nrhm-mis.nic.in/UI/RHS/RHS%202010/RHS%202010/Rural%20Health%20Care%20System%20in%20India.pdf. Last accessed on 2 March 2012.
13. Ministry of Health and Family Welfare, Government of India (June 2010). National Urban Health Mission: Framework for Implementation (Draft for Discussion). Available at www.mohfw.nic.in. Last accessed on 12 Feb 2012.
14. Ramani, K.V. et al. (2007), 'A GIS Approach to Plan and Deliver Healthcare Services to Urban Poor', *International Journal of Pharmaceuticals and healthcare Marketing*, 1 (2), pp. 159–172.

15. Agarwal, Siddharth, The State of Urban Health in India: Comparing the Poorest Quartile to the Rest of the Urban Population in Selected Cities and States. Available at http://www.uhrc.in/downloads/Publications/Articles/EAU.pdf. Last accessed on 10 Mar 2012.
16. WHO Report, India Country Health Profile: Country Health System Profile, India. Available at www.searo.who.int/en/Section313/Section1519_10852.htm. Last accessed on 3 Mar 2012.
17. Mahal, Ajay; Debroy, Bibek and Bhandari, Laveesh (2010), *India Health Report 2010*, Indicus Analytics: BS Books.
18. Ibid.
19. Government of India (Sep 2010), Annual Report, Ministry of Health and Family Welfare, Government of India, New Delhi.
20. Ibid.
21. Ramani, K.V. et al. (2007). 'A GIS Approach to Plan and Deliver Healthcare Services to Urban Poor', *International Journal of Pharmaceuticals and Healthcare Marketing*, 1 (2), pp. 159–172.
22. Government of India (Sep 2010), Annual Report, Ministry of Health and Family Welfare, Government of India, New Delhi.
23. Ibid.
24. (07 Apr 2008). India needs 600,000 more doctors: Plan Panel. Available at http://www.rediff.com/money/2008/apr/07panel.htm. Last accessed on 28 Mar 2012.
25. Annual Report, Government of India, Ministry of Health and Family Welfare, December 2011.
26. Mahal et al., (2010), *India Health Report 2010*, Indicus Analytics: BS Books.
27. Annual Report, Government of India, Ministry of Health and Family Welfare, December 2011.
28. Ibid.
29. WHO Report, India Country Health Profile: Country Health System Profile; India. Available at www.searo.who.int/en/Section313/Section1519_10852.htm. Last accessed on 3 Mar 2012
30. Government of India (Sep 2010), Annual Report, Ministry of Health and Family Welfare, Government of India, New Delhi.
31. India Reports (7 Nov 2009). Doctors per one hundred thousand people in India. Available at http://india-reports.in/future-growth-global-transitions/economy-in-transition/doctors-per-one-hundred-thousand-people-in-india/. Last accessed on 1 Mar 2012.
32. WHO, Country Office for India. (2007). Not Enough Here… Too Many There… Heath Workforce in India. Available at www.searo-who.int/en. Last accessed on 1 Mar 2012.
33. WHO Report, India Country Health Profile: Country Health System Profile; India. Available at www.searo.who.int/en/Section313/Section1519_10852.htm. Last accessed on 3 Mar 2012.
34. Mahal et al., (2010), *India Health Report 2010*, Indicus Analytics: BS Books.
35. Government of India (Sep 2010), Annual Report, Ministry of Health and Family Welfare, Government of India, New Delhi.
36. Hospital beds per 1000 people. Available at http://www.nationmaster.com/graph/hea_hos_bed_per_1000_peo-beds-per-1-000-people. Last accessed on 1 Mar 2012.

part 2

Hospital Management Challenges

CHAPTERS

3. Hospital Management: Service Quality
4. Hospital Management Functions
5. Hospital Management Support Systems

OBJECTIVE

The main focus here is to highlight the managerial challenges in delivering hospital services. The ultimate objective of hospital management is to utilize the hospital resources effectively and efficiently to provide good quality services at affordable prices to the community.

chapter 3

Hospital Management: Service Quality

CHAPTER OUTLINE

CHAPTER OBJECTIVE

The main objective of this chapter is to provide a general introduction to hospital management and the issues in hospital service delivery and service quality. We also provide a basic understanding of managing the hospital queuing systems to address the issues in service delivery and service quality.

3.1 AN INTRODUCTION

Any organization has four basic resources:

1. Human resources
2. Financial resources
3. Material resources
4. Machines and equipments

The management of any organization is responsible and accountable to utilize its resources to deliver products and/or services to meet its policy goals and objectives.

Management is all about effective and efficient utilization of the available resources to produce goods and services.

We begin this chapter with an introduction to management concepts and apply them to hospital management in the subsequent sections. Managing a service organization like hospitals is more challenging than a production unit, because of the simultaneity, intangibility and heterogeneity characteristics in service processes.

Hospitals play a vital role in delivering a wide range of healthcare services. Service quality is of utmost importance due to customer presence and participation in service delivery. We highlight certain important issues and managerial challenges in hospital service delivery by providing illustrations from real life.

Queues are formed in any service system because of mismatch between the rate of demand for service and the rate of service delivery. A basic understanding of managing queuing systems is, therefore, necessary for the hospital managers to ensure quality service delivery.

The ultimate objective of hospital management is to ensure good quality services at minimum cost. Poor quality of service not only wastes resources, but is positively dangerous to the health and welfare of the patient and the community at large.

3.2 BASIC CONCEPTS IN MANAGEMENT

Organizations have certain resources and are expected to produce goods and/or services, by utilizing their resources.

Organizational resources include:

- Human resources
- Financial resources
- Material resources
- Machines and equipments

Management is all about effective and efficient utilization of available resources to achieve the desired outputs.

Effective utilization of resources indicates the ability of the organization to achieve the desired outputs.

Efficient utilization of resources indicates the ratio of input resources utilized to produce one unit of output.

Effectiveness and efficiency together indicate an optimal utilization of resources to achieve the desired outputs.

Management of resources to produce goods and/or services involves coordinating several activities such as purchase, production, inventory, marketing, finance, and so on. Most of the organizations in India follow the traditional grouping of activities into functional departments (as opposed to grouping the activities into re-engineered value-added processes) such as:

- Production department
- HR department
- Finance department
- Purchase department
- Marketing department
- Sales department

The responsibility of each functional department is to utilize its resources to produce its deliverables. Since the utilization of resources is central to all functional departments, it would be useful to relate the functional departments with resource management functions such as:

- Operations management: Utilization of machines and equipments
- HR management: Utilization of human resources
- Financial management: Utilization of financial resources
- Materials management: Utilization of materials
- Marketing and sales: Generating demand and sales of goods/services

A well-designed organizational structure (also called organizational chart or organogram) facilitates inter-departmental coordination of the management functions to deliver goods and/or services. An organizational structure displays the formal management structure, responsibility and accountability of all the departments in the overall functioning of the organization. It also illustrates the hierarchical relationships between employees at various levels in an organization. An illustrative organizational structure is shown in Figure 3.1.

Managers at each level in the organizational structure take important decisions to ensure proper utilization of resources to achieve the deliverables. Managerial decisions can be broadly classified into:

- Policy decisions
- Strategic planning decisions
- Operational planning decisions
- Monitoring and control decisions

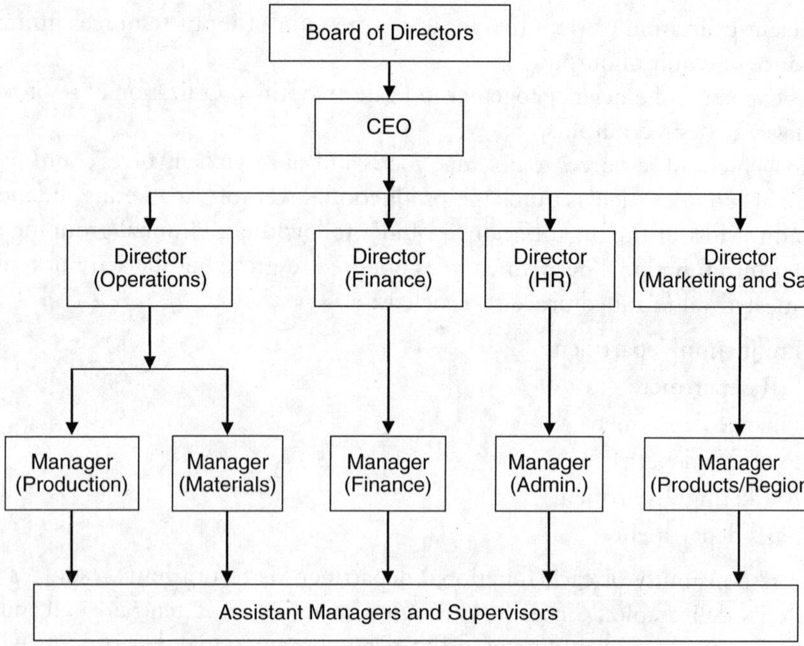

Figure 3.1 An Illustrative Organizational Structure

Policy Decisions: Policy decisions reflect the organization's goals and objectives derived from its vision and mission statements.

Strategic Planning Decisions: Strategic decisions give directions to translate the organization's policy goals into deliverables. Strategic planning deals with estimating the resource needs of the organization to meet its goals and objectives, and, if necessary, augment its resources by buying, leasing and/or contracting arrangements. Strategic planning also involves cost reduction strategies to deliver goods and/or services.

Operational Planning Decisions: Operational decisions focus on developing a detailed plan to implement the strategic decisions. Operational planning involves allocating the resources to various activities as per their needs assessment. Operational planning also deals with reacting to unplanned/ad-hoc events such as shortage of staff due to transfer and promotion, longer periods of machine breakdowns for want of spare parts, and so on.

Monitoring and Control Decisions: Monitoring and control decisions involve monitoring the implementation of the operational plan and making appropriate interventions whenever necessary. Monitoring the utilization of resources is essential to check if each planned activity produces its planned output. If not, it is necessary to exercise appropriate controls (interventions) as and when necessary so as to ensure the attainment of organizational objectives. Please note that monitoring without exercising appropriate controls is a waste of organizational resource.

Lack of monitoring or poor monitoring would lead to underutilization of organizational resources leading to underachievement of organizational objectives. For example, underutilization of human resources could have very adverse consequences. Employees could develop a casual approach to their professional commitment leading to lack of motivation, increased absenteeism, reduced working hours, compromise on product/service quality and resorting to unethical practices, all resulting in under performance. Over a period of time, lack of monitoring would even weaken the role of operational and strategic planning and, thereby, result in under achievement of the organizational goals and objectives.

Monitoring vs Evaluation: It would be useful at this point to understand and appreciate certain basic differences between monitoring and evaluation.

Monitoring is a continuous on-going activity to ensure that each activity is executed as originally planned, if required, by exercising control through appropriate interventions whenever necessary. Monitoring should be done at different levels in an organization to facilitate taking immediate corrective measures.

Evaluation, on the other hand, is an audit function done at periodic intervals (usually every half yearly or annually) and, therefore, does not facilitate on-line interventions. It is a statutory requirement, which through an audit of what happened in the past, provides useful information for future planning.

Table 3.1 highlights the basic differences between monitoring and evaluation.

Table 3.2 relates the types of managerial decisions and the decision makers in an organization.

Table 3.1 Monitoring vs Evaluation

Monitoring	Evaluation
Continuous on-going activity	Periodic activity
Live activity, under continuous observation	Audit function, examines the past at the end of each period
Identifies 'out-of-control processes' immediately	Identifies 'out-of-control processes' only at the end of evaluation period
Being a live activity, facilitates on-line interventions immediately	Being a periodic function, intervention has to wait till the next period starts
Like a patient in ICU, brings the activity under control immediately	Like post-mortem, useful lessons for the future from the past
Managerial requirement	Statutory requirement

Table 3.2 Managerial Decisions and Decision Makers

Managerial Decisions	Examples of Managerial Decisions	Decision Makers
Policy decisions	Factory location, size, deliverables (products, services), capital investment	The board of directors
Strategic planning decisions	Capacity planning, staffing, market segment, pricing, cost reduction	CEO in consultation with functional directors and other senior executives
Operational planning decisions	Product mix, media planning, transfers and promotions	Functional directors in consultation with functional managers
Monitoring and control decisions	Machine break-downs, quality of materials, staff absenteeism	Functional managers in consultation with assistant managers and supervisors

To summarize, the management of any organization deals with the task of utilizing its resources to deliver products and/or services. A good management utilizes its resources effectively and efficiently to deliver good quality products and/or services at minimal cost.

Effective utilization of resources is a measure of output.

Efficient utilization of resources is a measure of input resources to output.

Together, effectiveness and efficiency reflect an optimal utilization of resources in the delivery of goods and/or services.

Beginning the next section, we initiate our discussions on hospital management concepts and challenges.

3.3 HOSPITAL MANAGEMENT

3.3.1 Introduction to Hospital Management

Hospitals have become complex organizations as they consume vast amount of resources in delivering a wide range of healthcare services. Increased cost for medical care, ageing population and the potentially declining levels of service threaten the quality of service delivered. Liberalization of the medical insurance sector has added a new dimension to the delivery and pricing of healthcare services. Poor quality of services not only wastes resources but is positively dangerous to the health and welfare of the patients and the community at large.

> The health sector in India needs an additional 3 million hospital beds to achieve the world average of 3.6 beds per 1,000 population.

The resources of any hospital are as given in Table 3.3.

Table 3.3 Hospital Resources

Organizational Resources	Hospital Resources
Human resources	Medical, para-medical and administrative staff Regular and on-contract service
Financial resources	Income from patient care, donations, grant, and so on.
Material resources	Medical, surgical, laboratory items, office stationeries, house-keeping items, and so on.
Equipment and devices	Medical equipments, devices and instruments

Hospital services can be broadly classified into:

- Outpatient services
- Inpatient services[i]

Clinical departments such as the department of medicine, general surgery, cardiac care, and so on are responsible for providing outpatient and inpatient services. In providing clinical services, these departments are ably assisted by the investigation departments, namely, the clinical laboratory and the radiology/imaging departments. Para-medical services are offered by the nursing department, physiotherapy, and so on. Administrative support for service delivery is provided by the general administration departments such as finance, HR, house-keeping, medical stores, medical records and bio-medical wastes.

In the next section, we highlight certain unique characteristics of service organizations and relate these to hospitals offering healthcare services.

3.3.2 Managing a Service Organization

There are certain basic differences between managing organizations which deliver services and those which produce goods. Since hospitals are service organizations, it would be useful to understand the characteristics of service organizations in general.[1]

> Service is an experience of a process of interaction between service providers and customers.

Most services are characterized by an encounter between service providers and customers. Service providers, therefore, have an opportunity to build personal relationships with customers unlike manufacturers who are isolated from the eventual end customer by a distribution channel of stockists, wholesalers and

[i] Certain clinical departments also provide daycare services. In this book, we are including daycare services under inpatient services.

retailers. Services are produced and consumed simultaneously unlike products which are mass produced and kept in inventory for future use. These and other distinguishing features of services explained below have implications on the measurement of service quality.

The distinguishing features of service processes from production processes are as follows:

- Customer presence and participation
- Simultaneity
- Intangibility
- Heterogeneity

Customer Presence and Participation: The most distinguishing feature of any service process from a manufacturing process is the presence of the customer in the service delivery system.

Active participation by customers in service delivery could also influence the effectiveness of service delivery. For example, honest and frank inputs from patients about their health conditions and lifestyles would make it easier for their attending physicians to make an accurate diagnosis leading to more effective treatment.

Because of the presence of customers in service delivery, *facility design* assumes more importance in service delivery than production of goods.

The design should provide basic amenities and good ambience in waiting areas, unlike the environment in a production factory.

Simultaneity: Services are produced and consumed simultaneously and, therefore, cannot be 'stored' for future needs.

The inability to 'store' services for future needs makes the task of estimating the demand for services more challenging than estimating the demand for goods. Unmet demands for services are lost forever, while overestimating the demand could result in underutilization of resources. For example, unmet demand for cardiac care services in a hospital could lead to opportunity loss of revenues and increased customer dissatisfaction. On the other hand, overestimating the demand for cardiac care services could indicate poor investment decisions as setting up cardiac care facilities is very expensive.

The simultaneity characteristic of services also makes interventions for quality control impossible. Quality of manufactured products can be evaluated before, during or after delivery, while the quality of services delivered cannot be guaranteed. For example, how can you measure the quality of service for taking blood pressure? Another example, quality of surgical services in a hospital cannot be measured, even though infection rate after hospital discharge could be an indicator. It is not easy to establish whether the infections developed after hospital discharge are hospital acquired infections or not.

Intangibility: Services are intangibles, since service is an experience of a process of interaction between the service providers and customers. Products can be seen, felt and even tested for quality before purchase, but not hospital services.

Heterogeneity: The intangible nature of services, simultaneity, customer's presence in the service delivery system and the design of service facility introduce variability in service quality from customer to customer. The heterogeneity in service provision could be easily understood if we consider the process of blood collection. Even though blood collection procedures are well laid out, it is more difficult to draw blood from some people, especially children and old people. Different patients go through different experiences in getting the same service.

While a poor quality product can be recalled and replaced, poor quality of healthcare service could have adverse effects on patients' health.

In view of the above distinguishing characteristics of service processes, managing a service organization is more challenging than managing a manufacturing/production unit.

In the words of J. Willard Marriott, the founder of the Marriot Hotel Chain, 'In the service business, you cannot make happy guests with unhappy employees'.

In the next section, we discuss issues and challenges in hospital service delivery.

3.4 HOSPITAL SERVICE DELIVERY

3.4.1 Issues and Challenges

A brief introduction to hospital services would provide a better insight into the issues and challenges faced by the hospital management in the delivery of services.

Outpatient Services: Each clinical department offers outpatient services. The outpatient service process starts with registration followed by consultation, investigation and medication. Outpatients visit the outpatient department (OPD) clinics 2–3 times; first visit as new patients and follow up visits as repeat patients. Many hospitals handle a large number of OPD patients as no patient can be turned away, and, thereby, raise issues on service quality and turnaround time.

Inpatient Care: The inpatient care process starts with hospital admission under the care of a doctor, followed by medical and/or surgical care with special attention to customer[ii] satisfaction. When the treatment is complete, the inpatient

[ii] Customers include patients, their attendants, relatives and the community at large.

is discharged. Issues in the process of inpatient care delivery are on admission process, length of stay, bed occupancy, cost vs revenue, service quality (technical and patient satisfaction), dietary and discharge processes.

Operation Theatre (OT) Services: OTs consume a very large portion of all the hospital resources, high investment in OT infrastructure, highly skilled staff, expensive surgical materials and high overheads. Hence, a clear understanding of the cost incurred by the hospital for providing surgical services is necessary to arrive at a rational pricing for its services. Cost control is a major issue and options available include optimal scheduling of surgical procedures to minimize the idling of OT resources, adopting standard operating procedures, and so on.

Clinical Lab Services: Almost 60–70 per cent of major decisions on admission, treatment and discharge are based on laboratory test results. Lab tests can be classified into biochemistry, hematology, clinical pathology, microbiology, histo-pathology, and so on. Lab services start with collecting samples (pre-analytic), analysis of samples (analytic) and test report dissemination (post-analytic). Issues here focus on minimizing lab errors (arising from transcription errors, insufficient sample, and so on) to ensure sample integrity and, thereby, the reliability and timeliness of test results.

Imaging Services: Radiology or imaging services provide useful information to the clinicians regarding the body structure. There are a wide range of investigative modalities; X-ray (e.g., bone image), USG and CT Scan (e.g., soft tissue image), MRI (e.g., tumour size image, neuro image), Colour Doppler (blood flow image in heart chamber), PET Scan (image of body form and function), Gamma Camera (nuclear medicine imaging scans), and so on. Interpreting the images requires highly skilled staff. Issues here focus on achieving the maximum utilization from costly investments, pricing of imaging services, and so on.

Stores and Purchase: Hospital stores and purchase management are responsible for vendor selection, purchase, storage and distribution of drugs, medicines, reagents, and so on to the user departments. Hospital purchases account for 20–30 per cent of the total expenses incurred by any hospital, but account for 80–90 per cent of the total variable expenses. Overstocking and understocking of materials are, therefore, major issues here in order to achieve cost reduction without any compromise on service quality.

Medical Records: Medical records division manages the records of all inpatients. This is a herculean task for any hospital, especially large hospitals. Many hospitals even in developed countries still maintain manual records of their patients, as electronic patient records (EPR) systems are not practised by many doctors. With increasing dependence on hospital insurance, EPR systems would become a necessity in the future for handling medico-legal issues.

Billing: The billing department in any hospital is probably the only department which interacts with all its inpatients/attendants. It is responsible for collecting the registration fee, advance payment and the final settlement of all bills for inpatient services. In doing so, it has to interact with many supporting departments such as nursing station, pharmacy, and so on, as well as with outside parties such as the third party administrators (TPA) and insurance companies for insurance claims.

Nursing Station: Nursing stations are busy 24 × 7 throughout the year providing nursing care. Major issues here are non-availability of emergency medicines and basic materials for nursing care. Nursing stations are responsible for ensuring delivery of services ordered by the doctors, such as making the necessary arrangements for lab investigation, medicines, and so on, in addition to monitoring their patients' health status.

Facility Design: Facility design is an important determinant of service quality. Hospital entrance, admission desk, waiting areas, and so on should be designed so as to provide a good, clean and comfortable environment for the patients and their attendants.

Hospitality: Hospitality goes a long way in customer satisfaction. Sick patients who come to the hospital for medical care have to be treated with respect, dignity and compassion. Hospital communication is an important issue in patient care.

Bio-medical Support: Technology and medical equipments are gaining more importance. Bio-medical support is very vital for clinicians and managers to ensure healthcare delivery. Bio-medical support plays a critical role in sourcing equipments, testing for feasibility of local environment, in-house support, and calibration and ensuring preventive maintenance. Unforeseen medical equipment downtime would adversely affect safe, effective and timely service delivery.

Teaching and Research: Medical Council of India (MCI) and the National Board have laid down the resource requirements in teaching hospitals. These requirements are based on a given number of annual admissions to under graduate and post graduate courses. The MCI guidelines for teaching hospitals can be used as benchmarks for non-teaching hospitals as well. Main issues here are compliance with the norms to deliver teaching, research and patient care services.

Bio-medical Waste: Bio-medical waste management is a social responsibility. Hospitals generate a large amount of hazardous bio-medical wastes every day. Major contributors of hospital waste are the departments of orthopedics, gynecology and obstetrics, surgery, clinical laboratory, and so on. Main issues here are segregation of hospital waste at source into respective coloured bins, safe transportation to incineration sites and safe disposal.

Table 3.4 Issues and Challenges in Hospital Management: Some Examples

Hospital Service	Issues in Service Quality
Outpatient services (OP services)	OPD turnaround time OPD load vs service quality
Inpatient care (IP services)	Admission process Bed occupancy, length of stay Cost of service vs revenue Nursing care, dietary, discharge processes
OT services	Cost of services Revenue from services Highly skilled staff Optimal utilization of OT resources
Clinical lab services	Reliability of test results Turnaround time for results Lab errors
Radiology/imaging services	Maximum utilization of costly machines Pricing of services Highly skilled staff
Medical records	Manual storage, retrieval and update of the medical records of all patients
Billing	Interaction with patients/attendants, supporting departments and outside parties such as TPA, insurance companies
Stores and purchase	Number of vendors, number of items Storage and distribution Optimal stock, cost reduction
Facility design	Reception, waiting area, ambience, and so on
Hospitality	Reception, communication, respect, empathy
Medical college hospitals	Lack of qualified teachers as per MCI/DNB norms Compromise between teaching and patient care
Hospital waste disposal	Social responsibility Safe and secure disposal

Table 3.4 summarizes our discussion on hospital services and the issues to be addressed in the delivery of these services.

In the next section, we look at hospital service quality from a provider's perspective.

3.4.2 Service Quality: Provider Perspective

Service quality is a difficult term to define and even more difficult to measure, since services are intangible and are also produced and consumed simultaneously.

In a hospital, service quality implies giving the most appropriate treatment to patients in a medically correct manner, keeping the patients informed as to what is happening, and treating them with care, compassion, dignity and respect. Hence, quality of healthcare service refers to both the medical quality of services as well as patient/customer satisfaction.

To the service provider, hospital service quality refers to the technical quality of medical services. Technical quality, a determinant of medical service quality from a provider's perspective, is difficult to measure, due to the difficulties in measuring the impact of medical services on patients' health outcomes. It is necessary to realize that a patient's recovery depends also on the patient's compliance over a period of time after leaving the hospital. There are studies which show surgical patients developing infections after hospital discharge, but it is very difficult to conclude if the infections were hospital acquired or not.

Since impact measurement of medical service is difficult, hospital management focuses on the processes of delivering medical services which impact the final outcome. Use of partograph in labour rooms to manage the process of childbirth is an example. Another example is the Shouldice process for hernia repairs[2] which has shown remarkable success rate in hernia surgeries (very low recurrence rate). It is logical to assume that the final outcomes (impact) on patients' health would be good, if the process of service delivery is well-planned and executed.

In the next section, we look at hospital service quality from a customer's perspective.

3.4.3 Service Quality: Customer Perspective

To the customers (service recipients and the community at large), service quality refers to happiness and satisfaction with service delivery.

'Customer service quality' is defined as the 'gap' between a customer's expectations of a service and his/her perception of the quality of service delivered. SERVQUAL is the most common instrument to measure service quality.[3] Customer's expectations of a service are based on several factors such as word of mouth, personal needs, past experience, and so on. Customer's perceptions of service quality, as measured by the SERVQUAL instrument is based on five indicators, namely, reliability, responsiveness, assurance, empathy and tangibles.

1. **Reliability** is an indicator of the ability of an organization to deliver its promised services on time with dependability and accuracy (e.g., clinical lab test results).
2. **Responsiveness** is an indicator of the ability of an organization to respond to customer needs and provide services promptly (e.g., emergency services).
3. **Assurance** is an indicator of the ability of an organization to deliver services with courtesy, respect and effective communication (e.g., inpatient admission).

4. **Empathy** is an indicator of the ability of an organization to provide services with care, compassion and individualized attention to customers (e.g., labour room).
5. **Tangibles** such as the physical infrastructure and ambience are evidences of the care and attention to details exhibited by the service provider (e.g., waiting room for patients' attendants).

The measurement of the gap between expectations and perceptions of service delivery is usually done by collecting regular feedback from the customers using SERVQUAL instrument.

In the next section, we turn our attention to issues in quality control and provide a brief introduction to Six Sigma methodology.

3.4.4 Quality Control

3.4.4.1 Six Sigma Methodology: Traditionally, service quality management relied on the use of Three Sigma control charts to monitor and control service quality. For example, one could construct Three Sigma control charts to monitor the average waiting time for OPD consultation, inpatient discharge, and so on by collecting actual data on their waiting times. However, a Three Sigma quality level means that only 93 per cent of the times the service quality is 'acceptable'. Would you be happy with a hospital which has a success rate of 93 per cent in cesarean delivery section? There is a need to go beyond the Three Sigma level of quality. Hence, service quality management is moving towards the Six Sigma approach, widely used in the manufacturing sector.

Let us understand what Six Sigma means in a hospital setting, say, managing a hospital clinical lab. Lab performance is usually measured by estimating the turn-around time and quality, defined as the time elapsed between sample collection and reliable report generation. As a result, many labs in their pursuit to deliver test reports as quickly as possible may not be paying attention to lab errors.

Lab errors could occur at the time of sample collection (pre-analytic phase), sample analysis (analytic phase) and also at the time of giving the test result reports (post-analytic phase). Phlebotomy errors account for a majority of errors in the pre-analytic phase, lack of quality assurance could lead to wrong test results in the analytic phase, while misidentification errors are common in the post-analytic phase. Lab errors also occur at various stages; before centrifugation (e.g., insufficient sample quantity), after centrifugation (e.g., hemolysed[iii] sample), after test results are obtained (e.g., certain readings are extreme, out of range), and so on.

[iii] Hemolysis is the breakage of red blood cells causing the release of hemoglobin and other internal components into the blood serum or plasma. Hemolysis is an undesirable condition that influences the accuracy and reliability of test results.

Many lab managers believe that lab errors are infrequent in their lab and, therefore, there is no need for a continuous monitoring and/or recording of all lab errors. Such an assumption has serious drawbacks, as wrong lab reports could have adverse impact on the patients' health.

A Three Sigma quality level means 66,807 errors out of a total of 1,000,000 reports, or equivalently 933,193 reliable reports out of 1,000,000 reports, which means 93.32 per cent reports are reliable. In other words, seven reports out of every 100 test reports are likely to be erroneous. Is this level of performance acceptable to the management?

A Four Sigma quality level means 6,210 errors out of a total of 1,000,000 reports, which means 99.38 per cent of the reports are reliable. In other words, a lab operating at Four Sigma level produces six errors out of every 1,000 reports. This means about 20 error reports each day from large labs which do about 3,000–4,000 tests every day. Is this level of performance acceptable to the management?

A Six Sigma quality level would mean three error reports out of 1,000,000 test reports. Is the management targeting for this level of performance?

Six Sigma is all about increasing the profitability of operations by minimizing errors and, thereby, ensuring highly reliable and accurate outputs.

Lab errors, as and when detected, call for sample rejection. Any rejected sample calls for repeat sample collection and analysis, and, hence, additional costs to the lab, besides delayed reports which impact service quality and customer satisfaction. It is also possible that some lab errors could even go undetected and, thereby, could adversely affect the patients' health due to incorrect treatment protocol. Hence, controlling lab errors is very central to an effective and efficient management of lab activities.

Lab errors may not be seen as a big concern if the management feels that errors occur only occasionally. But, when all the lab errors are taken together, their combined impact on costs, profitability and customer satisfaction could be very serious. The Six Sigma approach to managing is all about helping the management identify the errors, understand their impact on lab performance and take appropriate error control measures so as to manage the lab activities effectively and efficiently. In other words, the Six Sigma methodology helps the management to eliminate most errors, reduce repeated sample collection and testing, minimize total costs and thereby achieve higher levels of profitability and customer satisfaction.[4–6]

For more details, interested readers could refer to Chapter 5, where we discuss the experience of Gangaram Hospital in its efforts to reduce clinical lab errors.[7]

3.4.4.2 NABH: National Accreditation Board for Hospitals and Healthcare Providers (NABH) is a constituent board of the Quality Council of India (QCI), set up to establish and operate accreditation programme for healthcare organizations. NABH has been established with the objective of enhancing health system and promoting continuous quality improvement and patient safety. NABH is an institutional member of the Accreditation Council of the International Society for Quality in Healthcare (ISQua), a founder member of the proposed Asian Society for Quality in Healthcare (ASQua), being registered in Malaysia, as well as a member of the International Steering Committee of WHO Collaborating Centre for Patient Safety as a nominee of ISQua Accreditation Council. Hospitals are assessed for compliance of standards for patient-centred activities and standards for organization-centred activities. Currently, accreditation is a voluntary option, but it is expected that the Indian healthcare sector would gravitate towards mandatory accreditation like in many developed countries.

In the next section, we highlight the importance of queuing systems management in the delivery of hospital services. Queues are always formed in any service system because of mismatch between the rate of demand for service and the rate of service delivery.

3.5 HOSPITAL QUEUING SYSTEMS

3.5.1 Simple Queuing Systems

Waiting for service (queuing) is a common sight, be it for banking, payment of bills, checking out in super markets, waiting for your luggage at airports, traffic intersections or hospital services. Waiting for hospital services should be seen differently from waiting for other services, since any unnecessary delay in the provision of healthcare services could have serious consequences on the health of the patients, and, thereby, impact the customer's perception of the hospital's service quality. Customer satisfaction is an important attribute of any hospital service delivery.

Any service manager has to manage the waiting line (queue) of customers waiting for service. Queues get formed due to mismatch between the rate of arrival for service and the rate of service delivery.

Any hospital service is a combination of several specialty services, each specialty service is handled by a specialty department. Each specialty department handles its own waiting line of customers. Managing hospital service delivery, therefore, involves managing multiple interdependent queues. An understanding of hospital queuing systems is central to hospital management. It requires proper coordination of all the activities involved in the service delivery process.

Hospital services are interdependent. An interdependent queuing system would have a 'bottleneck resource' which constraints the system throughput.

The system throughput (number of services completed in any given period of time) is constrained by the service which takes the maximum amount of time. Services which constrain the system throughputs are called 'bottlenecks' in the system of service delivery. Identifying bottlenecks in interdependent queuing systems and managing them to achieve optimum throughput from the system are critical managerial challenges in the delivery of hospital services. We discuss all these issues and more in this chapter.

Queues for services get formed when the demand rate (arrival rate) exceeds the service rate for any service.[8,9] Managing hospital customers (patients and/or their attendants) is far more critical than managing customers in a bank or restaurant. This is because patients waiting for hospital services are sick and very anxious. Unfortunately, such concerns of the customers are not clearly understood by the hospital service managers, who handle queues every day. Long waiting times would be an indicator of customer dissatisfaction and poor quality of service delivery.

Let us take a simple example of hospital service to understand the challenges in the management of queuing systems.

OPD Registration Services: First, let us take a simple queuing system; the case of outpatients waiting for registration to get an appointment for consultation services[iv]. OPD patients can be broadly classified into two categories, namely, new patients and repeat patients. The requirements of hospital resources are different for new and repeat patients. New patients take more time for consultation than repeat patients. Also, new patients could be assigned to any doctor on OPD duty, while repeat patients should be assigned to the same doctor who saw them first. Hence, the OPD registration counter entertains two types of customers: each type of customer demands different services. How does the hospital manage the waiting lines (queues) for a mix of services?

- **Option 1:** The hospital maintains two separate queues, one queue for new patients and another queue for repeat patients. Each queue has a dedicated registration clerk (server) for service.
- **Option 2:** The hospital maintains one long combined queue for both types of customers, new and repeat patients, and keeps two registration clerks in

---

[iv] This service is similar to banking services we are all familiar with. Let us take two banking services, namely, cash withdrawals and deposits. One bank may maintain different queues for different services; one queue for cash withdrawals and another queue for deposits, with a dedicated clerk for each service. Another bank may maintain only one long queue for both cash withdrawals and deposits with a single clerk. The management practices followed by the two banks are different, and, therefore, the costs to the bank management for service provision and the service levels to their customers would be different.

the registration counter. The patient in front of the queue would be served by either of the two clerks, whoever becomes free first. In this case, both the registration clerks (servers) can serve any type of patient.

- **Option 3:** The hospital maintains two queues, and any customer (new or repeat patient) can join any queue. Each queue is served by a dedicated registration clerk.

Consequences on Service Quality: In the first option, utilization of the two servers may not be uniform. It is possible that while one registration clerk is busy, the other clerk is idle, since the arrival rates of new and repeat patients are different and also repeat patients would be 2–3 times the number of new patients. Underutilization of hospital resources (registration clerks) is not a desirable characteristic for the service provider.

In the second option, there is uniform utilization of both the registration clerks as any clerk can serve any patient. What would be the implications on the average waiting time for each type of patient? This is because of a single queue with different types of customers (new and repeat) who demand different levels of service.

In the third option, the patients (or their attendants) are free to join any queue they choose. What would be the implications on patient waiting times and utilization of the two staff resources? (Such situations often arise in banks and airports. How many times have we ended up choosing the wrong queue? Personally, the queue I choose for checking in at airports always ends up moving slower than the other queues).

In the next section, we discuss more complex queuing systems, known as interdependent queuing systems, which are very common in hospitals.

3.5.2 Interdependent Queuing Systems

A queuing system is said to be interdependent if the performance of any queue in the system of service delivery influences the performance of any other queue in the system.

There are two types of interdependent queuing systems:

1. Sequentially interdependent queue
2. Pooled interdependent queue

Sequentially Interdependent Queuing Systems: A queuing system is said to be sequentially interdependent if the rate of completion of one service (service rate) influences the rate of demand (arrival rate) for the next service.

Let us explain this with a simple example.

Inpatient Discharge: The inpatient discharge process[v] starts as soon as the doctor orders discharge. This is followed by preparation and signing of the discharge summary, returning unused medicines to the pharmacy and purchasing new medicines prescribed in the discharge summary, settling all accounts with the billing department, and, if necessary, calling for ambulance. Usually, the doctors give discharge orders during their morning rounds around 9 am, but patients wait 'endlessly' for all the hospital formalities for discharge to be completed. Private hospitals have a tendency to blame the cashless medical insurance providers for the delay, but such excuses are not true as we will see in our case studies in the following chapters.

If the discharge procedures can be better streamlined, the patients could go home early (don't we want to be home soon, if we are patients) and the patients' attendants could go back to work and avoid losing another day's salary. Unnecessary waiting has both health and financial implications on the patients and their attendants. Moreover, unnecessary delay in the discharge process constraints the hospital from allotting the 'discharged' beds to new patients.

Pooled Interdependent Queuing Systems: A queuing system is said to be pooled interdependent if a pool of experts working independently coordinate (interdependence) their activities in providing a given service.

Let us explain this with a simple example. Take the case of surgical services in an OT. Surgical services require pooling of several independent services such as surgical procedures, anesthesia and nursing services. Here, each specialized service is done independently and in coordination with other services, and all services pooled together in some pre-defined order (not sequentially) would complete the surgical procedure.

If we add pre- and post-surgical procedures on patients and post-surgical activities (cleaning the OT before taking the next patient in, and so on) to the delivery of surgical services in OT, we have a mix of sequential and pooled interdependent queuing systems.

---

[v] Discharge process in a hospital is a sequentially interdependent queuing system, like the process of getting a driver's license at the Regional Transport Office (RTO). In the RTO, the customers go through the process of registration, digital photograph and test driving. RTO clerks in the registration counter accept the completed application forms and do the necessary processing. Following the registration, the applicants go to the digital photograph department and then go for test driving. After the driving test, the applicants leave the RTO and await driving license to be delivered at home by post. Long queues for registration, digital photograph and test drives are common due to the mismatch between their arrival rate and service rate.

If the pooled interdependent surgical services can be managed well, the service time for each surgery can be minimized without any compromise on service quality. By doing so, the surgical department would be able to perform more surgeries per day, and, thereby, the waiting time of surgical patients can be brought down. Optimal scheduling of surgical services is one way to achieve higher levels of throughput, without additional resources[vi].

Bottlenecks in Interdependent Queuing Systems: In managing an interdependent queuing system, managing any resource in the chain of service delivery would have implications on the management of all other resources. This means that managerial decisions for utilization of resources are taken by considering all the resources (staff, finances, materials and machines) together and not any resource in isolation, since all resources are required to provide any service.

In order to understand the importance of managing an interdependent queuing system, it is necessary to understand the concept of bottleneck resources in service delivery.

A resource is said to be a *bottleneck resource* in a chain of service delivery if its maximum output capacity is the least among all resources. A bottleneck resource, thus, puts constraints on the total throughput of the system over a unit of time. A bottleneck resource would, therefore, lead to underutilization of some or all other resources in the system. It is important to realize that augmenting a bottleneck resource irrationally to increase throughput would lead to another resource becoming a bottleneck. Capacity management is an important concept in the management of interdependent queuing systems.

[vi] To understand how to achieve increased throughput without adding resources, let us take an example in daily life. Consider the case of traffic waiting for clearance at busy intersections. Assume the traffic is allowed to flow either in east–west directions (both ways) or north–south directions (both ways). The cycle time for the traffic signalling scheme is 180 seconds; i.e., the cycle of traffic clearances repeats every 180 seconds. The phase time for clearance is equally divided by giving 90 seconds for traffic in north–south directions (both ways) and 90 seconds for traffic in east–west directions (both ways). If the phase time for north–south traffic (both directions) clearance is increased to 100 seconds to minimize its waiting time, then longer queues would be noticed for the east–west traffic (both directions), if we keep the cycle time unchanged. On the other hand, if both north–south and east–west traffic clearance times are increased to 100 seconds, then the signalling scheme should be designed to provide a longer cycle time of 200 seconds. Does this rescheduling of cycle time and phase time increase the total traffic cleared on any given day? Here, the traffic management has to manage the trade-off between cycle time and phase time, but no additional resources are required to increase the throughput!

3.5.3 Computer Simulation

Computer simulation is a very useful tool to study the behaviour of complex queuing systems.

Computer simulation is a useful tool to analyse capacity utilization in complex queuing systems.

Computer simulation is an experimental tool to evaluate the consequences of decision alternatives, when analytical methods are not available. Computer simulation models are experimental models which allow users to evaluate various options under several 'what-if' scenarios. Computer simulation models, therefore, do not guarantee optimal solutions, but they do give feasible and better solutions.

Computer simulation calls for a large volume of data for 'experimentation'. A computer simulation model requires as inputs, all the characteristics, parameters and descriptions of the working of the real system. A study of system characteristics and parameters is first undertaken through data collection. These data are then analysed to estimate the system characteristics and parameters and fed into a computer programme which simulates the working of the real system. A computer simulation model, thus, designed and developed is then used to evaluate the system performance under a number of alternate 'what-if' scenarios.

Computer simulation of queuing systems, if understood correctly, could be very effectively applied to manage hospital queues which are complex and interdependent.

Let us start with a familiar example.

A computer simulation model would choose the best feasible option for implementation from among several options experimented with. Hence, optimality of simulation results is not guaranteed.

Consider the case of traffic simulation mentioned earlier. Traffic control in any major city road is very challenging since it involves not only managing queues in each intersection, it also involves synchronizing the traffic flow from one intersection to the next. It would be dangerous to try evaluating various options for traffic clearance by actually trying them out in busy intersections. Computer simulation models are, therefore, extensively used for designing traffic signalling schemes. Implied in this approach is the fact that a computer simulation model, while providing a better solution (than the current solution) to improve system performance, may not give you the optimum solution. This is because computer simulation approach essentially is an experimental approach, to try various trials (options) under 'what-if' conditions, evaluate the consequence of each trial and choose that option which is best among the various options evaluated for implementation.

In the context of hospital service delivery, computer simulation could be used as a methodology to improve OPD service delivery, increase the throughput of surgical services, better management of inpatient discharge process, and so on.

STAR HOSPITAL

MINI CASE 3.1

The management of Star Hospital is concerned about the OPD service quality. The OPD process starts with registration, followed by consultation, investigations and medication.

OPD hours at Star Hospital start at 9 am. On an average, 100 outpatients arrive every day by 12 noon. The hospital maintains a single queue with three clerks for OPD registration services, which close at 12 noon. Each clerk takes an average of five minutes per patient.

The hospital has three doctors and each doctor sees an average of four patients an hour. Consulting hours are from 9 am to 1 pm. Following the lunch break from 1 pm to 2 pm, the doctors are busy with ward visit, administrative work, and so on.

The pathology laboratory has two technicians who work from 9 am to 2 pm for sample collection from OPD patients. Usually, sample collection in many hospitals would be closed by 2 pm, so as to complete analysis of all samples collected the same day. Each technician takes an average of 12 minutes per patient for sample collection.

There are two pharmacists for dispensing medicines; each pharmacist takes an average of 15 minutes per patient for dispensing medicines and drugs. Note that the pharmacists are not dedicated to OPD patients, they serve all their customers round the clock.

Case Analysis

The Problem: The management of Star Hospital is concerned about the OPD service quality. The OPD process[vii] starts with registration, followed by consultation, investigations and medication.

The service rate for each service influences the queue length for the next service. For example, the service rate for registration influences the queue length for consultation, while the service rate for consultation influences the queue length for investigation and medication. Table 3.5 summarizes the characteristics of OPD queuing system.

[vii]The OPD service process in hospitals is another example of sequential interdependent queues, involving registration, consultation, investigation and medication.

Table 3.5 Characteristics of OPD Queues: Star Hospital

OPD Activities	Characteristics of OPD Queues
Registration	Arrival rate: 33 patients per hour (100 patients in three hours) Service rate: 36 patients per hour (12 persons served by each clerk: C1, C2 and C3)
Consultation	Arrival rate: 36 patients per hour (output from registration is the input load for consultation) Service rate: 12 per hour (Four patients seen by each consulting doctor: D1, D2 and D3)
Investigation	Arrival rate: 12 persons per hour (output rate from consultation) Service rate: 10 per hour (Five patients by each nurse, N1 and N2)
Medication	Arrival rate: 12 per hour (*) Service rate: 8 per hour (Four patients by each pharmacist: P1, P2)

*Some repeat patients skip investigation.

The hospital has to complete all the services for its 100 outpatients who are already in the system. When would the last patient leave the hospital after collecting his/her medicines? What is the workload on the hospital doctors? What is the service level offered by the hospital? What is the level of customer satisfaction defined by the turnaround time from arrival for registration to exit from the hospital after availing of all the services? Please note that the mismatch between the arrival rate and service rate at each service window would result in queue formation, the queue length for each service would be different.

The registration department receives 100 outpatients from 9 am to 12 noon, and serves 36 patients per hour, on an average. Accordingly, the queue length for registration service is pretty much under control (queuing theory tells us that queues get formed even when the arrival rate and service rate are the same for any service).

The consultation department receives 36 patients per hour (hourly output from registration department) and serves 12 patients per hour. Thus, the queue length for consultation would keep building up from 9 am onwards. This mismatch between the arrival and service rates for consultation leads to long queues for consultation. There would be about 64 patients waiting for consultation by 12 noon, when the registration counter closes for the day (36 out of 100 registered patients would have completed consultation by 12 noon). Since all the registered patients have to be seen the same day, doctors would have to work beyond their four-hours OPD or the hospital should employ more doctors or reduce the consultation time per patient.

Similarly, the mismatch in the arrival rate and service rate for investigation and medication services would result in queues for each of these services. Patients who were seen by the doctors after 2 pm would have to come the next day for investigation, as the sample collection closes by 2 pm.

What are the options available to the hospital management to manage the OPD queues better? The manager has to make a trade-off between minimizing the waiting time of patients vs additional costs for employing one more doctor for consultation, without compromising on the service quality. (Is consultation the bottleneck resource?)

In the next section, we discuss a case study on the management of a bottleneck resource, which is very common in dealing with queuing systems.

A-ONE SURGICAL HOSPITAL — MINI CASE 3.2

A-One Surgical Hospital specializes in general surgery. It has 110 beds, five OTs working for 12 hours per day in two shifts: 6 am to 12 noon and 1 pm to 7 pm, Monday through Saturday. A team of 11 surgeons and two anesthetists is ably supported by other OT staff. Any surgeon can perform any general surgery, which takes an average of two hours including pre- and post-operative services. On any given day, one out of the 11 surgeons (on rotation) would be doing administrative duties, while the remaining 10 surgeons would be busy with clinical work, six hours in OT (either in the morning shift or the afternoon shift), one hour lunch break, and three hours doing OPD and ward visits.

Patients are admitted one day before the date of the planned surgery, Monday through Friday and Sunday. No admission is entertained on Saturdays since OTs remain closed on Sundays. Upon arrival at the hospital between 1 pm and 5 pm (Monday through Friday and Sunday), each surgical patient first goes through the process of admission, which consists of registration, an advance payment for hospital services and is allotted a bed. One of the two hospital receptionists assists the patients with their admission process which takes about 12 minutes per patient, including taking the patient to his/her room.

After the patient is admitted, one of the four doctors on duty examines the patient, makes a case sheet, orders some investigations and medications, all of which take about 30 minutes per patient. Examinations are done between 2 pm and 6 pm.

Following the examination, the nursing station takes the responsibility for arranging medications and sample collection for investigations. Three nurses are dedicated to this activity from 3 pm to 6 pm; each nurse can take care of four patients an hour.

The morning after admission, the patient is taken to an OT room for surgery which takes about two hours, including pre- and post-surgical procedures.

After the surgery, the patient is taken back to his/her bed, health conditions are monitored for the next two days and, if satisfied, the surgeon orders patient discharge the following day. The average length of stay in the hospital for a surgical patient is four days.

The hospital has a long waiting list of patients, and is, therefore, exploring options to augment its resources. As a management consultant to the A-One Hospital, what are your recommendations?

Case Analysis

The Problem: The problem here is to estimate the capacity of hospital resources, to identify the bottleneck resource and augment the bottleneck resource.

Step 1 Analysis: Let us understand the bottleneck resource in this hospital for surgical services. This requires an estimation of the maximum capacity that can be handled by each of the following departments, namely:

- Admission department
- Examination department
- Investigation department
- OTs

The following is the detailed computations involved in identifying the bottleneck resource in A-One Hospital:

- **Admission**

  Service time per patient = 12 minutes
  Number of admissions with one staff = 5 patients/hour
  = 20 patients/day (4 hours/day)
  = 120 patients/week (6 day/week)
  Maximum capacity with two staff = 240 patients/week

- **Examination**

  Examination time per patient = 30 minutes
  Number of exams with one doctor = 2 patients/hour
  = 8 patients/day (4 hours/day)
  = 48 patients/week
  Maximum capacity with four doctors = 192 patients/week

- **Investigation**

  Number of investigations with one staff = 4 patients/hour
  = 12 patients/day (3 hours/day)
  = 72 patients/week
  Maximum capacity with three staff = 216 patients/week

- **Surgery**

Time for each surgery	= 2 hours
Number of surgeries	= 3 patients/OT/shift
	= 6 patients/OT/day (2 shifts)
Maximum number of surgeries	= 30 patients/day (5 OTs)
	= 180 patients/week
Maximum capacity of admission department	= 240 patients/week
Maximum capacity of examination department	= 192 patients/week
Maximum capacity of investigation department	= 216 patients/week
Maximum capacity of OT	= 180 patients/week

The above calculations are summarized in Table 3.6.

Table 3.6 Estimates of Maximum Capacity: A-One Surgical Hospital

Service	Main Resources	Service Time	Max. Capacity
Admission	Two receptionists	12 minutes per person per staff 1–5 pm, six days per week Monday to Friday, Sunday	240 patients per week
Examination	Four doctors	30 minutes per patient 2–6 pm, six days per week	192 patients per week
Investigation	Three nurses	Four patients per hour 3–6 pm, six days per week	216 patients per week
Surgery	11 surgeons Two anesthetists Five OTs	Two hours per surgery Two shifts; six hours per shift six days per week	180 patients per week

From the above calculations, it is obvious that the hospital cannot perform more than 180 surgeries per week, even though other departments can serve more patients.

Question: Is it possible to achieve this maximum capacity of 180 surgeries per week? To answer this question, we have to compute the maximum capacity of any other resources required for surgical services.

Let us look at the bed capacity.

Bed Capacity: The admissions department, with its available resources, could admit a maximum of 240 patients per week. But are there enough beds in the hospital to accommodate 240 patients per week?

Number of hospital beds available = 110 beds∗6 days/week
= 660 bed days/week
Average length of stay (ALOS) = 4 days/patient
Max no. of inpatients accommodated = 660 bed days/4 days
= 165 patients/week

The above analysis has demonstrated an important concept in capacity management. Even if the hospital can handle a maximum of 180 surgeries per week, its inpatient wards can accommodate *only* 165 patients per week, given that the average length of stay of each patient is four days.

Hence, the number of beds is the bottleneck resource in the hospital and not the OT.

Next, let us undertake the analysis for Step 2.

Step 2 Analysis: Here, we have to calculate how many beds the hospital should add.

For example, maximum number of surgeries = 180
Number of surgeries possible with 110 beds = 165

(Since only 165 inpatients can be admitted per week with a capacity of 110 beds).

Question: Should the hospital add 180 – 165 = 15 beds?

What would be the implications if the hospital decides to add 15 additional beds, in the hope of doing 180 surgeries per week, and, thereby, achieve the maximum utilization of expensive OT resources?

If the hospital adds 15 beds, then

Number of hospital beds available per week = 125 beds ∗ six days
= 750 bed days/week
Average length of stay (ALOS) = 4 days/patient
Number of patients who can be accommodated = 750 bed days/4 ALOS
= 188 (say)

Hence, if the hospital were to add 15 more beds, then the maximum capacity in each department is as follows:

Admissions department:	Maximum capacity	= 240
Examinations department:	Maximum capacity	= 192
Investigations department:	Maximum capacity	= 216
OT:	Maximum capacity	= 180
Inpatient ward beds:	Maximum capacity	= 188

We summarize these results in Table 3.7.

Table 3.7 Estimates of Maximum Capacity After Adding 15 Beds: A-One Surgical Hospital

Sr. No.	Department	Max. Capacity Patients Per Week
1	Admissions	240
2	Examinations	192
3	Investigations	216
4	OT	180
5	Ward beds	188

Please note that if we add 15 beds (bottleneck resource), then the bottleneck resource is not the number of beds, but the number of surgeries. This means an underutilization of bed capacity.

Question: Would adding any more surgeons help the hospital to do more surgeries, so as to make the maximum utilization of 125 beds?

The hospital has 11 surgeons and five OTs. Ten surgeons do surgery every day, five surgeons in the morning shift, one in each OT and another five surgeons in the afternoon shift, one in each OT. The 11th surgeon (on rotation) looks after the administrative tasks. Therefore, no OT is available for a new surgeon, if employed.

The number of OTs has now become the bottleneck capacity. Hence, increasing the number of surgeons or any OT staff would not increase the number of surgeries done on any given day.

Question: If OT is a bottleneck capacity, should the hospital add one more OT?

Note that adding one more OT calls for additional resources, namely, finances, staff, materials and machines.

Therefore, augmenting the capacity (hospital resources) in any one department has consequences on the management of other resources. This is because we have followed an integrated approach to resource management. This is a characteristic of interdependent queuing systems.

To summarize, the hospital management should not focus on the management of any resource in isolation, but on an integrated management of all its resources.

We end this chapter by displaying (Figure 3.2) a summary of the issues in delivering hospital services and the challenges in managing the hospital queuing systems for service delivery.

3.6 SUMMARY

In this chapter, we have discussed issues in hospital service delivery and the management queuing systems to achieve higher throughput. We also introduced Six Sigma methodology for quality management.

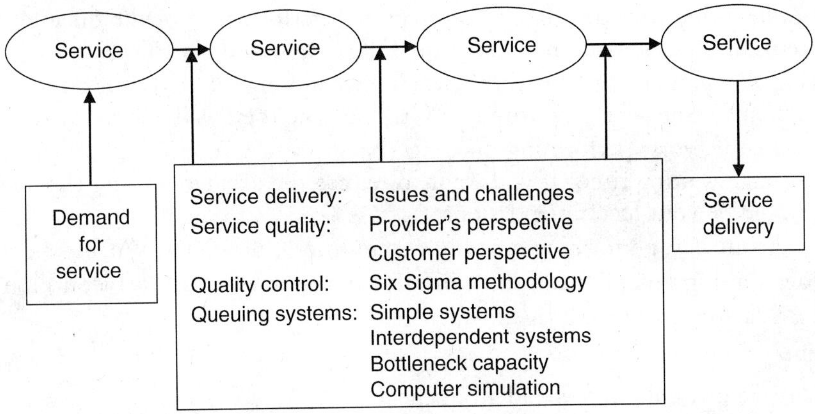

Figure 3.2 Hospital Service Delivery, Quality and Queuing Systems

In the next chapter, we discuss more concepts in hospital management focussing on hospital management functions: operations management, finance management, HR management and materials management.

QUESTIONS

1. How is managing a service organization different from managing an organization which produces goods?
2. What is hospital management? Explain a few differences between managing a hospital and managing any other service?
3. What is the basic difference between monitoring and evaluation?
4. Take any hospital service. What are the activities you would be monitoring in delivering this service? What are the activities you would be evaluating?
5. Identify issues in service delivery in any two clinical departments. What would you do to address these issues?
6. Identify issues in service delivery in any two supporting departments (paramedical). What would you do to address these issues?
7. Identify issues in service delivery in any two administrative departments. What would you do to address these issues?
8. What is meant by service quality?
9. Explain what is meant by provider service quality.
10. Explain what is meant by customer service quality.
11. Explain Six Sigma methodology. Can you find two suitable applications of Six Sigma methodology in a hospital setting?
12. List five simple queuing systems in hospitals.
13. What data would you collect from each of the above queuing systems in order to understand the 'performance' of each system?

14. Collect the necessary data to estimate the performance of the queuing systems in Question 12 and answer the following questions 15, 16 and 17.
15. How do you rate their performance? Which among the above simple queuing systems is the 'worst' performer? Which among them is the 'best' performer?
16. Take the worst performing queuing system from Question 12. What is the average waiting time? If you want to reduce the average waiting time, what would be your recommendations?
17. Take the best performing queuing system from Question 1. What is the average waiting time? What is the utilization of the server? Is the server utilization satisfactory for the management?
18. Explain what is meant by
    (a) Sequential interdependent queue
    (b) Pooled interdependent queue
    (c) Sequentially pooled interdependent queue
19. List two sequentially interdependent queuing systems in hospitals. Collect the necessary data to understand the interdependencies.
20. List two pooled interdependent queuing systems in hospitals. Collect the necessary data to understand the interdependence.
21. List two pooled interdependent sequential queuing systems in hospitals. Collect the necessary data to understand the interdependence.
22. What is meant by bottleneck capacity? How would you identify it in a system?
23. Take any hospital service which involves a sequential interdependent queue. Identify the bottleneck. Explain how would you increase the throughput of this service. What data do you need to collect?
24. Take any hospital service which involves a pooled interdependent queue. Identify the bottleneck. Explain how would you increase the throughput of this service. What data do you need to collect?
25. Take any hospital service which involves a pooled sequential interdependent queue. Identify the bottleneck. Explain how would you increase the throughput of this service. What data do you need to collect?

REFERENCES

1. Fitzsimmons, James and Fitzsimmons, Mona (2009), *Service Management*, 5th ed., Tata McGraw-Hill Publishing Company Limited.
2. Harvard Business School Case, 9-683-068 (1983), Shouldice Hospital Limited.
3. Parasuraman, A.; Zeithaml, V.A. and Berry, L.L. (Spring 1988), 'SERVQUAL: A Multiple-item scale for measuring consumer perceptions of service quality', *Journal of Retailing*, 64 (1), pp.12–40.
4. Jane-Ellen, Robinet (2003), *The Americal Society for Quality*, Nebraska Medical Centre.

5. Heuvel, Jaap van den (2005), 'Dutch Hospital Implemets Six Sigma', *Six Sigma Forum magazine*.
6. Gras, Jeremie M. Philippe, Marianne (Feb 27, 2007), 'Application of Six Sigma Concept in Clinical Laboratories: A Review', *Clin. Chem. Lab Med*, pp. 789–796.
7. Goswami, B.; Singh, Bhawna; Chavla, Ranjana and Venkatesan, Mallika (2010), 'Evaluation of Errors in a Clinical Laboratory: A One-year Experience', *Clinical Chemistry Laboratory Medicine*, 48 (1), pp. 63–66.
8. Wagner, Harvey M. (1977), *Principles of Operations Research*, 2nd ed., Prentice Hall of India, New Delhi.
9. Hillier, Fredericks S. and Lieberman, Gerald J. (1974), *Introduction to Operations Research*, 2nd ed., Holden Day, San Francisco.

chapter 4

Hospital Management Functions

CHAPTER OUTLINE

CHAPTER OBJECTIVE

The main objective of this chapter is to discuss the basic management functions responsible for hospital service delivery, namely, hospital operations, finances, human resources (HR) and materials.

4.1 AN INTRODUCTION

The activities in a hospital for processing its resources into service delivery could be conceptualized into five major management functions, namely:

Hospital management functions describe the activities involved in transforming the hospital resources into service delivery.

1. Operations management
2. Financial management
3. Cost management
4. HR management
5. Materials management

1. **Operations Management:** It focuses on managing the basic activities (operations) of the hospital in the delivery of services. A clear understanding of the processes and procedures in transforming the hospital resources into service delivery is required to address the managerial challenges in operations management, such as capacity management, cost reduction strategies, service quality, and so on.
2. **Financial Management:** It deals with challenges in the utilization of financial resources of the hospital for acquisition, allocation and control of assets in the delivery of services.
3. **Cost Management:** It is fundamental to managerial decisions on pricing of services, and, hence, on the profitability of the hospital.
4. **HR Management:** It is the design and development of formal systems to ensure maximum productivity from hospital employees in the delivery of services. A good coordination between the HR and operations management is the key to achieve maximum utilization of resources. Many organizations consider its HR as an investment for growth potential.
5. **Materials Management:** It deals with the tasks of procurement, transportation and maintaining optimal stock of materials for service delivery. Understocking and over-stocking of materials have a direct impact on the financial performance of the hospital and service delivery. The managerial challenges are in ensuring timely availability of good quality materials to support the basic operations in delivering hospital services.

We discuss each of these management functions in detail in the following sections, starting with hospital operations management in Section 4.2.

4.2 OPERATIONS MANAGEMENT

Operations management is the management of the basic activities (operations) of an organization in the production of goods and services.

A hospital uses its resources to process sick patients in order to better their health outcomes. For example, outpatient services, surgical services, and so on are some of the hospital services in order to improve the health status of sick patients. A slightly different example is that of a pathology laboratory which accepts blood samples from patients and generates test result outputs, which in turn would be used by the physicians to offer healthcare services.

> Hospital operations management focuses on managing the hospital activities to deliver services.

The ultimate performance indicator of operations management is the efficiency and effectiveness in delivering good quality services: minimize the turnaround time, maximize the capacity utilization and employ cost reduction methods.[1–7]

> 1. Service quality
> 2. Turnaround time
> 3. Cost reduction
> 4. Capacity management

4.2.1 Service Quality

Service quality, from a provider perspective or from a customer perspective, can be defined across three parameters, namely:

1. Speed of service delivery
2. Dependability of service
3. Flexibility of service

Speed of Service Delivery: Speed is an indicator of timeliness of service provision. It determines the time interval between the demand for service and the service delivery.

As an example, consider the turnaround time of outpatients in a busy hospital. Minimizing the waiting time of sick patients for consultation in the OPD cycle of services would be a good indicator of service quality. Both the service provider and the outpatients would benefit if the outpatients leave the hospital as quickly as possible after completing all the OPD services.

Another example of a hospital service is the speed (or lack of speed) of inpatient discharge process. Generally, the discharge process in any hospital takes 3–5 hours after the consultant orders discharge, as it involves obtaining clearances from the hospital pharmacy, insurance agencies, billing section, and so on. Unnecessary delay in discharge procedures leads to customer dissatisfaction and a loss of potential income to the hospital from new admissions.

Dependability of Service: Dependability refers to consistency in service delivery. One example would be a dependable emergency ambulance service, which ensures emergency care and transportation of seriously ill patients to hospitals quickly.

As another example, take the role of investigation services in hospitals. Investigation services have become very critical in hospital management, since more than 60–70 per cent of all decisions on admission, discharge and medication are based on laboratory test results. Dependability on investigation services means hospital doctors are assured of receiving reliable and accurate test results consistently in order to take evidence-based decision for medical services.

Flexibility in Service Delivery: Flexibility in service delivery is an indicator about the readiness of the hospital system as a whole to respond to any unforeseen demand for its services.

As an example, the emergency department in a hospital has to be flexible in its service delivery since each emergency case is likely to demand a different level and type of service. In case of a road accident, a large number of injured patients would be brought to the hospital, each demanding immediate attention, not necessarily of the same type; some patients may demand specialist cardiac care; some may demand orthopedic services, and so on.

4.2.2 Turnaround Time

The turnaround time of service delivery is an important indicator of service quality. A faster turnaround time indicates the effectiveness and efficiency in service delivery by the hospital, which calls for effective management of waiting lines and efficient management of its resources. From the patients' point of view, a faster turnaround time means minimizing the loss of productivity in the workplace for the patients as well as their relatives/attendants.

For example, turnaround time of OPD service delivery depends on the management of a sequentially interdependent queuing system, which calls for synchronizing the patient flow through the OPD system of registration, consultation, investigation and medication.

As another example, take the case of turnaround time of inpatient services. This calls for managing the sequence of activities starting with registration, admission, medical services and discharge process. Long waiting time for the discharge process of inpatients could lead to opportunity loss of income to the hospital arising from non-availability of beds for new admissions.

4.2.3 Cost Reduction

Cost reduction in service delivery is a very attractive proposition for the management to achieve higher profitability. There are several ways to achieve cost reduction.

For example, consider the case of costs vs revenue from hospital beds. Revenue from bed occupancy is the maximum in the first 2–3 days of an inpatient's stay in the hospital, since almost all investigations and any interventions, if necessary, are done during the initial days of hospitalization. Hospital costs for any additional day of bed occupancy is much more than hospital revenue. For example, orthopedic patients spent 2–3 weeks after surgery, and patients in burns and plastics spent 2–3 months for recovery. Opportunity costs are very high for longer length of stay. Minimizing the length of stay without compromising on service quality, thus, offers an ideal opportunity for the hospital to achieve cost reduction in providing inpatient care.

Cost reduction strategies could focus on maximizing the throughput in a given period of time. For example, the Aravind Eye Hospital, Madurai, has achieved substantial cost reduction on its services through increased productivity from its surgeons; the productivity of its surgeons is more than double the international norms.[8]

Process reengineering could also result in cost reduction. For example, the Gujarat Cancer Research Institute, Ahmedabad, has achieved cost reduction by reengineering its stores and purchase procedures.[9]

Cost reduction strategies in Western countries discussed in the literature include implementing care pathways (e.g., cardiac care, orthopedic services), replacing higher skilled staff with lower skilled staff (e.g., replace nurses by phlebotomists for blood collection), besides reducing the length of stay, empowering the nurses, and so on.[10–12]

4.2.4 Capacity Management

Capacity management is an important activity in hospital operations management. For example, managing the operating theatre (OT) capacity is very challenging. OT resources are expensive, in terms of both capital expenditure and operating expenses. Optimal utilization of OT resources means maximum throughput within a period of time, which means more surgical procedures can be done per shift of OT working hours with the same OT resources.

CITY CARDIAC HOSPITAL — MINI CASE 4.1

City Cardiac Hospital is a super specialty hospital with 50 beds. The hospital has two cath labs and two consultants. Any consultant can do any procedure in any cath lab. Whenever a consultant is not doing a procedure, he/she is either at the post-intervention CCU with his/her patients or doing OPD consultation. Currently, the hospital follows the first-come first-served (FCFS) rule to schedule the interventional procedures. Is there a better scheduling rule? A better scheduling rule could be the one which uses less resource and/or completes all the procedures earlier than the current schedule.

This is an ideal case for a simulation experiment, since it is not possible to evaluate different scheduling rules in the real cath lab. Therefore, can we simulate the cath lab activities on a computer and examine the impact of different scheduling rules on cath lab productivity?

> Since computer simulation models are experimental, it is necessary to rely on a large database to simulate the real system.

In building a simulation model, it is necessary to collect a large amount of data for experimentation. We have, therefore, collected data on total number of cath lab procedures for 100 days; Table 4.1 depicts the cath lab data for a sample one day (1 February 2012 for illustration). This table gives complete details on the daily load for each cath lab procedure for the sample day—procedure name, the consultant who did the procedure, cath lab reference, the time each patient was brought in the cath lab and the time each patient was shifted out of the cath lab.

Using the cath lab data we collected for 100 days, we can simulate cath lab data and provide answers to the following questions:

How many procedures are done each day? How many procedures of each intervention on each day? Which consultant did what procedure and in which cath lab? How long did each procedure take?

Table 4.1 City Cardiac Hospital Cath Lab Procedure Schedules: 1 February 2012

Sr. No.	Date	Patient ID	Name of Procedure	Consultant	Patient in at	Patient out at	Cath Lab
1	1/2/12	305239	PTCA[1]	Dr X	1.30 pm	2.05 pm	1
2	1/2/12	305368	CAG[2]	Dr X	3.55 pm	4.00 pm	1
3	1/2/12	288787	BMV[3]	Dr X	5.05 pm	5.20 pm	1
4	1/2/12	305367	CAG	Dr Y	5.45 pm	5.55 pm	1
5	1/2/12	305334	BMV	Dr Y	2.00 pm	2.15 pm	2
6	1/2/12	305333	CAG	Dr Y	3.00 pm	3.06 pm	2
7	1/2/12	305348	CAG + PTCA	Dr Y	3.20 pm	4.15 pm	2
8	1/2/12	305344	CAG + PTCA	Dr Y	4.25 pm	5.10 pm	2
9	1/2/12	305337	CAG	Dr Y	5.45 pm	5.50 pm	2

[1] PTCA: It is a therapeutic procedure by which the identified coronary artery disease is rectified by putting a wire mesh (stent) in order to restore normal flow in the compromised/diseased artery.

[2] CAG: It is a diagnostic tool in which a contrast (radio opaque dye) is being injected via catheter into the heart coronary arteries in order to investigate the condition of the heart.

[3] BMV: It is a therapeutic procedure where a BMV balloon is sent inside a narrowed (stenosed) valve and inflated at the origin to bring the valve to its normal size.

To answer the above question, we proceed as follows:

Part 1: Generate a monthly load for cath lab procedures.
Part 2: Evaluate different scheduling rules to handle the monthly load of cath lab procedures.

Part 1: We start with simulating the number of procedures on any day, and then generate the number of each procedure on that day and the time for each procedure. We repeat this for 30 days and, thereby, generate the cath lab load for a month.

We describe below the Monte Carlo simulation methodology.

We start with simulating the total number of procedures daily.

Step 1: Construct a frequency distribution for the number of procedures daily.

Assume that frequency for the number of procedures based on cath lab data for 100 days as given in Table 4.2.

Table 4.2 Frequency Distribution: Number of Procedures

Total Number of Procedures Daily	Frequency
7	15
8	17
9	18
10	16
11	17
12	17
Total Frequency	**100**

Step 2: Extend the above frequency distribution to a cumulative frequency distribution (Table 4.3).

Table 4.3 Cumulative Frequency Distribution: Number of Procedures

Total Number of Procedures Daily	Frequency	Cumulative Frequency
7	15	15
8	17	32
9	18	50
10	16	66
11	17	83
12	17	100
Total Frequency	**100**	

Step 3: Convert the cumulative frequency distribution into a cumulative probability distribution (Table 4.4).

Table 4.4 Cumulative Probability Distribution: Number of Procedures

Total Number of Procedures Daily	Frequency	Cumulative Frequency	Cumulative Probability (*)
7	15	15	0.15
8	17	32	0.32
9	18	50	0.50
10	16	66	0.66
11	17	83	0.83
12	17	100	1.00
Total Frequency	**100**		

(*) Cumulative probability = cumulative frequency/total frequency.

Step 4: Generate a value from the uniform distribution [0, 1],[13] and identify the frequency which just exceeds this value. This frequency is the simulated frequency of the variable, namely, the total number of procedures daily.

For example,

1. If the uniform random number drawn is say 59, then
   the frequency which just exceeds this value is 10, and, hence
   the simulated frequency of the total number of procedures that day = 10
2. If the uniform random number is say 10, then
   the frequency which just exceeds this value is seven, and, hence
   the simulated frequency of the total number of procedures that day = 7

Step 5: Repeat steps 1–4 for 30 days to generate a simulated value for the total number of procedures done daily for 30 days.

Step 6: Repeat steps 1–5 for generating 'number of each procedure each day' from the distribution of 'total number of procedures each day' obtained in Step 5.

We now have simulated the number of each procedure for each day for a 30-day period.

Next, we have to simulate the time taken for each procedure.

Step 7: Based on the cath lab data collected for 100 days, construct a frequency distribution of the time for each procedure. Repeat steps 1–5 for each procedure on each day for a period of 30 days.

We have now simulated the daily load for each cath lab procedure for a 30-day period.

Part 2: Our next step is to evaluate alternate scheduling rules to the current FCFS rule for scheduling the cath lab procedure. This requires developing a computer programme which captures the working of the current system; this task is beyond the scope of this book. Interested readers are advised to consult any book on computer simulation[14,15] or use any simulation software package.[16]

METROPOLITAN SURGICAL HOSPITAL (A)[17] MINI CASE 4.2

Metropolitan Hospital is an ultramodern, multi-specialty tertiary care hospital in a large metropolitan city. It offers a comprehensive set of services covering investigation and diagnosis to therapy, surgery and post-operative care.

With an average load of 35 surgeries per day, the Metropolitan Hospital management was curious to explore using computer packages for OT scheduling. About 60 consultant surgeons perform various types of surgeries ranging from minor to supra major surgeries. An average of 30–35 surgeries is performed every working day, with 20–30 per cent of surgeries being referrals from outside. Surgical patients account for almost 60 per cent of bed occupancy.

What are the challenges in OT scheduling?

OT Scheduling: The OT management at Metropolitan Hospital starts with the preparation of a daily schedule for each OT. Most of the patients who were advised to undergo surgeries at the hospital booked the date for their surgery and their preferred consultant surgeons before being admitted as inpatients. This helped the hospital to estimate the load of each surgeon and, thereby, allocate specific time slots on preferred dates for each OT to the surgeons.

OT scheduling was done based on:

- The resources required for each surgery
- The duration of each surgery

Once the resource requirements for each surgery was estimated, the next task was to schedule feasible time slots for surgeries, based on statistics such as:

- Average case loads
- Schedules for outpatient consulting
- Schedules for inpatient care

Some slots were kept open to accommodate unscheduled and emergency surgeries. Preparation of OT schedules started two weeks before the scheduled surgery date, showing the booked and open time slots in a master OT schedule (Table 4.5) indicating the availability of specific OTs at specific times for each day of the week. This master schedule was prepared after ensuring the availability of all resources such as:

Table 4.5 Metropolitan Surgical Hospital OT Slot System

		Slot System			07/08/2002	
OT	**Monday**	**Tuesday**	**Wednesday**	**Thursday**	**Friday**	**Saturday**
1	8.00–18.00 Dr V	8.00–11.00 Dr KTR	8.00–18.00 Dr C	9.00–20.00 Dr B	8.00–10.00 Dr D	8.00–13.00 Oncology
		11.00–18.00 G.I. Surgery			10.00–18.00 Dr U	13.00–17.00 Dr K
	18.00–20.00 Open	18.00–20.00 Open	18.00–20.00 Open		18.00–20.00 Open	17.00–20.00 Open Slot
2	8.00–13.00 Dr J	8.00–12.00 Dr KTR	8.00–10.00 Open	9.00–11.00 Open	8.00–10.00 Open	8.00–17.00 Urology
	13.00–18.00 Dr S	12.00–18.00 Dr S	10.00–17.00 Dr M	11.00–15.00 Dr Sh.	10.00–13.00 Dr Km	
				15.00–17.00 Open	13.00–17.00 Dr S	
	18.00–20.00 Unclean cases	8.00–20.00 Open	17.00–20.00 Open	17.00–20.00 Dr S.M.	17.00–20.00 Open	17.00–20.00 Open
3						
4						
5						
6						
7						

- Consultant surgeons
- Consultant anesthetists
- Special requests of surgeons (e.g., presence of a histopathologist, RBC packets)
- Time engagements of shared equipment like C-arms, microscope, laparoscopes, and so on.

The total number of surgeries to be scheduled on a given day also depended on the estimated time required for each surgery based on the requirements of each surgery.

All the open slots indicated in the master schedule were filled one day before finalizing the OT schedule. The finalized OT schedule was then posted in all the wards, labs, radiology centres, OT stores and so on by 7 pm the day before the scheduled date for surgery. Any emergency surgery meant rescheduling of planned surgeries the same day; no planned surgery was postponed to the next day.

Can you think of a better approach to OT scheduling? Is it possible to simulate a rough OT master schedule through a computer model?

In the next section, we discuss the concepts on financial management, cost management, capital budgeting, and their applications in hospital management.

4.3 FINANCE AND COST MANAGEMENT

4.3.1 Finance Management

Finance and cost management are important managerial functions to understand the utilization of finances, costing and pricing of services which affect the profitability of the hospital.

Financial statements of a firm provide very useful information to satisfy the varied information requirements of all its stakeholders. For example, the shareholders use the financial statements to know how well their capital is managed by the firm. Banks and other lending agencies use the financial statements to assess the credit worthiness of a firm. Managers use the financial statements to understand the firm's operational performance. Statutory bodies examine the firm's financial health from its financial statements.

Financial management:

1. Balance sheet
2. Profit and loss statement
3. Cash flow statement

We start our discussion on financial management with a brief introduction to the three basic financial accounting statements, namely, balance sheet, profit and loss statement and cash flow statement.[18–23]

These statements are prepared following the generally accepted accounting principles.

Financial management of a firm starts with (i) gaining an understanding of the three basic financial statements, (ii) analysis of these statements and (iii) identifying areas for managerial interventions.

It is useful to think of managing the financial health of a hospital as similar to managing our physical health. There are three important steps to manage our health:

- A health check-up once a year
- Properly carrying out our daily activities
- Taking care of changes in health status to remain healthy

Similarly, the financial management of your hospital starts with:

- An annual check-up of your hospital's financial health status (balance sheet)
- Properly managing the daily delivery of services (profit and loss statement)
- Taking care of changes in the cash flow of your hospital in order to remain financially healthy (cash flow statement)

4.3.1.1 Balance Sheet: The balance sheet of an organization summarizes its financial health at the end of every financial year. It 'balances' the hospital's assets (what it owns) and liabilities (what it owes). The difference between assets and liabilities is the owner's equity, also known as shareholders' funds/equity. Hence, the total assets would always equal total liabilities plus equity.

$$\text{Assets} = \text{Liabilities} + \text{Equity}.$$

OTs, beds and MRI machines are some of the assets a hospital owns. In order to acquire these assets, the hospital would have borrowed some money from banks or other sources (liabilities) and the remaining amount financed by the (owners') equity.

Current Assets and Fixed Assets: Assets can be broadly classified into current assets and fixed assets. Current assets are those assets which can be converted into cash within the accounting year, such as accounts receivable (e.g., receivables from insurance providers for the services rendered to the cashless insurance policy holders). Fixed assets are those that cannot be easily converted into cash, such as land, buildings, MRI machines, and so on. The value of fixed assets (except land) depreciates over a period of time due to wear and tear, and, thus, the concept of depreciation.[i]

Current Liabilities and Long-Term Liabilities: Liabilities can be broadly classified into current liabilities and long-term liabilities. Current liabilities are those which must be paid by the hospital within the accounting year, such as accounts payable (e.g., payments by hospital to its vendors for purchases of medicines and drugs). Long-term liabilities are those which may take years to repay, such as the capital component of bank loans. The interest component of bank loans to be paid annually would be an expense.

Working Capital: It is the difference between current assets and current liabilities. Working capital increases and decreases depending on the nature and level of operations. Financial managers are often concerned about the level of working capital to be maintained. Too little working capital may force the hospital to delay paying its suppliers. Frequent delays on payments to suppliers would lead to uncertainty in the lead time for deliveries in future and, thereby, affect service quality. Too much working capital, on the other hand, would affect the hospital's profitability by having 'idle cash', higher inventories and/or receivables.

---

[i] Depreciation is a non-cash expense that effectively reduces the balance sheet value of an asset over its presumed useful life. Depreciation is a way of recognizing that certain assets wear out or gradually lose their productive value.

Important Concepts: Current assets, fixed assets, depreciation, current liabilities, long-term liabilities, working capital, capital employed.

4.3.1.2 Profit and Loss Statement: Unlike the balance sheet which gives a snapshot of the financial health of an organization at a point in time, the profit and loss statement reflects the financial performance of operations over a specific period of time. For a hospital, its profit and loss statement for a period (say monthly, quarterly, yearly, and so on) would display the *total income* from patient care and other sources as well as the *total expenses* in providing healthcare services, and, thereby, reflect a profit or loss for that period. Hence, a profit and loss statement is also called income and expense statement.

A profit and loss statement provides very useful information on the profitability of the hospital. Profitability has to be understood from different angles: *gross profit, operating profit* and *net profit.*

Gross Profit: It is the profit before depreciation, interest and tax (PBDIT).

PBDIT = gross income – cash expenses[ii]

PBDIT is also known as EBDIT (Earnings Before DIT)

Operating Profit: It uses only operating income (income from operations only).

For example, operating income for a (non-teaching) hospital would be only the income from patient care.

Operating profit = operating income – operating expenses[iii]
PBIT = PBDIT – depreciation expenses

PBIT is also known as EBIT.

Net Profit: It is the profit after tax (PAT).

PAT = PBIT – interest – tax

Important Concepts: Gross income, operating income, operating expense, gross profit (PBDIT), operating profit (PBIT), net profit (PAT).

[ii] Cash expenses include fixed and variable expenses. (It does not include depreciation which is a non-cash expense). Fixed expenses are those which do not vary with volume (e.g., salaries and wages). Variable expenses are those which vary with volume (e.g., medicines and drugs).
[iii] Operating expenses include cash and non-cash expenses. Depreciation on fixed assets can be claimed as non-cash expenses. Suppose a hospital purchased an MRI for ₹5 crores, and its useful life is say five years. An annual depreciation of ₹1 crore can be claimed towards operating expense on account of using the MRI for rendering services.

4.3.1.3 Cash Flow Statement: A cash flow statement is like a bank passbook; it shows the change in cash flows between two time periods; say cash at the beginning of the year and cash at the end of the year.

$$\text{Change in cash flow} = \text{cash flow from operations} + \text{other sources of cash} - \text{uses of cash}$$

Changes in cash flow occur due to three activities: change in operations, change in financing the operations (change in liabilities such as borrowings or capital) or change in investments (e.g., acquisition of assets). A cash flow statement, therefore, has three sections:

1. Cash flow from operating activities
2. Cash flow from financing activities
3. Cash flow from investment activities

Changes in cash flow may not have an impact on the daily activities. However, a cash flow statement would indicate whether the hospital is turning its accounts receivables into cash within a reasonable period of time, and, thereby, indicates *liquidity or solvency*. Solvency is the ability to pay when bills are presented.

A positive cash flow from operations is an indication that the hospital's operations are profitable. The profits generated could be used for investments (fixed assets such as cath lab, bank deposits, and so on) or for accounts payable.

Hospital managers must pay special attention to the cash flows as it indicates the ability of the hospital to meet its financial obligations. It is possible that a hospital makes profit, but struggles for cash. Profit and net cash flows are, thus, two different indicators.

Important Concepts: Cash flow from operations, cash flow from investments, cash flow from financing, liquidity/solvency.

So far, we have only discussed accounting terminologies appearing in the three basic financial statements. Financial statements reveal only the essentials, they conceal a lot.

In order to assess the financial performance of a firm, we get into the discussion of financial ratios. Many financial ratios use information from more than one financial statement, so as to provide an integrated picture of the financial health. An integrated picture of financial performance should provide an analysis of operational efficiency, investment efficiency and financing leverages.

In the next section, we discuss certain commonly used financial ratios to assess the financial performance.

4.3.1.4 Financial Performance: Ratio Analysis: Ratio is a mathematical relation between two quantities. Relations expressed as ratios make comparisons meaningful and simple. For example, operating profits per se may not be comparable across years, since it depends on the level of activity which could be different across years. Therefore, we use operating profit margin as a ratio of operating profit to operating income and, hence, comparable across years.

Financial ratios can be broadly classified into three categories:

1. Profitability ratios
2. Liquidity/solvency ratios
3. Activity ratios

1. Profitability Ratios: From the shareholders' interest in your hospital, the most common indicator used is the Return on Equity (ROE). It indicates how the hospital has utilized its shareholders' funds.

- ROE = net profit/equity

  Denominator is the average of shareholders' equity in the beginning of the year and end of the year. This is necessary since shareholders' equity may change during the course of an accounting year.

  ROE = net profit/equity
  = (net profit/income) × (income/assets) × (assets/equity)

  ROE, thus, reflects operational efficiency, investment efficiency and financing efficiency.
- Return on Assets (ROA) = net profit/total assets.

  ROA is a measure of effective utilization of resources, irrespective of how the resources were acquired.
- Return on Investment (ROI) = (PBIT – tax)/capital employed
- Operating Profit Margin (OPM) = operating profit/operating income
- Net Profit Margin (NPM) = net profit/operating income
- Earnings per Share (EPS): When the shareholders hold different number of shares, it is meaningful to look at EPS.

  EPS = PAT/N; where N is the number of shares outstanding at the end of the relevant period.

A comparison of operating profit margin[iv] and net profit margin over a few years would produce useful information to the management on its management

[iv] Some firms use total income which includes income from sources other than operations. Similarly, some firms define operating profit as PBDIT. As long as a firm consistently uses the same accounting practices across years, it is safe to compare performances across years. Please note that comparisons across years for a firm or comparisons across firms for a given year would be misleading if different accounting practices are used.

of costs and revenue (income). If the operating profit margin shows an increasing trend over the last few years, it could be due to several reasons: increased revenue from services (increased revenue from increased demand or from increased pricing is a reflection of the quality of service), decreased cost for providing services (better control on cost management) or both. A decreasing trend of OPM would be a great concern for the management.

2. Liquidity/Solvency Ratios: Liquidity/solvency ratios help to assess the solvency status of a hospital.

A. Short-term liquidity ratios:

(i) Current ratio = current assets/current liabilities
A current ratio of less than one indicates negative working capital

(ii) Quick ratio = Quick current assets/current liabilities
Quick current assets are those which can be converted into cash quickly. Inventories are the most difficult to be converted into quick cash, and, hence, not used for computing quick ratios.

B. Long-term liquidity ratios:

(iii) Debt-equity ratio = long term debt/equity
Debt-to equity ratio is a useful indicator to assess the financial leverage of a hospital. Financial leverage refers to the use of borrowed money for asset acquisition. A hospital would be highly leveraged if its percentage of debt is much higher than the capital invested by its shareholders.

3. Activity Ratios: Activity ratios indicate the challenges in cash management during the activity cycle. Most common indicators are:

A. Average collection period for accounts receivable
B. Average payables period for accounts payable
C. Average inventory conversion period

All the above ratios are indicators of working capital management.

(i) Average collection period = average accounts receivables/income from operations per day

Collection period is an important determinant of working capital requirement. A longer collection period calls for more working capital than a shorter collection period.

(ii) Average payables period = average accounts payable/operating expenses per day

(iii) Inventory conversion period = operating expenses/average inventory

We have mentioned only a few commonly used financial ratios, interested readers are requested to consult Luecke (2002).[24]

4.3.2 Cost Management

Cost management is an important challenge for hospital managers as it is fundamental to managerial decisions on pricing of services and, hence, on the profitability of the hospital.

Managers must pay special attention to costs of products/services in order to develop a rational basis for pricing their products/services to identify costs that need to be controlled and to assess which products/services are profitable and which are not.

Costs of products/services can be classified in several ways. For example, costs can be classified based on changes in output, activity levels or volume. Another classification of costs is based on their traceability to the product/service at sub-unit levels (e.g., department, service). Functional classification of costs, costs for control, and so on are other ways of cost classification. In this section, we briefly discuss the first two types of cost classifications.

4.3.2.1 Fixed Costs and Variable Costs: Costs are broadly classified into fixed costs and variable costs, when cost classifications are based on changes in output, activity levels or volume.[v]

Fixed Costs are those costs which do not depend on the service load, namely, the number of patients handled in a hospital. For example, salaries and wages to hospital employees would be a fixed cost, since a fixed salary is paid to the employees irrespective of the number of patients served.

Variable Costs are those costs which depend on the service load. For example, hospital purchase of medicines and drugs vary with the number of patients served, and, therefore, the costs of hospital purchases would be a variable cost.

For illustrating these cost concepts, we reproduce the income statement of City Kidney Hospital in Table 4.6.

1. Can you identify the fixed costs and variable costs?
2. What are your comments on cost management at City Kidney Hospital?

4.3.2.2 Direct Costs and Indirect Costs: Costs are classified into direct costs and indirect costs based on their traceability to the product/service at sub-unit levels (e.g., department, service).

Direct Costs are those which can be allocated to specific activities, while *indirect costs* cannot be traced to any specific activity. Indirect costs are also called overheads. For example, salary to the gynecologists in a hospital is a direct cost for the gynecology department since a gynecologist renders services only to the

[v] Fixed costs and variable costs are discussed again in the next section in connection with our discussions on the concept of break-even volume.

Table 4.6 City Kidney Hospital Income Statement

City Kidney Hospital Income Statement: 1997–98 ₹ in Lacs							
Sr. No.	**Fees**	**Avg./Mth 1994–95**	**Avg./Mth 1995–96**	**Avg./Mth 1996–97**	**Avg./Mth 1997–98 (Apr–Nov)**	**Total 1997–98 (Apr–Nov)**	**% Variation**
1.	Consulting	0.49	0.52	0.54	0.73	5.87	35.67
2.	X-ray	1.47	1.81	2.33	2.92	23.33	24.98
3.	Laboratory	5.28	5.67	7.06	7.74	61.88	9.54
4.	Stay	2.29	2.62	3.02	3.57	28.52	17.88
5.	Operation	7.55	8.92	9.48	8.79	70.31	–7.32
6.	Kidney transplant	3.77	2.39	2.65	2.79	22.30	5.35
7.	Theatre (other charges)	3.06	3.41	4.94	4.61	36.86	–6.67
8.	Anesthetic	0.44	0.48	0.57	0.76	6.09	33.16
9.	Dialysis	2.11	2.80	3.99	4.36	34.87	9.11
10.	E.C.G.	0.13	0.13	0.16	0.16	1.30	–0.51
11.	Urodynamic	0.34	0.45	0.70	0.71	5.65	1.50
12.	Misc.	1.02	1.07	0.99	0.89	7.13	–9.59
13.	Special consultation	0.09	0.11	0.14	0.13	1.06	–5.92
14.	Stone clinic	2.47	3.56	2.85	2.34	18.71	–17.76
15.	Kidney care clinic	–	–	0.00	0.00	0.00	–100.00
16.	Andrology fees	–	–	0.02	0.01	0.09	–28.95
17.	Surcharge	0.00	4.19	0.00	0.00	0.00	–
	Total income	**30.50**	**38.12**	**39.45**	**40.50**	**323.97**	**2.67**
	Free ship	1.08	1.56	2.20	1.83	14.65	–16.70
	Net income	29.42	36.56	37.25	38.67	309.32	3.81
	Total expense	26.24	32.84	34.98	38.11	304.91	8.95
	Surplus/deficit	3.18	3.72	2.26	0.55	4.41	–75.65
Other Income							
1.	Rent	0.01	0.01	0.01	0.00	0.03	–43.75
2.	Interest (bank)	0.08	0.03	0.04	0.03	0.21	–35.71
3.	Interest (corpus)	1.52	2.21	3.06	3.08	24.65	0.72
4.	Insurance claims	0.15	0.29	0.48	0.00	0.00	–100.00
5.	Patient bill recovery	0.02	0.02	0.01	0.02	0.18	68.75
6.	Disposal of scraps	0.07	0.03	0.07	0.05	0.36	–39.33
	Total other income	**1.86**	**2.59**	**3.68**	**3.18**	**25.43**	**–13.50**

gynecology department. However, salary to staff nurses is an indirect cost as nurses are usually rotated among various departments. Overhead costs like rent, electricity charges, and so on are also indirect costs. Indirect costs arise due to common resources shared by many departments/services.

Indirect Costs are very high in service provision, especially in the delivery of hospital services. Costs of surgical procedures fall in this category. The cost of surgeons and anesthetists can be traced to their respective departments, and, hence, are direct costs. These costs would not occur if the OT is not working. But OTs do utilize the services of other departments such as house-keeping, information systems and billing. The costs for supporting services are indirect costs, as their services are utilized by several departments. In other words, support services are *shared resources*. It is not easy to trace the share of support services used by each department.

Allocation of indirect costs is an important component of cost measurement at the sub-unit level. Cost allocation assists the managers to arrive at rational pricing decisions.

4.3.2.3 Traditional Method of Cost Allocation: In the traditional method of costing, allocation of indirect costs to sub-unit levels is, in many cases, done by assuming average utilization of resources by all 'shared' products/services. Such an approach of uniform allocation of indirect costs across all competing products/services could lead to cost distortions. Cost distortions could have serious adverse implications on price distortions. We explain these with examples of hospital services.

Example 1: Some hospitals allocate the total hospital overhead costs of inpatient services to each department based on the average number of inpatient days for the hospital (average length of stay, i.e., ALOS). This assumption ignores two basic facts: (i) it does not differentiate longer inpatient stay from shorter inpatient stay in the same department and (ii) it does not recognize wide variations on average length of stay across departments; average length of stay for orthopedic inpatients would be 2–3 weeks, while the average length of stay for medical inpatients would be only 2–3 days.

Example 2: Let us take another example of hospital services. Surgical services in many government hospitals are classified into two categories, namely, minor procedures and major procedures. Major surgeries cover a wide range of procedures from simple hernia to complex pancreatectomy procedures. But, all major services carry the same charge, even though it is known that any major complex surgery performed over three hours definitely consumes more costly resources than a simple hernia surgery. Therefore, very costly surgeries in many government hospitals are highly subsidized. The management may be aware of subsidy, but not aware of the extent of subsidy.

4.3.2.4 Activity Based Costing Methodology: The cost distortions in allocating indirect costs to all shared products/services are addressed to a large extent by resorting to activity based costing methodology. The main objective in activity based costing is to allocate indirect costs of shared resources to products/services in proportion to the utilization of the shared resources by the products/services. An excellent example of the application of activity based costing is the primary care unit at the Cambridge Hospital Community Health Network.[25]

Central to activity based costing methodology is the concept of cost drivers.

Activity based costing identifies the activities in an organization and allocates the costs to activities through cost drivers. Since cost drivers are related to activities, they occur at many levels. Cost drivers can be defined as activities which cause a change in costs (drive the costs) over a period of time. The activities which generate costs should be matched to the level bases used to assign costs to products/services.

4.3.3 Capital Budgeting: A Perspective

Capital budgeting focuses on planning for financial resources for your proposed project and evaluating various possible options for return on investments under different future scenarios. Investments in fixed assets could also provide a marketing edge to hospitals to attract more specialist doctors and patients. Asset expansion requires considerable expenditure and, hence, calls for raising finances from external sources over and above the shareholders' funds.

The financial analysis of capital investment proposals consists of estimating the capital outlay and assessing the benefits of the proposed project through a detailed analysis of cash flow statements under uncertainty over a period of time.

Suppose you want to build a hospital or commission an MRI in your oncology centre. What steps should you take in order to ensure that your dream project becomes a reality within certain cost and time constraints? What rate of return would you accept on the proposed investment in the light of uncertainties, such as demand for services and sales revenues? Demand and sales revenues (which depend on pricing of services) are market sensitive and could change drastically if the level of competition changes in future.

All these concerns on uncertainties do impact your expected rate of return on current investments over a period of time in future. Time value of money is, thus, an important concept in evaluating investment options. Time value of money recognizes that the value of money invested today is more than the same amount of money to be received in the future.

For example, an amount of ₹10,000 invested today for one year in a bank at 10 per cent interest is worth ₹11,000 one year from now. Alternately, ₹9090.90 invested today for one year in a bank at 10 per cent interest would have a value of ₹10,000 one year from now, and ₹11,000 two years from now. In other words, the present value of ₹9090.90 has a future value of ₹10,000 one year from now and a future value of ₹11,000 two years from now at 10 per cent interest. In finance parlance, the interest percentage is called the discount rate.

Present Value: It is the monetary value today of a future payment (cash flow) discounted at some annual compound rate.

Net Present Value (NPV): It is the present value of one or more future cash flows less the initial investment. The NPV of ₹10,000 invested today at 10 per cent interest (discount rate) is, therefore, ₹11,000 one year from now.

Internal Rate of Return (IRR): It is that discount rate for which NPV equals zero.

IRR is a useful tool to evaluate investment options. For example, suppose your hospital has made a PAT of ₹4 crores. Should you invest this amount in a bank earning 10 per cent interest or invest this amount for acquiring an MRI? The answer lies in computing the IRR for the proposed investment in an MRI. If the IRR for investment in an MRI is greater than the 10 per cent interest from bank, it would make perfect sense to invest in an MRI. In fact, you may even take some risk in an MRI investment even if the IRR for the MRI investment is less than the interest offered by the bank, if you are convinced that an MRI in your hospital would fetch many benefits other than just financial benefits. For example, an MRI in your hospital could be perceived as an indicator of improved service quality. This brings us to discuss the concept of a hurdle rate. *Hurdle rate* is the minimal rate of return on an investment that you wish to achieve. You would, therefore, invest in an MRI if the IRR in MRI investment exceeds the hurdle rate, even though the IRR in MRI investment is less than the assured returns from the bank deposit. Of course, the expected IRR for MRI investment is subject to several uncertainties such as the demand for and revenue from MRI services. It is important to realize that 'your investment' could be a combination of the shareholders' funds and long-term interest bearing bank loans.

In order to address the concerns on uncertain demand and sales revenue, we introduce the concept of *break-even analysis*. Break-even analysis helps us to determine the volume level at which the *contribution* margin from sales revenue would cover the total fixed cost of delivering services/products. Contribution margin is the difference between sales revenue and the variable costs of delivering services/products. In other words, contribution margin is the money that every unit sold contributes to paying for fixed costs. Hence, we can represent break-even volume as follows:

Fixed cost = break-even volume × unit contribution margin, and, hence,
Break-even volume = fixed costs/unit contribution margin

Going back to our discussion on MRI investment, we could, therefore, conclude that the proposed investment in MRI would be financially beneficial only if the demand for MRI services is likely to exceed the break-even volume at the proposed price for MRI services. It may not be fair to assume that your hospital would achieve the break-even volume in the very first year of commissioning the MRI unit. It would take a few years to break-even. Capital budgeting would provide an analysis of cash flows from the year of investment to the useful life of the MRI under various scenarios for demands and sales of services.

In this section, we have provided an overview of capital budgeting. Interested readers are requested to consult standard references on healthcare financing.

METROPOLITAN SURGICAL HOSPITAL (B) MINI CASE 4.3

Besides OT scheduling, the Metropolitan Hospital management faced several other challenges. The management realized that the input costs for surgical procedures keep increasing regularly and, therefore, would like to revise its pricing of surgical services.

The management wants to get a better understanding of the costs for its OT services and identify areas for cost control.

A basic understanding of the working of OTs would be necessary to understand the process of costing OT services. The OT management consists of six important activities:

- Preparation of the OT complex
- Pre-operative procedure on patients
- Anesthesia procedures
- Surgical procedures
- Post-operative patient care
- Post-operative OT work

The above activities are shown in Figure 4.1, which highlights the management of a pooled interdependent queuing system in the delivery of surgical procedures.[26]

Below, we explain a few important concepts in the application of activity based costing methodology to surgical procedures. In this case, we have to identify cost drivers at two levels, as can be seen from Figure 4.2:

- **Level 1:** Identify cost drivers to allocate the total OT costs (expenses) to the OT activities
- **Level 2:** Identify cost drivers to allocate OT activity costs to OT services

Besides providing assistance in a rational allocation of indirect costs, the insights on activity costs provided by activity based costing methodology would be of immense help to the managers to manage costs and, thereby, address profitability of operations.

Can you identify the cost drivers for levels 1 and 2?

In the next section, we provide a perspective of HR management in the context of hospital management.

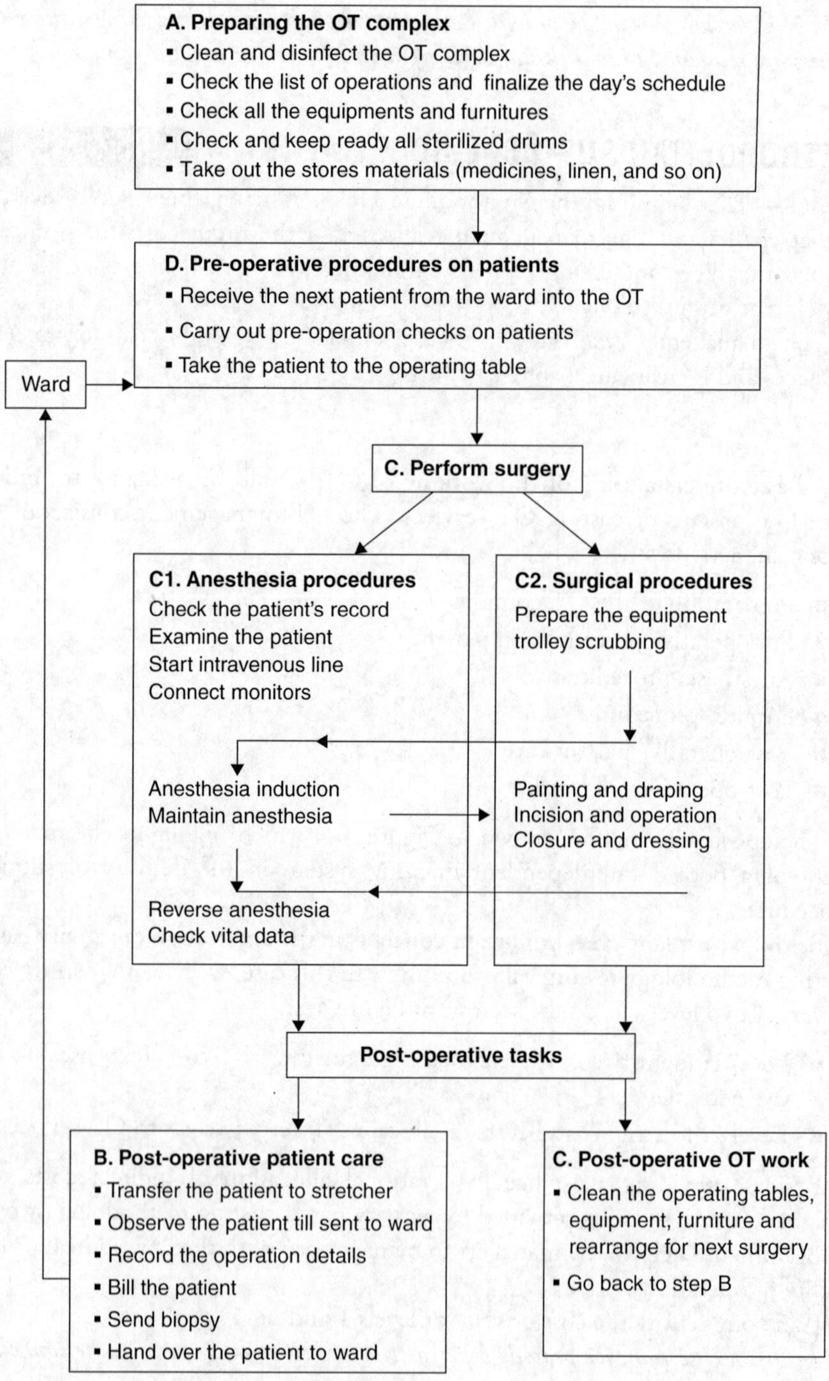

Figure 4.1 OT Activities

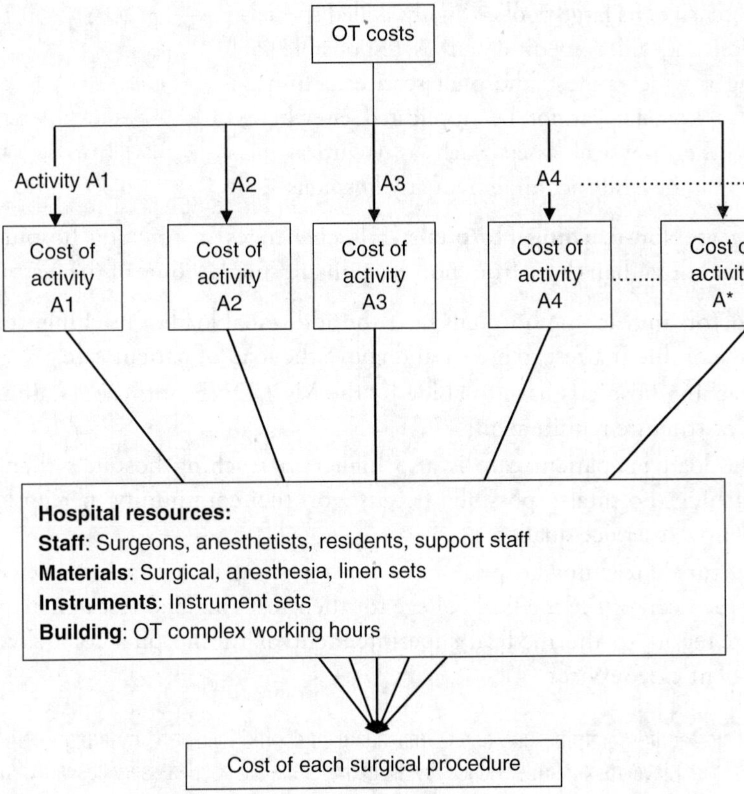

Figure 4.2 OT Activity Based Costing Methodology

4.4 HR MANAGEMENT

Since all healthcare services are ultimately delivered by people, HR management in hospitals plays a vital role in the success of effective and efficient healthcare service delivery. Acute shortages of doctors and nurses in our country make HR management in hospitals very challenging.[vi]

> All healthcare services are ultimately delivered by people and, hence, the importance of HR management in hospitals.

HR managerial challenges can be broadly described across four basic themes, as shown in the box.[27–32] HR is an important 'asset' to any hospital as hospitals are

[vi] As mentioned in Chapter 2, India has a shortfall of 1 million physicians, 2 million nurses and 3 million hospital beds to achieve the world average of 1.7 physicians, 3.3 nurses and 3.6 beds per 1,000 people.

labour-intensive. Its large pool of highly skilled specialist medical and allied medical staff is responsible for delivering a wide range of hospital services. Human assets of a hospital cannot be duplicated elsewhere, whereas other physical assets such as facilities and machines can be easily acquired by many hospitals.

1. HR planning and development
2. Staffing
3. Work systems design
4. Reporting relationships

Teaching vs Non-teaching Hospitals: HR challenges in teaching hospitals are more demanding than those from non-teaching hospitals. Some of the reasons are:

- Doctors in teaching hospitals have the additional load of teaching, training and conducting research over and above the load of patient care.
- Teaching hospitals have to abide by the MCI/DNB norms on staffing and infrastructure requirements.
- The load on patient care is also higher in teaching hospitals than non-teaching hospitals, possibly because of the community perception of improved service quality.
- Doctors in teaching hospitals have dual reporting relationships. They report to the dean of the medical college for their teaching and research activities, and report to the medical superintendent of the hospital for delivery of patient care services.

HR policies and programmes in hospital management should focus on 'investing in human assets' to achieve maximum productivity from its staff, as hospital services are highly labour-intensive.

Government vs Non-government Hospitals: The complexity of HR issues also differs between government hospitals and private hospitals, in areas such as:

- Minimum qualifications of staff
- Procedural requirements for staff recruitment
- Government rules on transfers and promotions

Instead of discussing general issues on HR management, we propose to take up HR issues that are specific to teaching hospitals and government hospitals.

4.4.1 HR Planning and Development

The most critical component of HR management is planning for HR. HR planning should ensure that the hospital has an optimal number of staff with the required skills. Aggregate planning focuses on estimating the total staff requirement, while succession planning focuses on filling up vacant positions, arising from retirements, resignations, transfers and promotions.

HR planning should be sensitive to the frequent changes in service delivery due to medical technology developments, information technology developments, higher expectations by the community, increased competition, and so on.

One of the important areas for HR planning in teaching hospitals (government or private) is to schedule the activities of the doctors. This is an area which has not received much attention. In the absence of any schedule, certain activities end up getting less attention, such as research activities. Promoting and acknowledging research contributions by faculty are integral to HR development. A well-designed HR plan would lead to identifying the developmental needs of the employees. HR development in hospitals should also address the interpersonal and communication skills as healthcare services touch human lives.[33] As mentioned earlier, hospital management should consider HR development activities as 'investments in human assets'.

4.4.2 Staffing

Teaching hospitals (government or private) have to abide by the MCI[vii] norms on staffing. MCI norms do not allow part-time faculty in teaching hospitals. HR management, therefore, should consciously address the different staff resource needs of teaching and non-teaching hospitals.

HR management should also consciously address the different staffing rules and regulations for government hospitals vs private hospitals. Staff shortages are very common in government hospitals. This could be due to a number of reasons:

- Sanctioned posts are less than the requirements
- Sanctioned posts lying vacant
- Procedural delays in staff recruitment
- Frequent transfer of staff, and so on

Staff shortages in private hospitals go unnoticed in the absence of any regulation of the private sector; there are many private hospitals which employ less qualified staff to address the shortage of skilled staff.

Acute shortage of specialist doctors is another reason why some private sector hospitals are opting for a mix of full time vs visiting specialist consultants, such as cardiologists, neurology surgeons, and so on. Some hospitals consider their specialist consultants as their valued clients as a part of their marketing strategy to attract patients.

All hospitals (government and private) could also address their staff requirements by contracting in and/or contracting out certain services. Several state

---

[vii] DNB teaching has its own requirements.

governments have a contractual agreement with E108 ambulance service providers. Many hospitals are contracting out certain non-core activities such as laundry, security, food services, and so on.

It is important to realize that the quality of contracted-out (outsourced) services depends very much on the supervision by the hospital managers, since the ultimate responsibility for providing hospital services rests with the hospitals. Unfortunately, many hospitals fail to do the necessary supervision and, therefore, the service quality of contracted-out services may deteriorate over a period of time.

> Performance management is the key to all hospital services, irrespective of who delivers the services, hospital staff, contracted in or contracted out.

The government of Gujarat addressed its shortages of government gynecologists/obstetricians by announcing the very popular scheme called Chiranjeevi Yojana for institutional deliveries. Under this scheme, the government of Gujarat pays a fixed amount to the private sector gynecologists/obstetricians for performing a package of 100 deliveries to handle both normal and complicated cases. This scheme has worked very well and there is evidence to suggest that it has led to reducing maternal mortality in the state of Gujarat.[34]

4.4.3 Work Systems Design

Work systems design involves identifying the tasks and responsibilities of each employee as well as groups of employees for delivering services.

Hospital services are labour-intensive and call for a fair amount of interaction and coordination among several departments. Take the case of designing a work system for doctors in teaching hospitals. This is a key managerial challenge[35] as the doctors in teaching hospitals are involved in teaching, research, patient care and administrative work. Similarly, work design for support staff is equally, if not more, challenging, because the support staffs in hospitals (physiotherapists, house-keeping staff, and so on) have to serve several departments with each department having its own special requirements. The support staffs also provide different types and levels of support based on the needs of service delivery. For example, the work system design of support staffs in an OT should facilitate a pooled interdependent[viii] nature of service delivery. On the other hand,

[viii]As mentioned earlier, in a work system with pooled interdependency, service provision requires pooling of independent services; here, individual employees work independently in doing their own specialized tasks, and coordinate with other skilled employees to deliver effective services.

the work system design of support staffs in OPD services delivery should facilitate a sequential interdependent[ix] nature of service requirement.

Work system design should motivate the staff to give the maximum productivity and improved levels of service. Unfortunately, the practice of rotating staff nurses between departments in government hospitals works contrary to this concept. Consider the case of an OT skilled nurse shifted to pediatrics department, and a staff nurse with no OT skills replacing her in OT. Similarly, consider a trained midwife shifted from maternity ward into an orthopedic unit and her post in labour room being filled by a nurse from geriatrics department!

4.4.4 Reporting Relationships

Work system design does influence the organizational structure design and, thereby, the reporting relationships. Reporting relationships between employees at different levels are best represented by the organizational structure. The organizational structure is defined as a formal system of interaction and coordination that links the tasks of individuals and groups to achieve organizational goals (Pugh et al.). While certain large hospitals maintain a formal organizational structure, many medium-to-small hospitals in India do not have a formal system of reporting.

Dual reporting relationships are common in both teaching and non-teaching hospitals. In the case of teaching hospitals, doctors report to the dean of the medical college for all matters related to teaching and research. But on matters related to patient care services, they report to the medical superintendent of the hospital.

In the case of all hospitals (teaching, non-teaching, government, private), dual reporting relationships is faced by many functional support staff. The functional staff members provide support to the medical departments seeking their services, and, thereby, end up reporting to the head of the medical departments they serve in addition to their own functional head. In order to overcome this concern, some hospitals have formed multi-disciplinary teams (by drawing skilled staff from different support departments into a multi-disciplinary unit) to provide patient-focussed multidisciplinary services. These teams report only to the head of their multi-disciplinary unit.

What is a better option for hospitals: maintaining a centralized pool of support staff who can provide services to medical departments or should the support

[ix] In a work system with sequential interdependency, service provision consists of a sequence of work flows; here, the output from one service station forms an input to the next service station. HR management in such a situation should focus on efficient work flow.

staffs be grouped into multi-disciplinary units? Please note that each option has its own implications on the HR needs, costs and service quality. A centralized pool of support staffs could be cost-effective because of shared resource utilization. On the other hand, groups of multi-disciplinary staffs could improve service quality, since multi-disciplinary groups are 'patient focused'.

The dual reporting relationship is likely to create conflicting expectations and ambiguity in the working of the hospital staff. Performance appraisal of such staffs is, thus, very challenging.

METROPOLITAN SURGICAL HOSPITAL (C) — MINI CASE 4.4

The Metropolitan Hospital had a reputation for orthopedic services, especially the post-surgery rehabilitation services. Based on each surgeon's advice, a multi-disciplinary team was constituted to meet the individual rehabilitation needs of his/her patients. The rehabilitation support team consisted of a junior doctor, a physiotherapist and a nurse, each care giver drawn from his/her parent department. Each member of the rehabilitation support staff participated in 3–4 multi-disciplinary teams and looked after the needs of 5–6 patients every day. Each team met once or twice every week to review the progress and schedule the therapy plan for the following week.

The management felt the current system lacked patient focus. Under the current system, each care giver came as per his/her schedule, not necessarily a convenient schedule for the patient. The current system also called for enormous coordination between several departments.

An HR consultant suggested a 'patient-focused' approach which meant closing the physiotherapy unit and assigning the physiotherapists to various clinical units. Nurses continued to be assigned from the centralized nursing department.

Please comment on the HR consultant's suggestions.

4.5 MATERIALS MANAGEMENT

1. Purchase management
2. Inventory management
3. Stores management
4. Hospital pharmacy

Materials management is more than inventory management. It includes the management of materials in the pre-inventory (purchases), inventory and post-inventory (stores) phases.[36–43] The task of a materials manager is to control the costs of material management process without compromising on service quality. In the context of hospital management, materials would refer to medicines, drugs, surgical items, X-ray films, reagents, and so on.

4.5.1 Purchase Management

This includes the tasks of forecasting the annual demand for each material, selection of vendors, placing purchase orders and follow ups with the vendors for ensuring timely receipt of materials.

In the case of hospitals, demand forecasting for medicines, drugs, surgical items, and so on should start with an analysis of the consumption pattern of materials by each user department. Unfortunately, many hospitals do not maintain consumption reports of user departments properly. This practice has serious cost implications on under-ordering some items and over-ordering some other items. Additional complexity arises from developments in medical technology, obsolescence, expiry date, and so on.

Many hospitals select vendors based on technical qualifications and L1, L2 and L3 prices (L1 is the lowest quotation on prices). The selection process usually ends up in a large number of vendors, with many supplying only a few items. The 80:20 rule applies here, 80 per cent of all purchases are made from 20 per cent of the suppliers. Once the vendors are chosen on rate contracts, purchase orders are placed. Each order placed has to be followed up several times with the suppliers to ensure receipt of materials on time. Large number of vendors and more frequent purchase orders increase the clerical cost of follow up activities with vendors.

Vendor management is an important issue. Vendor management goes beyond vendor selection. It involves building a long-term relationship with vendors for a regular uninterrupted supply of good quality materials on time. It is necessary to keep the number of vendors as minimum as possible since the clerical costs associated with regular follow up and monitoring of purchase orders is very high, and generally overlooked by many hospitals.

> The task of a materials manager is to control the costs of material management process without compromising on service quality.

Purchase management calls for frequent interactions with the finance department so as to pay the vendors on time. Unnecessary delays in accounts payable to vendors would affect the quality of vendor services, often leading to delayed deliveries of hospital supplies, forcing the hospitals to resort to 'emergency purchases'. Emergency purchases should be properly monitored and audited as ad-hoc and unplanned emergency purchases would create many disturbances in the purchasing systems.

The tasks of purchase management, therefore, includes demand forecasts, selection of vendors, preparing purchase orders, arranging for the deliveries to be made, arranging for payments to vendors, purchase order follow ups, emergency purchases and keeping proper records of all transactions.

4.5.2 Inventory Management

Inventories always exist due to mismatches between the rates of supply and demand. If an organization can match its supply and demand rates, it will also succeed in reducing its inventory levels. In making decisions on purchase quantity, it is necessary to balance two sets of costs: ordering cost which is the cost associated with placing an order and inventory holding cost associated with holding the stock in inventory. Inventory holding cost includes not only the cost of purchase, but also the cost of storage and insurance.

An important consideration in inventory management is to identify optimal order quantity for each material per purchase order and the number of purchase orders. Many hospitals place purchase orders every month for almost all materials (except those to be imported or which require special clearances). In doing so, decisions on purchase quantity ignore the consumption rate and the lead time for procurement of materials, and, thereby, leading to under-stocking of some and over-stocking of some other materials.

In hospitals, stock-out costs are very undesirable, as services have to be provided when demanded. Many hospitals, therefore, end up over-stocking materials so as to ensure service delivery at all times. Over-stocking of materials leads to unnecessary inventory holding costs and, thereby, adversely affects the working capital.[x] Inventories are costly as they tie up considerable amounts of working capital.

Inventory planning decisions on 'how much to order' and 'when to order' each material, should take into account the lead time for procurement and storage capacity available.

Surgical departments in many hospitals do over-stock OT materials, so that no surgery is postponed, delayed or lost as surgical services are major revenue generating activities. Different surgeons may require different brands[xi] of the same materials for the same procedures, resulting in over-stocking of the same materials of different brands. Surgical materials usually account for almost 30 per cent of the total value of hospital supplies. Materials in surgical services would account for at least 25–30 per cent of total OT service charges.

It is not easy to account for materials used in surgical procedures. We would use an illustration to highlight this issue later in this section.

4.5.3 Stores Management

Upon receipt of items from vendors, the stores management takes the responsibility to inspect the items for quality and quantity, store the materials which

[x] Refer to our discussions on working capital in Chapter 4.

[xi] The author has observed different surgeons in a hospital indenting different brands of surgical needles and sutures for the same procedure.

pass inspection, update the stock-on-hand, authorize payment to vendors and issue the materials to user departments as per their indents. Each user department is expected to maintain its consumption register regularly, so as to facilitate preparing its monthly indents. While supplying the items to user departments, the store manager has the added responsibility to monitor the expiry date of medicines and drugs.

Hospital materials require different storage needs. Some materials take up a lot of storage space (e.g., dialysis solutions), some materials may require refrigeration (e.g., vaccines), while blood platelets need to be kept in an agitated condition at sub-zero temperatures.

Some hospitals do not have enough storage space in their central stores, and, therefore, storage is left to the individual user departments. This is not a healthy practice as it could give rise to pilferage of materials by user departments, since no monitoring of material usage is done by the central stores.

Some hospitals maintain a separate OT store. This practice is a safety precaution to ensure availability of OT materials at all times so as to avoid rescheduling of OT services for want of any material. The author has seen such practices resulting in overstocking of OT materials. In one hospital, the OT sub-store was always carrying the equivalent of 4–5 months of consumption at any point in time.

4.5.4 Pharmacy Management

The working of hospitals pharmacy varies between hospitals. Besides serving the outpatients, the hospital pharmacy caters to the needs of inpatient wards (ordered through the nursing stations), OT sub-store, and so on.

METROPOLITAN SURGICAL HOSPITAL (D)[44] MINI CASE 4.5

In the process of estimating the cost of OT procedures, the management of Metropolitan Hospital realized the difficulties in accounting for the materials consumed in each procedure. Difficulty for inventory accounting arises due to the nature of OT materials—disposable items, fully consumable items, semi-consumable items, implants, and so on.

The OT sub-stores at Metropolitan Hospital received their supplies from the pharmacy store, medical store and general store. The central store handled about 3,000 items. The OT sub-stores accounted for almost 30 per cent of the total value of hospital supplies.

Items handled by the OT sub-stores were classified as follows:

- Disposable items (IV sets, cannula, and so on)
- Fully consumable items (IV fluids, drugs and medicines, sutures, and so on)

- Semi-consumable items: These were mostly surgical items that could be sterilized by CSSD and used again. It was a common practice in knee surgery to try different types of screws before finding the one that fits well on the patient's body. Such items that were tried but not consumed in surgery were sent to CSSD by the OT nurse supervisor. The CSSD supervisor, after inspection, sent them for re-sterilization for future usage. Re-sterilized items were then passed on to the OT sub-stores by CSSD. The logistics planning to coordinate the OT-CSSD interaction was very important in order to understand the usage (and, hence, costing) of semi-consumable items in OT.
- Consignment items, which did not form part of the inventory, but stored by the supplier, to be purchased by the hospital as and when the need arose (implants like heart valves, knee joints, and so on). This helped the hospital reduce its inventory holdings, and also helped the supplier meet ad-hoc demands for such items.

Inventory accounting was not easy. Metropolitan Hospital followed the most widely used system of tray accounting, briefly described below. Based on the OT schedule for a given day, the stores supervisor prepared at least two trays of materials for each surgery—an anesthesia material tray and a surgical material tray—and handed them over to the OT nurse supervisor. In certain cases, a third tray was prepared such as a perfusionist's tray (cardiothoracic surgery) and a fourth tray containing materials for post-operative recovery rooms. Each tray was custom made for each surgery and each surgeon. Items were taken out of these trays during the surgery, and the unused items in their respective trays were returned to the OT stores after surgery. The issue of materials and their returns were recorded in specific registers. The difference between the issue of materials and their returns was assumed to be consumed. Such an assumption was not correct all the time, since the semi-consumable items missing in the tray need not have been consumed. Some items tried (considered used) during surgery might have been sent for re-sterilization for further use. Pilferage of OT materials (e.g., sutures) was another common complaint. As a result, inventory balancing of OT materials for each surgery could only be approximate. The difficulty to balance the inventory of OT materials at the end of each day was, therefore, very disturbing.[xii]

[xii]Instead of addressing these challenges in inventory balancing, many hospitals have now taken the easy way out by introducing disease-specific packages and a price for each package. Package prices are fixed mostly in consultation with insurance providers and not so much based on a clear understanding of costs for services listed under each package. The package rates are very high (play it safe approach by the hospitals) and package details totally blind to the customers.

Consumption of emergency material stored in the various operating rooms often goes unrecorded because of the rushed usage at the time of life-saving effort. Also, recording discrepancies occur because of incorrect identification of used materials due to visual similarities. For example, screws 1.1(M) and 1.2(M) for orthopedic surgery look similar but the latter costs several times the cost of the former. All these concerns lead to difficulties in reordering and variations precipitating in the annual stocktaking.

Question: How would you address the materials management challenges faced by the OT management at Metropolitan Hospital?

To summarize, materials management includes the functions of purchase management, inventory management, stores management and the hospital pharmacy.

4.6 SUMMARY

Figure 4.3 summarizes our discussions on hospital management functions.

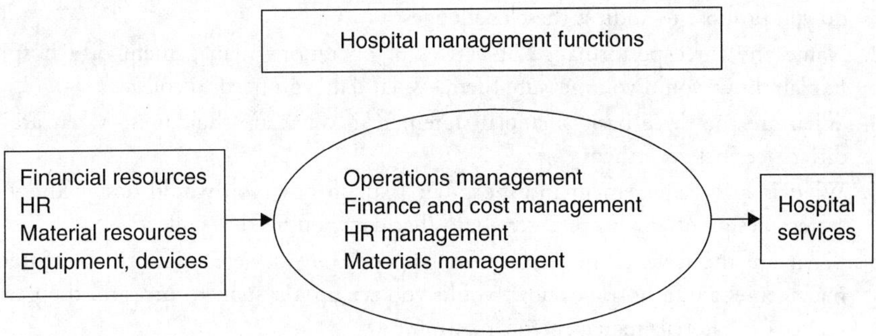

Figure 4.3 Hospital Management Functions

In the next chapter, we discuss the importance of hospital support systems, which form the backbone of any hospital service delivery.

QUESTIONS

1. Take any hospital service and describe its activities under the following management functions:
   (a) Operations management
   (b) Financial management
   (c) HR management
   (d) Materials management

2. Identify two critical challenges in the operations management in a hospital. How do you propose to address these challenges?
3. Identify two critical challenges in the financial management in a hospital. How do you propose to address these challenges?
4. Identify two critical challenges in cost management in a hospital. How do you propose to address these challenges?
5. How is activity based costing different from traditional method of costing?
6. What are the issues involved in pricing of a hospital service?
7. Explain the difference between fixed and variable cost.
8. Explain the difference between direct and indirect cost.
9. Give an example for each of the following:
   (a) Fixed and direct cost
   (b) Fixed and indirect costs
   (c) Variable and direct cost
   (d) Variable and indirect cost
10. Identify two critical challenges in the HR at your hospital. How do you propose to address these challenges?
11. Identify two critical challenges in the materials management at your hospital. How do you propose to address these challenges?
12. Name any three performance objectives of operations management of a hospital. Explain how would you measure them. What data you need to collect?
13. What are the three basic financial statements? What are their uses? What are the differences between them?
14. What is HR management in a hospital? Explain how you would design the work system design of any hospital service. What data you need to collect?
15. What are the tasks in materials management? If you were in charge of materials management in a hospital, how would you set up a system to measure the performance of materials management function?
16. What are the objectives in hospital waste management?
17. Why is bio-medical waste management a social concern?
18. Describe the steps to be adopted in a hospital for bio-medical and general waste management. How would you rate your hospital practices for waste management?
19. What is computer simulation? Identify two service delivery systems which are ideal for computer simulation in hospitals.
20. Collect the data for any service delivery system you have identified for computer simulation in hospitals and simulate the monthly load for these services.
21. Refer to the simulation of cath lab services. You are now told that the cath lab has to manage emergencies as well as planned procedures. What additional data would you need to handle emergencies?
22. With reference to Question 21, describe Monte Carlo Simulation approach for simulating the average daily load of planned and emergency cath lab services.

REFERENCES

1. Chase, Richard Jacobs; F. Robert and Aquilano, Nicholas J. (2005), *Operations Management for Competitive Advantage*, 10th ed., Tata McGraw Hill, New Delhi.
2. Gaither, Norman and Frazier, Greg (2002), *Operations Management*, 9th ed., Thomson South Western, Australia.
3. Greasley, Andrew (2006), *Operations Management*, John Wiley and Sons, England.
4. McLaughlin, Daniel B. et al (2008), *Healthcare Operations Management*, PHI Learning Pvt. Ltd., New Delhi.
5. Metters, King-Metters and Pullman, Walton (2006), *Service Operations Management*, South-Western: Cengage Learning 2010.
6. Slack, Nigel; Chambers, Stuart; Harland, Christine; Harrison, Alan and Johnston, Robert (1998), *Operations Management*, 2nd ed., Pitman Publishing, London.
7. Waters, Donald (2002, 2nd ed.), *Operations management: Producing Goods and Services*, Prentice Hall, Harlow.
8. Case, IIMA/BP 0299 (2004), Aravind Eye care System: Giving the Most Precious Gift; Indian Institute of Management, Ahmedabad.
9. Ramani, K.V. and Dileep Mavalankar (2006 a), 'Health System in India: Opportunities and challenges for improvements', *Journal of Health Organization and Management*, 20 (6), pp. 560–572.
10. Harvard Business School Case, 9-696-015 (1997), Massachusetts General Hospital: CABG Surgery (B).
11. Harvard Business School Case, 9-898-172 (2000), Reading Rehabilitation Hospital: Implementing Patient Focused care.
12. Harvard Business School case; 9-696-015, (2004), Massachusetts General Hospital: CABG Surgery (A).
13. Watson, Hugh (1981), *Computer Simulation in Business*, John Wiley & Sons.
14. Ibid.
15. Law, Averill M. and Kelton, David W. (1982), *Simulation Modeling and Analysis*, McGraw-Hill Book Company.
16. Lennon, J. (1992), 'Simulation of the Design and Planning of Emergency Departments', In Hilbert, J.E. and Dixon, A.J., *Simulation in Education for Business Management and MIS*, Society for Computer Simulation, San Diego, pp. 93–97.
17. Case, CMHS 0021, (2012), PDHN Hospital, Indian Institute of Management, Ahmedabad.
18. Baker, J.J. and Boyd, G.F. (1997), 'Activity Based Costing in the Operating Room at Valley View Hospital', *Journal of Healthcare Finance*, 24 (1), pp. 1–6.
19. Richard, Luecke, *Finance for Managers*, Harvard Business Essentials Series, Harvard Business School Press, 2002.
20. Ramachandran, N. and Kakani, Ram Kumar (2011), *How to Analyze Financial Statements*, Tata McGraw Hill Education Pvt. Ltd.

21. Miller, John A. (1996), *Implementing Activity Based Management in Daily Operations*, John Wiley & Sons, New York.
22. Lal, Jawahar (2009), *Cost Accounting*, 4th ed., Tata McGraw Hill, New Delhi.
23. Sharan, Vyuptakesh (2009), *Fundamentals of Financial Management*, 2nd ed., Pearson Education, New Delhi.
24. Richard, Luecke, *Finance for Managers*, Harvard Business Essentials Series, Harvard Business School Press, 2002.
25. Harvard Business School Case, 9-100-054 (2002), Cambridge Hospital Community Network-The Primary Care Unit.
26. Ramani, K.V. (2004), 'A Management Information System to Plan and Monitor the Delivery of Healthcare Services in Government Hospitals in India', *Journal of Health Organization and Management*, 18 (3), pp. 207–220.
27. Mathis, Robert L. and Jackson, John H. (2002), *Human Resource Management*, 10th ed., South Western College Publications, Australia.
28. Mello, Jeffrey A. (2002), *Strategic HR Management*, South Western, A Division of Thomson Learning.
29. Niles, Nancy J. (2012), *Basic Concept of Healthcare Human Resource Management*, Jones & Bartlett Learning, Burlington.
30. Pugh, Richard (2007), 'Dual relationships: personal and professional boundaries in rural social work', *British Journal of Social Work*, 37 (8), pp. 1405–1423.
31. Rowley, Chris and Jackson, Keith (Eds.) (2010), *Human Resource Management: The Key Concepts*, Routledge, New York.
32. Storey, John (2007), *Human Resource Management, A Critical Text*, 3rd ed., Thomson Learning, London.
33. Gvan, Servellen (2009), *Communication Skills for the Healthcare: Professional Concepts, Practice and Evidence*, 2nd ed., Jones & Bartlett Learning, New Delhi.
34. Mavalankar, D. and Ramani, K.V. (2012), 'A Study of Mortality Impact Evaluation of Chiranjeevi Scheme of the Government of Gujarat', *Report of IIM Ahmedabad*.
35. Ramani, K.V. (2002), 'Scheduling Doctor's Activities at a Large Teaching Hospital', *Production and Inventory Management Journal*, 43 (1 and 2), pp. 56–62.
36. Arnold, Tony; Chapman, Stephen and Ramakrishnan, R.V. (2007); *Introduction to Materials Management*; 2nd ed., Pearson Education, New Delhi.
37. Chopra, Sunil; Meindl, Peter and Kalra, D.V. (2010), *Supply Chain Management; Strategy, Planning and Operation*, 4th ed., Dorling Kindersley (India) Pvt. Ltd, New Delhi.
38. Crandall, Richard E.; Crandall, William R. and Chen, Charlie C. (2010), *Principles of Supply Chain Management*, Special India Edition, Charlie C. Chen CRC Press, Boca Raton.
39. Hillier, Fredericks S. and Lieberman, Gerald J. (1967), *Introduction to Operations Research*, 2nd ed., Holden Day, San Francisco.

40. Ramani, K.V. (2001), 'DSS-enabled Materials Management Process at MP Trust Hospital', *Production and Inventory Management Journal,* 42 (1).
41. Ramani, K.V. (2006 b) 'Managing Hospital Supplies: Process Reengineering at Gujarat Cancer Research Institute, India', *Journal of Health Organization and Management,* 20 (3), pp. 218–226.
42. Sahney, V.K. and Rupp, L.B. (1988), 'Henry Ford hospital improves scheduling, inventory, communications', *Journal of Industrial Engineering,* pp. 58–65.
43. Wagner, Harvey M. (1977), *Principles of Operations Research,* Prentice Hall of India, New Delhi.
44. Case, CMHS 0021, (2012), PDHN Hospital, Indian Institute of Management, Ahmedabad.

chapter 5

Hospital Management Support Systems

CHAPTER OUTLINE

CHAPTER OBJECTIVE

The main objective of this chapter is to highlight the role of hospital support systems in service delivery. Support systems can be broadly grouped under clinical support, management information support (MIS) and administrative support.

5.1 AN INTRODUCTION

Support services to hospital health service delivery can be broadly classified under the following heads:

- Clinical services
- Information services: MIS
- Administrative services

Clinical Services

Clinical services form the backbone of hospital service delivery. Clinical laboratory services and radiology/imaging services provide very critical information to the clinicians for diagnosis and treatment. It is known that investigation test results contribute to more than 75 per cent of all decision making by the clinicians.

Information Services: MIS

MIS in any organization should be designed to support managerial decisions at all levels. Hospital MIS should, therefore, support the policy, strategic planning, operational planning and monitoring and control decisions to assist the operations management, finance and cost management, human resource (HR) management and materials management functions.

Administrative Services

Hospital administrative support services include stores and purchase, medical records maintenance, dietary services, house-keeping, ambulance services, bio-medical services, interaction with insurance providers, admission, discharge, hospital waste management, and so on. Even though some of these services may be outsourced, the ultimate responsibility for all administrative support rests with the hospital management.

We begin our discussion on hospital support systems with a detailed discussion on clinical lab support.

5.2 CLINICAL SUPPORT

5.2.1 Clinical Lab Services

The use of clinical laboratory test results in diagnostic decision making has become an integral part of clinical medicine. With increasing dependence on lab test results by the clinicians (physicians) for treatment, the reliability of laboratory testing and reporting is of utmost importance. Even though automation, standardization and technological advances have significantly improved the analytical reliability of laboratory tests, lab errors still do occur in the pre-analytical, analytical and post-analytical processes of the total testing process. It is the responsibility of the lab manager to minimize lab errors occurring at any stage of the testing process. Lab errors lead to sample rejection which in turn calls for repeat sample collection and analysis, and, thereby, cause delays in reporting the test results. Any delay in test results could have adverse consequences on the patients' health. Repeat sample collection and analysis also increase the cost of providing reliable test results and, thereby, affect the profitability of the laboratory and hence the hospital itself.

5.2.1.1 Total Testing Process:[i] An understanding of the most critical steps in the total lab testing process is a pre-requisite for setting up a plan for a corrective and preventive strategy aimed at minimizing lab errors and safeguarding the health of the patients. Total testing process is a multi-step process that begins and ends with the needs of the patients. It consists of three major phases:

1. ***Pre-analytical phase:*** The pre-analytical phase deals with collection of specimens from patients and submitting them to the lab.
2. ***Analytical phase:*** The analytical phase involves testing, examination, analysis and interpretation of the investigations.
3. ***Post-analytical phase:*** The post-analytical phase deals with giving the test reports to the clinicians and their patients.

It can be seen from Figure 5.1 that each of these phases can be further subdivided.

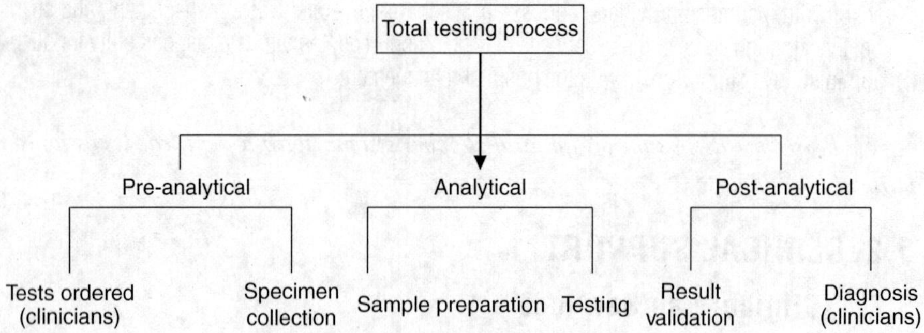

Figure 5.1 Total Testing Process

[i]We will discuss in detail the guidelines and actual practices in the total testing process in clinical labs. Our discussion would highlight the need for monitoring and control of lab activities in order to reduce lab errors and, thereby, improve the performance of lab management.

Tests Ordered (Clinicians): This phase starts when a clinician orders tests for her/his patients and ends when the lab receptionist prepares work orders for the phlebotomists for specimen collection.

Specimen Collection: This phase starts with the phlebotomists picking up their work orders from the lab receptionist, preparing bar-coded labels for each sample tube, collecting specimens from patients and submitting samples[ii] to the analytic section of the lab for testing.

Sample Preparation: Sample processing in the lab may involve centrifugation,[iii] aliquotting,[iv] pipetting,[v] dilution,[vi] and so on. Sample adequacy, a critical pre-analytic factor, affects test result accuracy and usefulness. Accepting samples unsuitable for analysis can lead to erroneous information that could compromise patient care.

Testing: After ensuring sample integrity, the lab technicians carry out tests and examinations of the samples as ordered by the clinicians.

Test Result Validation: This phase deals with activities within the laboratory including technical and medical validation of the test results, the production of test reports, interpretation of test results and their transmission to the requesting clinicians and their patients.

Diagnosis (Clinicians): These activities occur outside the laboratory such as the clinician's reaction to the report and interpretation and utilization of laboratory information for diagnosis and treatment.[1]

In the next section, we discuss lab errors occurring in each phase of the total testing process.

[ii] The literature uses the words 'specimen' and 'sample' interchangeably. Any biological material collected from the human body for testing is a specimen, and what is submitted for analysis is a sample. For example, blood is a specimen. Sometimes, blood is mixed with certain chemicals to prevent it from clotting and submitted as a sample for testing. At other times, blood specimen is submitted as sample for testing. Sample collection is the most commonly used term to refer to either specimen or sample.

[iii] Centrifugation is a process by which serum and plasma are separated from the whole blood.

[iv] Aliquotting is the process by which blood specimen or serum/plasma obtained from centrifugation is transferred into 2–3 tubes for different tests to be conducted in parallel. Aliquotting, though takes time to prepare, possibly saves time in reporting the test findings. This is especially useful when specimens should be sent to two different lab sections, such as biochemistry and microbiology.

[v] Pipetting is a process by which a small quantity of liquid is measured and transferred to another container.

[vi] Dilution is a process by which concentration of an active substance is diluted by adding a neutral agent.

5.2.1.2 Lab Errors: Many lab managers believe that lab errors are infrequent in their lab and, hence, there is no need for continuous monitoring and/or recording of labs errors. Such an assumption has serious drawbacks, as lab errors do occur and wrong lab reports could have adverse impact on patients' health.

Lab errors may be defined as 'any defect from ordering tests to reporting results and appropriately interpreting and reacting on these'.[2]

Lab errors occur in each phase of the total testing process.

Pre-analytic lab errors: Phlebotomy errors account for a majority of errors in the pre-analytic phase.

Analytic lab errors: Lack of quality assurance could lead to wrong test results in the analytic phase.

Post-analytic lab errors: Misidentification errors are common in the post-analytic phase.

Almost 70 per cent of all lab errors occur in the pre-analytic phase, when specimens fail to pass sample integrity, often leading to sample rejection.

Hemolysed[vii] blood is the most common reason (as high as 60 per cent) for sample rejection. Other major reasons for sample rejection are: insufficient sample quantity, lipemic,[viii] icteric[ix] and clotted samples.[3] Lab errors, as and when detected, call for sample rejection. Any rejected sample calls for repeat sample collection and analysis, leading to delayed reports, additional costs to the lab and, thereby, impacting service quality and customer satisfaction. Undetected lab errors could adversely affect the patients' health due to incorrect treatment protocol.

Consequences of lab errors, therefore, have implications on finances, service quality and additional training inputs to lab staff. In short, lab errors cut the profitability margin of the laboratory, and, therefore, minimizing lab errors is a major task in lab management.

[vii] Hemolysis is the breakage of red blood cells causing the release of hemoglobin and other internal components into the blood serum or plasma. It can occur both in-vitro and in-vivo. In-vitro hemolysis happens mostly as a result of inappropriate blood collection practices, and is easily detected by the presence of pink- or red-coloured specimens in the serum/plasma after centrifugation. Causes for in-vivo hemolysis are many, including hereditary, acquired conditions such as autoimmune hemolytic anemia and certain infections, e.g., falciparum malaria. Hemolysis is a very undesirable condition that influences the accuracy and reliability of lab tests.

[viii] Lipemia indicates the presence of fat in the blood serum. It is an inherent characteristic of the patient's blood. Lipemic sample can arise due to sample collection after heavy meals or the presence of some metabolic disorder. Lipemic samples become turbid, making it difficult for investigation.

[ix] Icteric blood means excess bilirubin in the blood and such a sample should be used for testing with caution as the deep yellow colour of serum may interfere with certain analyte measurements like false lower values of S. Creatinine in modified Jaffe's test. Bilirubin also interferes with glucose, cholesterol, triglyceride, phosphorus, uric acid and the total protein measurements.

Monitoring and control of errors is very crucial to an effective and efficient management of lab activities. Effective management is an indicator of producing reliable test results. Efficient management is an indicator of costs incurred for producing reliable test results.

5.2.1.3 Pre-analytical Phase: We begin our discussion on controlling lab errors by listing all the activities in the pre-analytical phase (Table 5.1).

Table 5.1 Pre-analytic Activities

Sr. No.	Activities	Source	Sub-activities
1	Tests ordered	Clinician	Tests ordered orally or handwritten
2	Work orders	Lab receptionist	Work orders prepared for each patient—inpatients, ICU patients, emergency patients, outpatients
3	Sample collection	Phlebotomist	Bar-coded labels for blood collection, identification Patient identification Blood collection Proper mixing Sample identification Disposal of used materials Submit the samples for testing

Activity 1: Investigations/Tests Ordered: Transcription errors are the most common errors in this phase as it involves processing the tests ordered by clinicians.

Oral orders: Many times, clinicians give oral orders to the nurses for investigations which are not correctly/completely heard or understood by the nurses while preparing written orders for investigation. For example, a nephrologist asked for iron profile with ferritin. This was a verbal request to the staff nurse in a hospital. The nurse in turn wrote the test request which did not include ferritin, and the test was done without ferritin.

Handwritten orders: At times, the handwritten orders for investigations by the clinicians/nurses are not legible and, therefore, the wrong test gets registered, leading to wrong work orders for the phlebotomists. For example, in a large hospital, the staff nurse received a handwritten order for testosterone from a clinician, but she wrongly read it as progesterone and, therefore, progesterone test was conducted, instead of testosterone test.

Activity 2: Work Orders: The lab receptionist prepares a separate work order for each patient for all tests ordered. It is the responsibility of the lab receptionist to highlight different priorities for sample collections; for example, tests ordered by the emergency department gets the highest priority than tests ordered by any other department.

The daily work schedule of a lab receptionist includes responding to queries on investigations, test reports, collection of payments for investigation from outdoor patients, in addition to preparing work sheets for investigations. As a result, she is under tremendous pressure to respond satisfactorily to all the demands on her from the hospital staff and patients' friends and relatives while she is busy preparing work orders for the phlebotomists. Continuous distraction of the lab receptionist might lead to wrong or incomplete work orders, not highlighting urgent requests, and so on. Transcription errors present in the preparation of work orders could lead to wrong identification of patients, wrong specimen collected, wrong tests done, and so on.

Activity 3: Specimen/Sample Collection: This phase starts with the phlebotomist picking up work orders from the lab receptionist and ends when she/he submits the patient samples to the analytic section of the lab for testing. It has been demonstrated that the most laboratory errors occur in this phase, primarily because of a lack of standardized protocols and the difficulty in monitoring the practices of all phlebotomists.

The pre-analytic phase accounts for almost 70 per cent of all lab errors.

Activity 3.1: Bar-code labels: As soon as a phlebotomist picks her/his work order, the immediate step is to prepare bar-code labels for each sample tube. The bar code on each sample tube provides a unique identity of the patient, clinician, tests ordered and sample details. The phlebotomist should be well trained in identifying the type of containers for specimen collection, based on the type of tests ordered.

Activity 3.2: Patient Identification: Correct patient identification is one of the first critical steps in ensuring correct laboratory results. Many factors may contribute to misidentification, such as issues related to the workload on the phlebotomist, the approach taken by the staff to confirm the identity of individual patients, and so on. Patients with identical (last) names present a unique challenge to acute healthcare settings. On an average, literature points out that one out of every 18 identification errors results in an adverse event affecting the patient's health result.[4]

Activity 3.3: Sample (Blood) Collection: Among pre-analytical variables, inappropriate procedure for collection of venous blood accounts for 60 per cent of the errors, highlighting the need for a more rigid and effective supervision of this pivotal and irreplaceable part of the diagnostic process.[5] The phlebotomist should be well-trained in the following:

- Use of gloves
- Site selection for appropriate venous access
- Site preparation for venipuncture
- Use of tourniquet
- Order of drawing samples for multiple sample collection
- Needle size selection
- Blood collection

Insufficient quantity of blood is the second most common cause of rejection. All blood collection tubes need to be filled to the correct volume. Every analytical process requires a fixed volume of serum/plasma for analysis.

Activity 3.4: Proper Mixing: After blood collection, the collection tubes are gently inverted several times (6–8 times) to allow effective mixing of blood and anticoagulant, but without provoking hemolysis or clotting.

Activity 3.5: Sample Identification: After proper mixing, bar code labels on the tube are pasted, before drawing the next specimen in order to provide a unique identity to the specimen.

Activity 3.6: Disposal of Used Materials: It is essential that the phlebotomist disposes of all the used materials before leaving the patient's bedside; for example, the phlebotomist should burn and throw all used needles in sodium hypochloride solution. All bio-medical wastes should be kept in appropriate coloured bags. Used materials should never be taken out of the patient's room.

Activity 3.7: Sample Submission to the Lab: Each sample type has standards for timely delivery and conditions for transport in order to maintain its integrity.

We end this discussion on pre-analytic process by referring to a recent study on lab errors in a clinical laboratory in India (Table 5.2).[6]

Table 5.2 Lab Errors: Pre-analytic

Types of Errors	Sample Frequency	Percentage	Causes of Error
Hemolysed sample	508	53.2	Wrong phlebotomy technique, incorrect transportation, centrifuging before sample is clotted
Insufficient sample	72	7.5	Lack of knowledge on volume required, difficult sampling pediatric, old patients
Illegible handwriting	69	7.2	Lack of knowledge/lax attitude of the phlebotomist/staff involved in sample collection and test ordering
Incorrect identification	44	4.6	
Order slip without sample	16	1.7	
Empty tube	10	1.0	
Lipemic sample	7	0.7	Collection under non-fasting state
Tube broken in centrifuge	6	0.6	Improper centrifugation technique
Physician's request order missed	4	0.4	Carelessness of the lab staff
Total pre-analytic	**736**	**77.1**	
Total analytic and post-analytic	**218**	**22.8**	
Grand Total	**954**	**99.9**	

Source: Goswami, B.; Singh, Bhawna; Chavla, Ranjana and Venkatesan, Mallika (2010), 'Evaluation of errors in a clinical laboratory: a one-year experience', *Clinical Chemistry Laboratory Medicine*, 48 (1), pp. 63–66.

It can be seen that hemolysed sample (53.2 per cent) is the most common cause of pre-analytical error, followed by insufficient sample (7.5 per cent), illegible handwriting (7.2 per cent) and incorrect identification (4.6 per cent).

5.2.1.4 Analytical Phase: We begin our discussions on analytic errors by first providing a conceptual view of the analytic process (Figure 5.2).

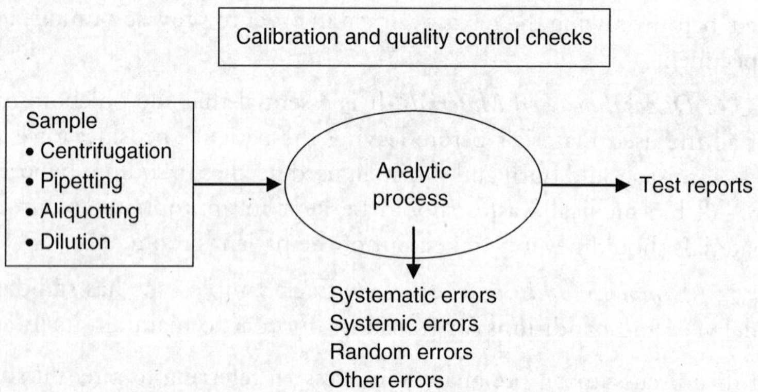

Figure 5.2 Analytic Process: A Conceptual View

Analytical Reliability: Analytical process focuses on the importance of providing reliable test results. Reliability of test results is measured across two important determinants of quality, namely, accuracy and precision.

1. **Accuracy:** Accuracy is the degree of conformity of a measured or calculated quantity to a reference value. Accuracy of any instrument is established through regular calibration of the instrument. Calibration is the act of checking or adjusting (by comparison with an acceptable value) the accuracy of a measuring instrument.
2. **Precision:** Precision refers to the closeness of agreement between independent test results obtained under varying operating conditions. Quality control is a measure of precision or how well the instrument system reproduces more or less same results over time. It is important to realize that repeated test results of a single patient sample do not produce the same result value for any analyte, but rather a range of values clustering around an average value of each analyte. This dispersion of values, known as analytic variation, is a measure of precision of the analytic process. Any process with a low-analytic variation would produce more reliable test results than a process with high-analytic variation.

Activities in the Analytic Process: Even though automation, standardization and technological advances have significantly improved, the analytical reliability of laboratory tests[7] and analytical errors still do occur.

Table 5.3 lists the various activities in the analytic process and explains the possible errors associated with each activity.

Table 5.3 Analytic Activities

Sr. No.	Activity
1	Sample processing before analysis (labelling, centrifugation, aliquoting)
2	System check
3	Calibration*
4	Quality control checks
5	Sample integrity (includes volume checks, clot detection)
6	Analysis
7	Report preparation

* Calibration is done less frequently than quality control checks. On those days when both calibration and quality control checks are to be done, first do calibration followed by quality control checks.

Activity 1: Sample Processing Before Analysis: This step involves verification of sample labelling, centrifugation and aliquoting. Sample processing involves verification of patient identification, tests ordered, relevant clinical information and time of collection with the information provided in the accompanying requisition form.

Centrifugation is the process by which serum and plasma are separated from the whole blood. Most of the tests are done on serum and/or plasma.

Aliquoting is the process by which serum/plasma obtained from centrifugation is transferred into 2–3 tubes for different tests to be done, in perhaps different sections of the lab. Aliquoting allows parallel processing and, thereby, facilitates quicker generation of test reports.

Activity 2: System Check: Before any test is carried out, the machine must be switched on and a full system check carried out to ensure that the instrument is in proper working condition. Common problems are wear and tear, improper shut down in the previous run, and so on.

It is equally necessary to ensure that reagents are stored in proper conditions. If storage conditions for reagents are disturbed due to power outage with rise in storage temperature, the reagents must be considered unreliable and discarded.

Activity 3: Calibration: Calibration is a measurable signal related to a substance concentration or other reported result. It requires testing of sample against one or more materials (calibrators) that behave similarly to the specimen and for which the true result is known. Calibration drift is a systematic change in measurement that occurs over a time period of unadjusted, continuous operation of a test instrument.

Activity 4: Quality Control (QC) Checks: QC checks are meant to establish precision of test results. QC checks are usually run at the beginning of each shift, after an instrument is serviced, when the reagent lots are changed, after calibration and when patient results seem inappropriate. Acceptability of QC result is established by estimating the variability or standard deviation of the process. It is the responsibility of the lab manager to perform calibration and QC runs as per protocol, and, thereby, ensure that the lab results are reliable.[x] Achieving accuracy and precision requires strict adherence to established protocols, rigorous use of controls, careful selection of reagents and the quality of specimens submitted for analysis. The quality of a laboratory's work can be no better than the quality of the sample and specimens submitted for analysis.

Activity 5: Sample Integrity: It is needless to emphasize that samples taken for analysis have to fulfil all the criteria for sample integrity. Pre-analytical problems (raising concerns on sample integrity) may not be discovered until the samples are examined in the lab, prior to testing. Volume checks, clot detection are also part of this activity.

Activity 6: Analysis: This is the technical component of testing process, and hence not discussed here, as we are concerned about management issues and not technical.

Activity 7: Report Preparation: Most of the automated analysers have built-in computers which generate reports after the testing is completed. It is the responsibility of the technical staff to ensure that reports are in order.

We end this section with a discussion on analytical errors.

Analytical Errors: For illustration, we reproduce in Table 5.4 the results of a one-year hospital study in India on the evaluation of errors in a clinical laboratory.[8] It can be seen that analytic errors accounted for 7.9 per cent of the total lab errors, while pre-analytical and post-analytical errors accounted for 77.1 per cent and 14.9 per cent, respectively. Even though the analytical process is less prone to errors than pre-analytical and post-analytical processes, it is necessary to understand the type of analytic errors and take appropriate measures to keep controllable errors at a minimum.

---

[x] Pre-analytical process focused on ensuring test worthy samples. Analytical process focuses on ensuring test worthy results.

Table 5.4 Lab Errors: Analytic

Types of Errors	Sample Frequency	Percentage	Causes of Error
Systemic error*: Probe malfunction, old lamp, blocked tubing	36	3.8	Inherent technical problem Routine wear and tear
Random error**	15	1.6	Unknown cause
Calibration drift	10	1.0	Reagent instability, reagent changeover, expiry of calibration data with time
Non-conformity with quality control	6	0.6	Old QC, improper storage
Reagent contamination	8	0.4	Reagent mix up, improper storage
Total Analytic	**75**	**7.9**	
Pre-analytic errors	736	77.1	
Post-analytic errors	143	14.9	
Grand Total	**954**	**99.9**	

* **Systemic errors:** Systemic errors are caused by inherent technical problems and/or by the wear and tear of the equipment and instruments.

** **Random errors:** Random errors are unavoidable since they arise from the limitations of physical measurements. Random errors can be caused by timing, temperature or pipetting variations.

It can be seen that systemic errors (3.8 per cent) due to inherent technical problems or routine wear and tear accounted for almost 50 per cent of all analytic errors. Random errors (1.6 per cent) due to unknown causes came next, followed by other causes such as reagent contamination.

5.2.1.5 Post-analytical Phase: In this phase, the most common mistakes are wrong validation, results that are delayed, not reported or reported to the wrong providers, and incorrect results reported because of post-analytical data entry errors and transcription errors.[9] The study of lab errors in an Indian hospital mentioned earlier[10] reported post-analytical errors at 14.9 per cent of all lab errors, with transcription errors (11.7 per cent) as high as 80 per cent of all post-analytical errors.

The post-analytical procedures performed within the laboratory (Table 5.5) include verifying laboratory results, feeding them into the laboratory information

Table 5.5 Post-analytical Activities

Sr. No.	Activity
1	Report validation
2	Communicating the results to physician or patient
3	Result interpretation by physicians

system and communicating them to the clinicians in a number of ways (in particular, by producing a report and making any necessary oral communications regarding 'alert' or panic results).

Activity 1: Report Validation: Review of laboratory reports requires checking the results for any instrument error codes, markedly abnormal (especially critical) results or specimen integrity issues; comparing multiple results on the same specimen if applicable; and determining appropriate commentary for inclusion in the final report. Most laboratories have some levels of review depending on the type of test and values in the report. At the first level, the technician or technologist analysing the specimen reviews the test results. Then, the supervisor (technologist) approves results for certain tests, reports the results to the clinician unless additional review by more senior professional staff is required. At the next level, a professional staff member (e.g., pathologist, microbiologist, biochemist) reviews and approves the test results for release. Senior level review and approval usually is performed when test results indicates abnormal values. Manual review of results is necessary in such instances as verification of anatomic pathology results and critical test results.[11]

Activity 2: Communicating the Results: Miscommunication can happen between physician and laboratory personnel, especially while reporting the results verbally and could lead to critical situations.

In most large clinical laboratories, test results are produced from and stored in the computerized lab information system (LIS). In these laboratories, test data may be entered manually into the LIS or automatically transferred to the LIS from automated systems. In the case of manual entry of the test data into the LIS, there are chances of transcription errors.

The production and release of the laboratory report is the crucial step in post-analytical procedures as its format, content and communication significantly affect the interpretation and utilization of laboratory data by clinicians.

Activity 3: Result Interpretation: The clinician, on receipt of the report, interprets the results and makes decisions on the basis of test report and an understanding of the patients' health condition. In fact, results released by the laboratory may not contain all the information needed by the clinician; the laboratory report may even contain information that the clinician considers superfluous or irrelevant.

Incorrect interpretation of results is a source of error that can severely affect the quality of patient care.

We end this section by reporting post-analytical errors in the Indian hospital (Table 5.6).[12]

In the next section, we discuss radiology and imaging support services .

Table 5.6 Lab Errors: Post-analytic

Types of Errors	Sample Frequency	Percentage	Causes of Error
Transcription errors	112	11.7	Manual error in copying numerical data from the printout onto the requisition slips
Prolonged turnaround time	31	3.2	Problems arising from inadequate water supply, irregular electricity, instrument problem, and so on.
Post-analytic errors	143	14.9	

5.2.2 Radiology and Imaging Services

Radiology and imaging services provide critical inputs to the clinicians regarding the body structure for diagnosis, prevention and treatment of diseases or health assessment. Images of the human body are generated by directing a variety of different energy sources into the body (like ultrasound) and using the returned energy to create images that can then be viewed either on film or on a computer monitor.

There are a wide range of investigative modalities:

X-rays	Bone image
USG, CT Scan	Soft tissue image
MRI	Tumour size image, neuro image
Colour Doppler	Blood flow image in heart chamber
PET Scan	Image of body form and function
Gamma camera	Nuclear medicine imaging scans

A Picture Archiving and Communication System (PACS) is a medical imaging technology which provides economical storage of, and convenient access to, images from multiple modalities. It consists of four major components: the imaging modalities (X-ray, CT, MRI, and so on), a secured network for transmission of patient information, workstations for interpreting and reviewing images, and archives for the storage and retrieval of images and reports.

Teleradiology is the transmission of radiological patient images, such as X-rays, CTs and MRIs, from one location to another for the purposes of sharing studies with other radiologists and physicians. Teleradiology provides an excellent solution in serving patients who are geographically far away. It would be possible for rural hospitals to transmit X-ray images over the Internet to a radiologist in an urban location, who can read, interpret the images and also recommend appropriate line of treatment. There are many hospitals in India who are already providing such services. Teleradiology can be made available 24×7 by hiring trained specialists to interpret images.

Radiology and imaging equipment are very expensive and pose managerial challenges for investment decisions. Investments in technology and medical equipments should be backed up with bio-medical engineering support. Bio-medical support plays a critical role in sourcing equipment, testing for feasibility of local environment, in-house support, and calibration and ensuring preventive maintenance. Unforeseen medical equipment downtime would adversely affect safe, effective and timely service delivery.

In the next section, we introduce the concept of hospital MIS to support the information needs of the management functions in service delivery.

5.3 INFORMATION SUPPORT: HOSPITAL MIS

Below, we discuss hospital management decisions at policy, strategic planning, operational planning, and monitoring and control levels and their implications on the hospital management functions.

MIS in any organization should support managerial decisions.

5.3.1 Hospital Management Decisions

The utilization of hospital resources to deliver services calls for important decisions by the hospital management. Managerial decisions can be broadly classified into the following:

- Policy decisions
- Strategic planning decisions
- Operational planning decisions
- Monitoring and control decisions

5.3.1.1 Policy Decisions: Policy decisions should emerge from an integrated evidence-based policy process. Evidence-based policy will lend credibility to the process of setting policy goals.

As an example, suppose you are interested in setting up a hospital. Table 5.7 lists a few policy decisions you should address at the time of conceptualizing the service delivery from the proposed hospital.

Hospital Location: Location is an important determinant of healthcare service delivery as it addresses issues on access to healthcare services. There are hospitals which are poorly located, making the access to their services very difficult; many such hospitals end up opening their city centres subsequently.

Hospital Type: Hospitals can be grouped into various categories based on the nature and type of services they provide: single vs multi-specialty hospitals,

Table 5.7 Some Examples of Policy Decisions

Sr. No.	Policy Decision
1	Hospital location
2	Hospital type
3	Hospital size
4	Investment decisions
5	Staffing policy
6	Public–private partnership

super-specialty hospitals vs general hospitals, teaching vs non-teaching hospitals, and so on. There are hospitals which started with a single super specialty such as cardiac care, subsequently expanded their services to include other specialties and super specialties.

Hospital Size: The number of beds in a hospital is an indicator of the hospital size. Decisions on hospital size should be based on an assessment of demand for each type of service, source of demand (market segment), support services required, and so on. There are hospitals with poor bed occupancy and there are hospitals which are overcrowded.

Investments: Investment decisions are taken at a policy level based on the requirement of hospital resources to provide its range of services. Investments are needed in medical technology, information technology (IT), buildings, and so on. Hospitals have a choice to own or lease medical equipments. For example, a hospital clinical laboratory can either buy an auto-analyser or take it on lease. Choice of auto-analyser technology (wet vs dry chemistry) is another important policy decision, since it has implications on lab management practices as well.

Staffing: The Medical Council of India has clearly laid down policy decisions on staff requirements, their qualifications and workload for teaching hospitals, both public and private. Similarly, each state government has laid down strict policy guidelines for staffing in non-teaching hospitals. However, policy guidelines are lacking in non-teaching private hospitals.

Public–private Patnership (PPP): PPP is very high on the government agenda for improving the quality of healthcare service delivery. A meaningful PPP requires a good understanding of the strengths and weaknesses of both the public and private sectors. While published data on public hospitals is available from government documents, published data from the private sector healthcare service providers is lacking.

> Regulation of the private sector (not control of the private sector) is essential for establishing and sustaining mutually beneficial PPPs.

It is important to realize that policy decisions are interlinked. For example, choice of a particular location may decide the hospital size and the range of services to be offered. Similarly, the choice of services to be offered would determine the investment required.

5.3.1.2 Strategic Planning Decisions: Strategic planning decisions are driven by policy decisions. They focus on evolving a clear strategy to translate the organizational goals and objectives to deliverables. Strategic planning decisions start with estimating the resource needs to achieve policy goals. Please note that failure to draw a strategic plan to meet the resource needs could lead to under achievement of the policy goals and poor quality of service. A few strategic planning decisions are given in Table 5.8.

Facility Planning: Service quality starts with facility design. Facility planning is an important strategic decision since it has an impact on the quality of medical service as well as on customer satisfaction. Unfortunately, this aspect is very often overlooked. Crowded waiting areas, poor location of medical records division, and so on are some of the consequences of poor facility planning.

New Service: Suppose a hospital has taken a policy decision to start a new service, say cardiac care services. The strategic planning required for translating this policy decision into service delivery starts with estimating the demand for each cardiac care service under cardiology and cardiothoracic departments. Based on the demand projections and an assessment of market competition for cardiac care services, the strategic planning unit identifies its market segments and then estimates the resources to provide services to meet its service quality goals.

HR Planning: HR planning to start a cardiac care unit includes estimating the required number of qualified in-house vs visiting cardiologists, cardiothoracic

Table 5.8 Some Examples of Strategic Decisions

Sr. No.	Strategic Decisions
1	Facility planning
2	Starting a new service
3	HR planning
4	Finance planning
5	Materials planning
6	Equipment planning
7	Pricing of services
8	TN medical services corporation
9	Cost reduction
10	Private vs general patients

consultants, anesthetists, technicians and other support staff. HR planning should be followed by HR development activities to keep the staff motivated for achieving higher productivity.

Finance Planning: Financial planning includes estimating the investment in capital expenditure (medical and IT support), fixed and variable expenses, working capital requirements, and so on for providing good quality healthcare services.

Materials Planning: Material requirement planning involves estimating the requirements of medicines, drugs and other consumables, disposables and semi-consumables. This involves purchase planning, inventory planning and stores planning.

Equipment Planning: This aspect of planning takes into account medical devices, equipment and machines for service delivery. It should also include planning for bio-medical engineering needs to ensure proper utilization of costly machines, equipment and devices.

Pricing: A major decision in any service delivery is the pricing of its services. Pricing decisions, though market sensitive, should be based on a clear understanding of the cost for providing services. There are cases where private hospitals took decisions on pricing their MRI services purely based on purchase cost recovery in 3–4 years. Many of these hospitals subsequently revised their pricing (both upwards and downwards) due to demand fluctuations arising from market competitions.

Never let your competitor dictate your strategies.

Tamil Nadu Medical Services Corporation: The Tamil Nadu government took a strategic decision in the 1990s to set up an autonomous Medical Services Corporation, headed by an IAS officer to handle the entire logistics of procurement, storage, and distribution of medicines and drugs to all the state government health facilities. By setting up such a corporation, the government had saved large amount of money (volume purchase discounts), established a transparent tendering and vendor selection process, in addition to delivering medicine and drugs on time even to the remotest health facility. Subsequently, it has also undertaken the task of procurement of medical equipment and devices, such as CT Scan for all government facilities.

Cost Reduction: Cost reduction strategies provide alternatives for hospitals to bridge the gap between its resource needs and the resources available. Minimizing the patient's length of stay in hospitals is a good cost reduction strategy. This is because most of the revenues from patient care come from the first 2–3 days of hospital stay, arising from consultation, investigation and interventions. Any length of stay beyond 2–3 days is not very profitable for hospitals. Other methods of cost reduction include achieving higher productivity from doctors (For example, Aravind Eye Hospital),[13] adopting BPR approach,[14] designing care paths, and so on.

Priority Customers: Certain Hospitals, like CMC Hospital, Vellore, maintain two types of OPD customers, private and general patients. Private patients come on appointments with their preferred consultant (less waiting time), while general patients wait for their turn for consultation with any doctor on OPD duty. Private patients are charged more than general patients for a differential level of customer service.

5.3.1.3 Operational Planning Decisions: Operational decisions provide a roadmap for implementing the strategic plan and, therefore, address the issues regarding the utilization of resources in the attainment of organizational goals. A clear operational plan of implementation requires a good understanding of project management, assessment of internal and external risks associated with implementation and contingency plans to deal with emergencies. Table 5.9 lists a few operational planning decisions.

Resource Allocation: Operational planning of hospital services starts with the allocation of hospital resources to the hospital units/departments (clinical and administrative departments) as per the assessed resource needs through strategic planning. For example, allocation of nursing staff to clinical ward given the acute shortage of nurses is a major operational planning decision.

Discharge Process: Operational planning of inpatient discharge is an important area for hospital management. It is necessary to complete the discharge process as quickly as possible, so that the discharged patients can go home and their attendants could go back to work. A quick discharge is good for the hospital also since the released bed can be allotted to new patients, as income from patient care is the

Table 5.9 Some Examples of Operational Decisions

Sr. No.	Operational Decisions
1	Resource allocation
2	Discharge process
3	OT management: OT schedules
4	OT management: billing for materials
5	Procedural delays
6	Unfilled posts
7	Frequent transfers
8	Lab errors

maximum in the initial period of 2–3 days of hospitalization. Hence, any delay in discharge activities due to procedural reasons should be avoided.

Operation Theatre (OT) Schedules: Operational decisions in the management of OT start with the preparation of a weekly master OT schedule, showing the booked time slots as well as open time slots for each OT. This master schedule is prepared after ensuring the availability of consultant surgeons and their special requests (e.g., presence of a histo-pathologist during surgery, RBC packets, and so on), time engagements of shared equipment like C-Arms. All open slots in the master schedule are filled one day before the date of planned surgeries.

OT Store: Managing the inventories in OT sub-store is important as it accounts for 40 per cent of the value of hospital supplies. It is important never to run out of any OT material. As a result, many OT sub-stores have a tendency to over stock materials; 3–4 months of stock of OT materials is common in many hospitals, even though the lead time for procurement is much less for many items.

Vendor Management: Vendor management is important to ensure timely receipt of good quality hospital supplies. Planning calls for special attention to maintain an agreed schedule for accounts payable.

Unfilled Posts: Procedural delays in filling up sanctioned posts are a major concern in operational planning. Non-availability of qualified staff is another reason for posts lying vacant. Many medical colleges (private, public) report shortfall of qualified teachers. Public sector hospitals face this challenge more than private hospitals, mainly due to the government processes and procedures for recruitment.

Procedural Delays (Government): Many government hospitals face delays in the receipt of funds already approved, due to lengthy government processes and procedures. Lack of funds for purchase of medicines and drugs, delayed receipt of allocated funds, logistics involved in procurement, storage, transportation and distribution are common events which adversely affect service quality. Since procedural delays are common in government hospitals, it is necessary to recognize this eventuality in the operational planning of resources.

Frequent Transfers (Government): Frequent transfers of government doctors to various locations is a major concern in government teaching hospitals. Rotation of special skilled nursing staff between departments within a hospital, leading to lack of skilled nurses in OT, ICU, labour room, and so on, affect service quality. Operational planning to address transfer and promotion in government hospitals is very challenging.

5.3.1.4 Monitoring and Control Decisions: Monitoring the utilization of hospital resources and making appropriate interventions whenever necessary are very essential to achieve the desired outputs from each hospital department. Table 5.10 lists a few monitoring and control decisions.

Table 5.10 Some Examples of Monitoring and Control Decisions

Sr. No.	Monitoring and Control Decisions
1	Staff absenteeism
2	Clinical lab errors
3	Equipment break-downs
4	Managing OPD queues for consultation
5	Managing inpatient discharge

Monitoring and control functions go hand-in-hand, as monitoring without control is a waste of resources.

Monitoring the progress of the operational plan is critical in order to relate the utilization of input resources to planned outputs. Any delay in the quantity and quality of outputs should be identified as quickly as possible, so that appropriate interventions can be undertaken to bring the activities 'under control'. Monitoring is, therefore, a continuous activity to facilitate timely and appropriate interventions to achieve organizational goals. Unfortunately, monitoring is the weakest link in many hospitals, especially in government hospitals.

Lack of monitoring or poor monitoring could adversely affect the service quality. For example, lack of monitoring and control on the hospital staff could lead to absenteeism of hospital staff and, thereby, loss of productivity from the hospital's skilled workforce, which in turn would affect the quality of patient care.

Staff Absenteeism: Staff absenteeism is common in hospitals. There are doctors who always report late for work. One of the private hospitals, by maintaining an open register to record the reporting time of surgeons for planned surgeries, has ensured better adherence by surgeons to their OT schedules.

Lab Errors: Unnoticed or undetected errors leading to wrong test reports could have serious consequences on patients' health. Monitoring the pre-analytic phase closely and controlling phlebotomy errors is very important to provide reliable test result reports. Some hospitals[15] have closely monitored the reasons for sample rejections and took necessary steps to control lab errors.

Equipment Maintenance: Take the case of poor monitoring and break-down of USG machines in the department of gynecology and obstetrics in government hospitals. Too frequent and long downtime of USG machines would force pregnant women to seek USG services from elsewhere, incurring high costs. Such events defeat the very policy goal of government hospitals to provide timely maternal care services at affordable costs to the poor.

Managing Queues: Many government hospitals have long queues for OPD services. Given the shortages of doctors working in public hospitals, the queue for consultation is usually very long. One of the teaching hospitals introduced a 'triaging system' to distinguish cases with common ailments from cases with serious ailments. The patients with common ailments were seen by junior doctors, while only the serious cases were referred to the senior doctors. This helped the hospital management tremendously to achieve better customer satisfaction.

Monitoring and control activities in a hospital can be compared with monitoring the life of a sick patient in an ICU. ICU patients are continuously monitored on different parameters by staff at different levels and timely appropriate actions are taken to save patients' life. It is important to realize that monitoring should be done only by those managers who can intervene quickly. For example, there is no point in immediate reporting of X-ray machine break-downs to the health secretary.

We summarize the understanding of hospital management functions and hospital management decisions in Table 5.11.

Table 5.11 Management Functions vs Management Decisions

Management Decisions → / Management Functions ↓	Policy Decisions	Strategic Decisions	Operational Decisions	Monitoring and Control Decisions
Operational management	Hospital size	Facility planning	OT scheduling	Clinical lab errors
Financial management	Capital investment	Pricing of services	Working capital	Accounts receivables
HR management	Staffing policy	HR planning and development	Filling up vacant posts	Staff absenteeism
Materials management	Purchase policy and procedures	Inventory planning	Vendor management	Expiry dates: drugs and medicines

5.3.2 Hospital Management Information System (HMIS)

Many hospitals maintain a computer database, but this is not a claim to having an MIS.

5.3.2.1 An MIS Perspective: Few areas of management have been more controversial than MIS. Many managers boast of MIS in their organizations. If you ask them to explain the use of MIS in managing their organization, many managers refer you to the head of computer division (IT division). This is an indication of the 'lack of use' of MIS reports by the managers, even though they should be the ultimate users of MIS reports, and *not* the head of the IT division. The head of the IT division would proudly show you hundreds of reports produced by the IT team and sent to the management regularly and claiming that they have done their job. The IT division would even claim that they can generate any report at any time, since they maintain a computer-based database. It is this feeling of 'owning a computer database' that makes organizations claim that they have an MIS. This is unfortunate, since not all computer-generated reports qualify as MIS reports.

It is possible to wake up those 'who do not know and know that they do not know'. How about those 'who do not know and do not know that they do not know?'

> The real success of an MIS lies in the use of MIS reports by the managers and *not* in the generation of 'MIS reports' by the IT department.

What is, therefore, an MIS?

> An MIS is a computer-based system which provides information to the managers for decision making.

Any report generated from a computer-based database need not necessarily be an MIS report, unless it assists the managers in decision making, mostly in the areas on planning and control. MIS systems should, therefore, be driven by the information needs of managers which would in turn suggest an appropriate database organization. The information needs of managers should be obtained from the managers and not left to the IT division head to articulate the information needs of managers. IT is a support activity and should, therefore, play a supporting role to provide information support for managerial decisions.

The strength of a computer, namely, its ability to handle large masses of data can become a liability if thought is not given to the information that needs to be reported. Data is not information, whereas analysed data is.

> There is a huge communication gap between the management executives and the IT department head regarding the information needs for managerial decision making. In the design of MIS, it is essential that the information needs should be clearly spelt out by the managers, and *not* by the IT head. Otherwise, MIS reports would not serve any real purpose.

Defining MIS: An MIS is an integrated man-machine system that provides information to support the planning and control functions of managers in an organization.[xi,16]

[xi] Emphasis on hospital MIS is more on support to planning and control decisions and less on policy decisions. This is because policy decisions are made not merely on hospital database, but on market demand and competition. On the other hand, planning and control decisions depend almost entirely on hospital data.

An MIS report to assist strategic planning should provide information on the resource needs to achieve the stated goals and objectives. MIS report to support operational planning should provide information to successfully translate the strategic plan to implementation. MIS reports for monitoring and control should focus on the utilization of resources against planned achievements.

5.3.2.2 Basic Characteristics of Hospital MIS: From the above discussions, it should be clear that owning a computer database is *not* a claim to having an MIS. Raw data in a computerized database is *not* information. Data should be analysed to generate information for managerial decision making.

Many hospitals have computerized the billing of their impatient and OPD services. It is important to realize that such an IT application does not necessarily constitute a component of HMIS, unless these IT applications also support analysis of data from these bills and provide useful information to the hospital authorities to improve service delivery.

Traditionally, analysis of hospital systems have focused on the working of various departments offering particular services, such as scheduling of appointments for outpatients,[17] planning of emergency departments,[18] shift-scheduling of nurses,[19] and so on. Activity based costing methodology was adopted for estimating the costs of surgical procedures.[20,21] Leicester Royal Infirmay NHS Trust, UK, re-engineered its procedures in coordinating the patient visits to various clinics in order to offer good services at low cost.[22] St James Hospital, UK, re-engineered its purchase and supplies departments by adopting a BPR approach.[23] MP Trust Hospital, India, replaced its legacy inventory systems for hospital supplies with a decision support system enabled materials management process.[24]

Many hospital departments have IT applications to meet their needs. However, an integrated approach has been lacking in many hospitals in order to assist the management in planning and controlling decisions for the hospital as an entity.

HMIS, therefore, should be designed to support the timely and reliable information needs for the following decisions:

- Strategic decisions
- Operational decisions
- Monitoring and control decisions

Performance Measurement Is Central to HMIS: The overall objective of HMIS is to provide information support to the hospital management to improve the hospital performance in the delivery of services. The design of performance indicators is very critical. Please note that performance indicators which cannot be measured are of no use. All performance indicators should be measurable so as to facilitate comparison of performance between comparable departments at a point in time or comparison of performance of a given department over time.

Performance of hospital services depend on the effective and efficient management of hospital resources. It is, therefore, necessary to identify effective and efficient performance indicators of each management function in addressing the issues and challenges facing service delivery (see Table 5.11). Indicators of effectiveness and efficiency together provide estimates of the performance of a hospital in offering quality healthcare services at minimum cost.

As a rule of thumb, any performance indicator should have a numerator and a denominator.

Data needs to be processed appropriately in order to generate indicators to analyse the performance of each activity undertaken by the hospital. For example, the number of OPD patients in medicine department is *not* a performance indicator, but the average number of OPD patients handled per hour is an indicator of performance of medicine OPD. A better indicator would distinguish between the average number of new OPD patients served vs the average number of repeat OPD patients served.

Statutory data such as OPD load and inpatient load are not part of HMIS reports, unless such data is analysed to reflect performance.

Many hospitals report average length of hospital stay (ALOS) as an indicator of hospital performance. This indicator could be very misleading since ALOS for a patient in the medicine department could be 3–4 days, while the ALOS for a patient in the orthopedics department could be 1–2 months, and ALOS for a patient in the burns and plastics department could be even longer. It is, therefore, necessary to assess the performance of each specialty department independently, since each specialty department offers a specialty service.

It is also necessary to realize that any hospital service (rendered by specialty departments) is a combination of services from many departments, both clinical and administrative departments. For example, outpatient services call for registration services, consultation services (could be cross referrals, if required), investigation services and medication services. Hence, the performance of outpatient services (e.g., turnaround time of an outpatient) depends on the performance of each participating department.

Performance Indicators Should Be Used For Planning and Control Decisions: Let us take the case of investigation services by the clinical laboratory department. The total turnaround time is a performance indicator in clinical lab management.

Regular monitoring and control of lab errors is the key to delivering cost-effective and reliable test results.

The turnaround time can be interpreted in three different ways:

1. Time interval between the receipt of test orders in the lab and the release of test results by the lab.
2. Time interval for each stage in the total lab testing process, namely, the interval from test order to specimen collection, specimen collection to sample submission and sample submission to test reports. This is done in order to determine the specific points at which delays occur.
3. A few laboratories also are expanding the scope of measurement by evaluating 'therapeutic turnaround time', the time from initiation of the test order to the implementation of clinical decisions (e.g., change in treatment).[25]

Ideally, lab performance should be measured by the turnaround time *for reliable test results,* and not merely test results per se. In order to achieve minimum turnaround time for reliable test results, it is necessary to achieve minimum rejection of test samples. This is because rejection of samples at any stage of lab operations, calls for repeat collection of samples and analysis, and, thereby, delays the delivery of reliable test reports.

Any control decision is based on monitoring.[xii] If the turnaround time has to be 'controlled', then it would be necessary to monitor the individual components of the total turnaround time. Total turnaround time is made up of the following components:

1. Time interval between the time doctor ordered investigations and the time samples were collected (time for pre-analytic phase).
2. Time interval between sample collection and sample analysis completed (time for analytic phase).
3. Time interval between completing the sample analysis and giving the test result reports (time for post-analytic phase).

Accordingly, the MIS reports for controlling the total turnaround time should provide estimates for the turnaround time at each phase of the lab testing process, namely, pre-analytical, analytical and post-analytical phases. This requirement of MIS report by the lab manager should be taken as an input by the IT team to design a lab database.

In order to control lab errors, it is obvious that lab errors should be monitored regularly. Monitoring lab errors calls for maintaining a detailed documentation of all errors and the causes for these lab errors. It is the responsibility of the lab manager to insist on her/his lab staff to record all errors and their causes as

---

[xii] Please recall that monitoring and controlling go together. Monitoring without exercising control is a waste of resources. Control decisions without monitoring would serve no purpose.

and when they occur. An analysis of documented lab errors and taking corrective actions to avoid such errors in future would go a long way to minimize sample rejections and, thereby, provide reliable test results within the shortest possible time.

As a second example, if the average number of OPD patients served per hour is very low, then the management has to plan for additional resources to achieve a higher throughput. While a higher throughput would indicate a higher effectiveness in OPD service delivery, what would be an efficient indicator of OPD service? If increased throughput calls for additional doctors to be assigned OPD work, then an efficient indicator could be the average throughput per doctor.

As another example of hospital services, the surgical OTs consume vast amount of resources and, therefore, their performance should be assessed by the quality of OT services (indicators of effective service delivery) as well as the costs for providing OT services (indicators of efficient service delivery) which in turn provide useful information to the management for decisions on pricing of OT services.

A Framework for HMIS: The output of HMIS is information that supports managerial functions of planning and control. We suggest the following framework (Figure 5.3) for HMIS, which is based on an MIS framework.[26]

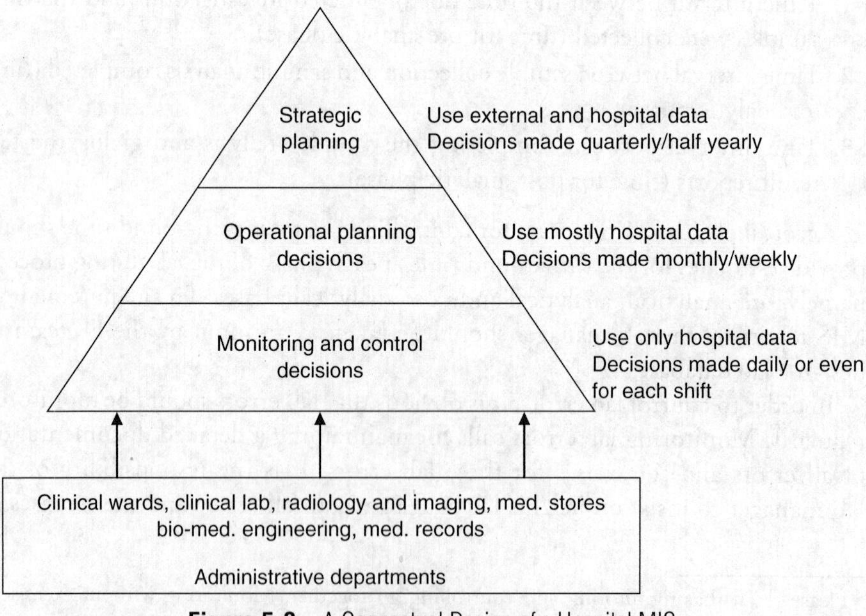

Figure 5.3 A Conceptual Design of a Hospital MIS

Frequency of Reporting: Frequency of reporting should be guided by the need for information by decision makers. Frequency of HMIS report generation should not be the same for all reports.

For example, monitoring and control reports should be generated daily, but not strategic planning reports.

Unfortunately, IT departments in many hospitals continue to generate all reports with the same frequency.

Also, information (MIS reports) should be sent only to those who can act on the information immediately. For example, if the X-ray machine in the radiology department is not working, this information should be immediately brought to the attention of the hospital superintendent who can make appropriate decisions for delivering X-ray services. Any delay in providing this information to the hospital superintendent would adversely affect the service delivery.

HMIS Reports Should Be Routine, Not Ad-hoc: An HMIS deals with information that is systematically and routinely collected in accordance with a well-defined set of rules. This implies that HMIS is a formal information network in a hospital. For example, daily reports on income from patient care for discharged patients from each ward form an important component of HMIS. However, one-time reports prepared by teaching hospitals for MCI inspections are not part of HMIS.

For example, every hospital has to plan and control the consumption of hospital supplies (medicines, drugs, disposables, and so on). A well-designed inventory system that provides information on consumption of hospital supplies by each department is, therefore, a component of HMIS. Inventory turnaround time is a common performance indicator of inventory management. It represents the average number of days of stock from the day of receipt (from vendors) to the day of issue (to hospital department). Inventory turnover is also an important indicator of working capital management.

Monitoring and control of lab errors is an excellent example to highlight the importance of monitoring and control function in MIS.

Any computer application that outputs the salaries and wages of all hospital employees every month is *not* an HMIS. On the same account, computer systems that provide statutory reports for government agencies are also not HMIS. Most of the statutory reports contain data and not information. For example, many hospitals report their service statistics, such as total number of OPD patients, total number of annual admissions, total number of radiology investigations, and so on. Please note that these are mere statistics. They do not reflect hospital performance. For example, a less load on radiology investigations could be due to several reasons—frequent break-downs of X-ray machines, absenteeism of X-ray technicians, shortage of X-ray films, and so on.

A well-designed HMIS would be of immense help for any hospital management for improving the service delivery, while a poorly designed HMIS would only consume hospital resources without producing any useful outputs.

5.4 ADMINISTRATIVE SUPPORT SYSTEMS

5.4.1 Medical Records Management

Medical record is a clinical, scientific, administrative and legal document containing information about each patient's health record, doctors' findings and the treatments given. The terms 'medical record', 'health record' and 'medical chart' are used interchangeably to describe the systematic documentation of a single patient's medical history and medical care across times.

Some major functions of medical records department are:

- Managing daily receipt of case sheets pertaining to discharged and expired patients from various wards
- Daily compilation of hospital census report
- Maintenance and retrieval of records for patient care and research study
- Computing various hospital statistics and preparation of different periodical reports on morbidity and mortality
- Providing epidemiological data
- Providing assistance to medico-legal issues

The advent of electronic medical records has not only changed the format of medical records but has provided immediate access to health-related information. The use of an individual dossier style medical record, where records are kept on each patient by name and illness type originated at the Mayo Clinic out of a desire to simplify patient tracking and to allow for medical research.

5.4.2 Bio-medical Waste Management

All healthcare facilities such as hospitals, nursing homes and clinical laboratories generate bio-medical waste every day. All the health facilities and other similar organizations (animal slaughter house, units producing biological products, and so on) have a social responsibility for proper disposal of the bio-medical waste they generate. The amount of bio-medical waste generated in India is estimated to be 1.5 kg/bed/day.

Bio-medical waste management starts from the point of generation and ends at the point of disposal. All organizations are financially liable for safe management of the wastes they generate; transport and disposal are usually contracted out.

All healthcare facilities and similar organizations have a social responsibility to properly manage the bio-medical waste they generate.

The World Health Organization (WHO) defines bio-medical waste as any waste that is generated during diagnosis, treatment or immunization of human beings or animals, in research pertaining thereto or in the production or testing of biologicals, animal waste from slaughter houses or any other like establishments.

Bio-medical waste generated by hospitals and other healthcare facilities can be broadly classified into two groups:

1. General waste (packaging material, food, paper, and so on) which accounts for almost 80 per cent of the total waste.
2. Hazardous and infectious waste (soiled dressings, used needles, syringes, and so on) which account for 20 per cent of the total waste.

Negligence on bio-medical waste management poses serious risks to human health, environment and public health in general. All those who generate, collect, separate, handle, package, store, transport and dispose waste are exposed to occupational risks. The community is exposed to blood-borne transmitted diseases like AIDS, hepatitis B, hepatitis C, cholera, and so on.

The WHO has estimated that in the year 2000, injections with contaminated syringes caused 21 million hepatitis B virus infections (HBV), 2 million hepatitis C virus infections (HBC) and 260,000 HIV infections, accounting for 32 per cent of all new infections, 40 per cent of all new infections and five per cent of all new infections, respectively.[27]

In many developing countries like India, hospital waste management practices are very poor. The results of a WHO study conducted in 22 developing countries in the year 2002 showed that the proportion of healthcare facilities that do not use proper waste disposal methods ranged from 18 per cent to 64 per cent. In many of these countries, bio-medical waste gets mixed with general waste and dumped in municipal bins or thrown out in the open. By doing so, the general waste also gets infected resulting in 100 per cent waste becoming hazardous and infectious.

Hospital waste management in India got highlighted in a writ petition in the Supreme Court. As per the court directives, the government of India notified the Bio-Medical Waste Management and Handling Rules on 27 January 1998 under the provision of the Environment Act, 1986. These rules regulate the bio-medical waste management at the local, regional and national levels.

The major activities in the management of bio-medical wastes are as follows:

- Segregation
- Handling
- Storage

- Transportation
- Treatment and disposal

Segregation is the act of separating the bio-medical waste into specific coloured containers based on the treatment and disposal option for various categories of waste. Categories of bio-medical waste are human anatomical waste, animal waste, microbiology and biotechnology waste, waste of sharps, discarded medicines, soiled waste, solid waste, liquid waste, incinerated ash and chemical waste. Disposal should be done within 48 hours.

Handling waste needs attention. Care should be taken to reduce the risk of needle prick injuries and infection. Overloading of wastes in coloured containers should be avoided while transporting them to the disposal site.

The storage locations in hospitals should be identified and marked clearly. Access to storage areas should be restricted only to the waste handlers.

The transportation of waste to disposal site should be only through vehicles authorized by the government for this purpose. Transportation logistics are very binding.

The treatment and disposal of wastes are based on the category of wastes. Treatment and disposal options include incineration, deep burial, autoclaving, microwaving and disinfection by chemical treatment.

Hospital superintendents are primarily responsible for ensuring safe segregation, handling and storage, and, therefore, play a vital role in planning, designing and implementing bio-medical waste management system. The task of transport and disposal of hospital waste is usually contracted out. Unfortunately, hospital management does not supervise the management of waste by the contractors. There are many reports highlighting the violation of norms by the contractors for transport and disposal of bio-medical waste and, hence, there is a real threat of spread of infectious diseases.

Contracting out the tasks of transport and disposal of bio-medical waste to contractors does not absolve the bio-medical waste generators of their responsibility for safe execution of these tasks. Outsourced contracts should be supervised by the hospital management, since the ultimate responsibility and accountability for waste management lies with the hospital management.

5.4.3 Other Support Systems

Other administrative support services include dietary services, house-keeping, ambulance services, bio-medical services, interaction with insurance providers, admission, discharge, and so on. Even though some of these services may be outsourced, the ultimate responsibility for all administrative support rests with the hospital management.

5.5 SUMMARY

In this chapter, we have discussed the hospital management support systems—clinical support, information support and administrative support.

A well-designed MIS should provide the necessary information support for planning, monitoring and control decisions.

For example, monitoring lab errors calls for maintaining a detailed documentation of all errors and the causes for these lab errors. For this, we analysed in detail the lab operations in each stage of the total testing process, namely, pre-analytical, analytical and post-analytical stages and highlighted possible errors at each step in the lab operations. Controlling lab errors is essential to minimize sample rejections, and, thereby, improve lab performance. In order to control lab errors, it is obvious that lab errors should be monitored regularly. It is the responsibility of the lab manager to insist on her/his lab staff to record all errors and their causes as and when they occur.

The examples of MIS support for planning include OPD management, inpatient discharge management, and so on.

Another area of MIS would be resource planning based on service delivery for a period of time; such data can be captured from the billing system by a suitable design of the billing database.

Hospital administration has a social responsibility to safely dispose all the biomedical waste generated in the process of service delivery, besides extending support for service delivery.

In chapters 6–10, real-life case studies from large hospitals have been analysed to understand the application of hospital management concepts to address managerial issues. Chapter 6 discusses case studies on operations management, Chapter 7 on finance and cost management, Chapter 8 on HR management, Chapter 9 on materials management and we conclude with case studies on hospital MIS in Chapter 10.

QUESTIONS

1. What are the causes of lab errors in a clinical laboratory?
2. Name any three steps in the pre-analytic phase of lab testing which require monitoring to control lab errors. What data should be recorded for monitoring and control of lab errors arising from the above three steps?
3. Name any two steps in the analytic phase of lab testing which require monitoring to control lab errors. What data should be recorded for monitoring and control of lab errors arising from the above two steps?
4. Name any three steps in the post-analytic phase of lab testing which require monitoring to control lab errors. What data should be recorded for monitoring and control of lab errors arising from the above three steps?

5. Take any hospital service and describe the managerial decisions involved:
   (a) Policy decisions
   (b) Strategic decisions
   (c) Operational decisions
   (d) Monitoring and control decisions
6. Suppose you want to start a 100 bed general hospital offering standard services, namely, medicine, surgery, pediatrics and gynecology. What are the steps you would take to determine the resource requirements?
7. Take any policy decision in a hospital. Explain its implications on service delivery and service quality.
8. Take any strategic decision in a hospital. Explain its implications on service delivery and service quality.
9. Take any operational decision in a hospital. Explain its implications on service delivery and service quality.
10. Take any monitoring and control decision in a hospital. Explain its implications on service delivery and service quality.
11. What are the basic characteristics of a hospital MIS?
12. What is the role of performance indicators in hospital MIS?
13. Take any hospital service and define its performance indicators for each level of decision making. Be sure that these performance indicators are measurable. Design a few MIS reports for this hospital service. Who are the intended managers for these reports? What should be the reporting frequency for each MIS report?
14. Take any clinical department in a teaching hospital. Design MIS reports for teaching, research and patient care. What are the data needs for MIS? Design suitable data collection formats for MIS reports.

REFERENCES

1. Plebani, M. (2006), 'Errors in clinical laboratories or errors in laboratory medicine', *Clinical Chemistry Laboratory Medicine*, 44 (6), pp. 750–759.
2. Plebani, M. and Carraro, P. (1997), 'Mistakes in a STAT laboratory: Types and frequency', *Clinical Chemistry*; 43, pp. 1348–1351.
3. Bonini, P.A.; Plebani, M.; Ceriotti, F. and Francesca, Rubboli F. (2002), 'Errors in laboratory medicine', *Clinical Chemistry*, 48, pp. 691–698.
4. Valentin, P.N.; Raab, S.S. and Walsh, M.K. (2006), 'Identification errors involving clinical laboratories: A college of American Pathologist Q-Probes study of patient and specimen identification errors at 120 institutions', *Archives of Pathology and Laboratory Medicine*, 130, pp. 1106–1113.
5. Lippi, G.; Salvagno, G.L.; Montagnana, M.; Frachini, M. and Guidi, G.C. (2006), 'Quality improvement in laboratory testing', *Clinical Laboratory*, 52 (1).
6. Goswami, B.; Singh, Bhawna; Chavla, Ranjana and Venkatesan, Mallika (2010), 'Evaluation of errors in a clinical laboratory: A one-year experience', *Clinical Chemistry Laboratory Medicine*, 48 (1), pp. 63–66.
7. Stankovic, A.K. (2004), 'The laboratory is a key partner in assuring patient safety', *Clinical Laboratory Medicine*, 24 (4), pp. 1023–1035.

8. Goswami, B., et al. (2010), *Clinical Chemistry Laboratory Medicine*, 48 (1), pp. 63–66.
9. Plebani, M. (2006), *Clinical Chemistry Laboratory Medicine,* 44 (6), pp. 750–759.
10. Goswami, B., et al. (2010), *Clinical Chemistry Laboratory Medicine*, 48 (1), pp. 63–66.
11. Wolcott, J. Schwartz and Amanda, Goodman C. (2008), 'Laboratory medicine: A national status report'.
12. Goswami, B., et al. (2010), *Clinical Chemistry Laboratory Medicine*, 48 (1), pp. 63–66.
13. Case, IIMA/BP 0299 (2004), Aravind Eye care System: Giving the Most Precious Gift; Indian Institute of Management, Ahmedabad.
14. Ramani, K.V. (2006 b), 'Managing Hospital Supplies: Process Reengineering at Gujarat Cancer Research Institute, India', *Journal of Health Organization and Management*, 20 (3), pp. 218–226.
15. Goswami, B., et al. (2010), *Clinical Chemistry Laboratory Medicine*, 48 (1), pp. 63–66.
16. Bhatnagar, S.C. and Ramani, K.V. (1991), 'Computers and information management: A primer for practicing managers', 2nd ed., Prentice Hall of India (P) Limited, New Delhi.
17. Brahimi, M. and Worthington, D. (1991), 'Queuing models for outpatient appointment systems—A case study', *Journal of the Operational Research Society*, 42, pp. 733–746.
18. Gabaeff, S.C. and Lennon, J. (1991), 'New computerized technology for the design and planning of emergency departments', *Proceedings of the American Hospital Association*, Anaheim: AHA, pp. 1–15.
19. Siferd, P. and Benton,W.C. (1994), 'A decision mode for shift scheduling of nurses', *European Journal of Operational Research*, 74 (3), pp. 519–27.
20. Baker, J.J. and Boyd, G.F. (1997), 'Activity based costing in the operating room at Valley View Hospital', *Journal of Healthcare Finance*, 24 (1), pp. 1–6.
21. Lakhia, T.S. and Ramani, K.V. (2001), 'Hospital logistics: Activity based costing for hospital services', *Proceedings of the First International Conference on Integrated Logistics*, 21–24 August, Singapore, pp. 359–364.
22. Newman, K. (1994), 'The single visit clinic: A case study in process reengineering', *Journal of Business Change and Reengineering*, 2, pp. 10–19.
23. Bence, V. (1995), 'St James hospital and Lucas engineering systems: A BPRC collaboration', *Journal of Business Change and Reengineering*, 2 (3), pp. 30–39.
24. Ramani, K.V. (2001), 'DSS-enabled Materials Management Process at MP Trust Hospital', *Production and Inventory Management Journal*, 42 (1).
25. Kilgore, M.L.; Steindel, S.J. and Smith, J.A. (1998), 'Evaluating stat testing options in an academic health center: Therapeutic turnaround time and staff satisfaction', *Clinical Chemistry*, 44 (1), pp. 1597–1603.
26. Anthony, Robert and Graham, Willard (2006), Management Control Systems; McGraw Hill, Irwin.
27. Bio-medical Waste Management—Self Learning Document for Doctors, Superintendents and Administrators (2004), prepared by Environment Protection Training Research Institute (EPTRI), Hyderabad, supported by WHO, India Country Office.

part 3

Hospital Management Case Studies

CHAPTERS

6. Hospital Operations Management
7. Hospital Finance and Cost Management
8. Hospital Human Resource Management
9. Hospital Materials Management
10. Hospital MIS

OBJECTIVE

The main objective here is to build skills in dealing with managerial issues faced by large hospitals:

CMC Hospital, Vellore (A) and (B)
Apollo Hospitals
ARAM Hospital (Apollo Group)
Bangalore Baptist Hospital
Majestic Hospitals
City Municipal Hospital
AMC Hospitals
MPS Hospital
MP Trust Hospital
Mahanagar Hospital
SJ Hospital
RD Clinical Lab

chapter 6

Hospital Operations Management

CHAPTER OUTLINE

CHAPTER OBJECTIVE

The main objective of this chapter is to apply the concepts (discussed in Chapter 4) to address operations management issues in three large hospitals through real-life case studies.

CMC HOSPITAL, VELLORE (A)* CASE 6.1

Dr Suranjan Bhattacharji, Director, CMC Hospital, Vellore was getting very concerned about the increasing load for OPD services over the years. While CMCH handled about 2,500 outpatients per day in 1998–99, the OPD load had increased to 5,000 outpatients per day by 2010. This trend was likely to continue in future also. The increased load on its OPD system was stretching the clinical resources as well as the support services beyond limits, leading to increased waiting time for outpatients in the clinics and their total duration of stay for OPD treatment. Almost 30 per cent of the outpatients came from the North-East, West Bengal and Orissa who had to incur out-of-pocket travel and stay costs for self and attendants/relatives, in addition to the hospital charges. For them, the total cost of their trip to CMC, Vellore, (travel and stay cost in addition to the hospital charges) was a critical component of their satisfaction with CMCH and their willingness to recommend CMCH to others.

Christian Medical College, Vellore

The Christian Medical College (CMC) Hospital, Vellore, was founded by an American missionary, Dr Ida S. Scudder. Born in South India, in 1870, she spent most of her childhood in the US and was educated there. Although her grandparents, parents, and most other members of her extended family served as missionaries in India, this was not the life that she wanted for herself. However, one night, while visiting her parents at their home in India, her life was turned around. Three well-to-do men came one after the other, with the same desperate story. Each of them had a young wife in the throes of childbirth, but unable to deliver. The traditional midwife had been unable to help. Would the young missy come and help deliver the baby? Ida had no medical training at that point, and suggested that her doctor father should go. However, owing to the social and religious customs of the day, each of these men went away sadly saying that it was impossible for another man to see their wives. With no doctor to look after them, these three women and their babies all died that night. Ida took this as a clear signal from God that she should strive to help the women and children

---

* Reproduced with the permission of the copyright owner.

Prepared by Dr K.V. Ramani of the Indian Institute of Management, Ahmedabad and Dr Vijay Kumar Aruldas of the CMC Hospital, Vellore.

Cases of the Indian Institute of Management, Ahmedabad, are prepared as a basis for class discussion. They are not designed to present illustrations of either correct or incorrect handling of administrative problems.

© 1999 by the Indian Institute of Management, Ahmedabad, Revised July 2012.

of India. She returned to the US to study and graduated from Cornell University Medical College in 1899 among the first batch of women. Soon Dr Ida S. Scudder returned to India and started her medical work with a one-bed clinic in Vellore in 1900.

The city of Vellore in Tamil Nadu, India, is about 140 km to the west of Chennai. It has a spectacular 'Golden Temple' at Sripuram, a nearby town, which attracts a lot of pilgrims. However, Vellore is known the world over as the home of the Christian Medical College—a centre of excellence in medical services, research, and education. Over the years, CMC Hospital, Vellore, has grown into a large multi-specialty teaching hospital. Many of the CMC faculty and alumni have received national and international rewards for their humanitarian efforts and research contributions. At the time of this study, CMC Hospital, Vellore, catered to nearly every specialty with over 2,500 beds across a number of campuses, with a dedicated staff of about 8,000 employees including 1,290 doctors, and 2,481 nurses.

The range of services offered by CMC included

- Medical services,
- Education and training, and
- Research (Exhibit 6.1).

Outpatient Services at CMCH

By the end of the year 2010, the hospital was handling close to 5,000 outpatients daily, across 40 different clinics covering a number of specialties, supported by a comprehensive range of investigation facilities (Exhibit 6.2).

Outpatients had the option of being private or general patients. Private patients paid a much higher registration fee (than general patients) and met their preferred consultant in the appropriate clinic by prior appointment. General patients were seen by any doctor available in the clinic on the day of their arrival. However, all outpatients, private or general, went through the same process of consultation and investigation, and received the same amount of care and attention. Every patient, private or general, made an average of two to three visits for Out Patient Department (OPD) treatment; first visit as a new patient and one to two repeat visits.

The outpatient service process at CMCH is shown in Figure 6.1. Every patient went through a sequence of processes, namely, registration, consultation, payment for investigation, investigation, and medication. The OPD process became more complicated when more than one doctor got involved for specialist consultation, in which case, the patient repeated the same cycle of processes with the referred clinical department. At the end of the outpatient visit, when a final diagnosis was

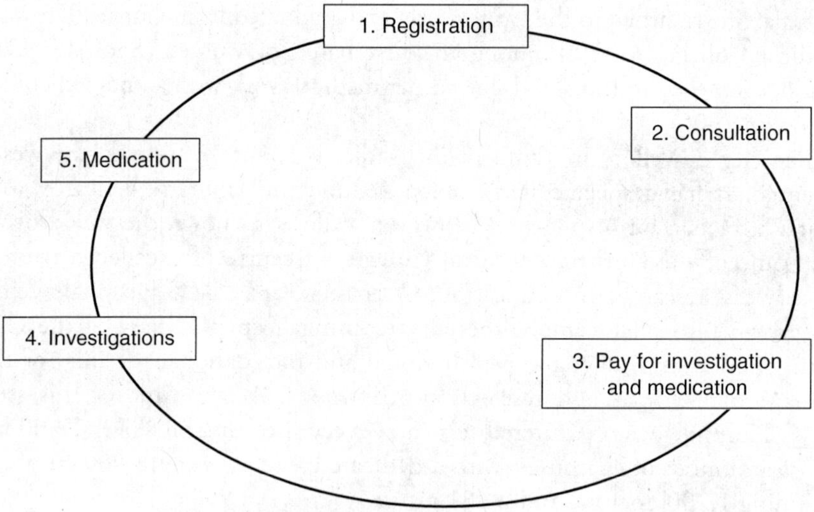

Figure 6.1 OPD Service Process

made and treatment recommended, the patient left the OPD system till the next follow up or the next illness episode.

Registration: Registration was the process by which a patient was given an appointment to see a doctor. Registration counters were open at CMCH from 8.00 am to 11.00 am, Monday through Saturday. The appointment specified the location of the clinic, the date, and approximate time of consultation. For private patients, the appointment specified the name of the consultant chosen by the patient. General patients were assigned to any doctors on OPD duty. In the case of repeat patients[i], the registration clerk ensured that they were assigned to the same doctor who saw them in their first visit. All visits to the doctor were only through registration, including repeat visits. The registration number which was a unique hospital number remained valid for one full year.

Consultation: On arriving at the clinic after registration, all patients were seated. The repeat patients ensured that their case sheets and medical records of previous visits were ready in the OPD clinic. Though the consultation hours were fixed from 8.00 am to 5.00 pm, many consultants stretched their OPD hours beyond

[i] Repeat patients were different from old patients. Repeat patients were those who were still in the OPD system receiving medical attention. Old patients were those who had completed their OPD treatment and were advised by their doctor for routine consultation at regular intervals, if required.

5.00 pm to ensure that all the registered patients were seen the same day. OPD working hours were also utilized for under graduate teaching.

In the case of new patients, consultation started with the preparation of case sheets, followed by physical examinations. After the examination, each patient was advised to do one or more of the following:

1. Investigations to aid diagnosis
2. Medication
3. Referrals: consult other specialists for opinion/evaluation
4. Return for a repeat consultation
5. Admitted for treatment as inpatient

For repeat patients, consultation started with a review of the patient's health based on their case sheets (prepared on their earlier visits) and the results of investigation reports, followed by physical examinations. If required, they were advised to go through any of the above steps (1 to 5). If any repeat patient did not require any further attention from the OPD system, the case was closed.

Each advice gave rise to its own sequence of events.

Investigation: Patients who were advised to undergo investigations, paid for the investigations at any of the common payment counters and then proceeded either to the sample collection centres or to the radiology section, which were open from 8.00 am to 1.00 pm.

For pathology investigations, the hospital maintained a common Central Sample Collection Facility (CSCF), where the samples for testing (blood, urine, and so on) were collected from the patients. Samples were then transported to the appropriate laboratory section (bio-chemistry, clinical pathology, and so on) for analysis. At the laboratory, the samples were processed and the results fed into the CMC Local Area Network (LAN). The medical records department accessed these reports, updated the respective case file of each patient, and kept them ready for repeat visits by the patients. The lab reports remained available for a limited period of time on LAN to the participating OPD clinics.

Requests for imaging services were handled differently. After initial processing, the films were sent to the radiologists and interpreted. The films along with the reports were sent to the clinics from which they were ordered, and kept in the CMC LAN for the consultants to view the images at the time of the patient's next visit.

Medications: All new and repeat patients were usually given prescriptions for purchasing medicines and drugs at the CMC pharmacy. Patients paid for medications at any of the payment counters and then went to the pharmacy to collect their medicines and drugs. The hospital pharmacy was open 24 hours every day.

Referrals: Referrals are very common in large multi-specialty hospitals. Based on the seriousness and nature of illness, the parent consultant referred their patients for specialist consultations in other clinical departments. For example, the medicine OPD referred some of their patients to the gastroenterology department for specialist consultation. Since not all clinical departments offered daily OPDs, referrals usually led to increased length of stay for the patients and their attendants at Vellore.

Repeat Consultation: All new OPD patients required one to two repeat visits to complete the OPD treatment cycle, which involved consultations, investigations, and medications.

Outpatient Stay: The duration of a patient's stay in OPD depended on:

1. Results of investigations ordered,
2. Outpatient schedule of the primary clinician,
3. Cross-referrals requested (and outpatient schedules of the clinicians referred to),
4. Number of revisits needed to complete the consultation and investigation process.

1. **Results of investigations:** The availability of investigation (test) results varied with the kind of tests ordered. Some test results were available within hours of the test being done; others took several days (e.g., microbiology tests required growing the culture for examination). In addition to the sample processing time, the work schedule of the laboratory and that of the Central Sample Collection Facility also affected the availability of test results.
2. **Outpatient schedule of the primary clinician:** The outpatient schedule of the primary clinician determined when he/she could review the investigations advised and the opinions requested from other doctors. As a teaching hospital, CMC doctors were involved in a number of activities (teaching UG and PG students, research meetings, seminar, special academic meetings, ward visits: split rounds individually and grand rounds with the entire unit, and so on) and, therefore, available for OPD consultation for only one day in a cycle of three days. The medicine department was organized into three units of three consultants each, with Unit 1 doctors having OPD on Mondays and Thursdays; Unit 2 doctors having OPD on Tuesdays and Fridays, while Unit 3 had OPD days on Wednesdays and Saturdays. The above systemic constraint also led to longer turnaround time for OPD services.
3. **Outpatient schedules of the clinicians the patient was referred to:** The clinician to whom the patient was referred (for specialist consultation) usually ordered additional investigations to aid diagnosis, leading to prolonging the turnaround time for OPD services.

4. **Number of revisits:** The nature and complexity of illness contributed to the turnaround time of OPD services. A patient with a more complicated problem needed a larger number of revisits before completing the treatment.

It was also possible for a patient to quit the OPD system without completing the process, if she/he was not satisfied with the care and attention, or due to the three day delay for repeat consultation: delays imposed by the three day cycle of doctors' schedule of activities at CMC.

After initial discussions the case writers had with the CMCH management, the medicine department was taken up for a detailed case study, since it handled the maximum OPD load in the hospital.

Medicine Department: The medicine department operated three units, namely, Medicine 1, Medicine 2, and Medicine 3. Each medicine unit had four consultants and an equal number of registrars (senior post graduate students). The weekly schedule of each medicine unit included two full days for OPD services; Medicine Unit 1 offered OPD services on Mondays and Thursdays, Unit 2 on Tuesdays and Fridays, and Unit 3 on Wednesdays and Saturdays. While the consultants took care of all private patients, the registrars were responsible for all general patients who were assigned on a First-Cum-First Served (FCFS) basis. Many doctors on OPD duty worked beyond their OPD hours to ensure that all the registered outpatients were seen the same day.

Management Concerns: The hospital management was wondering if there was any way to improve the service quality of its OPD services. The three day cycle of doctors' activities meant an interval of three days between consecutive OPD visits. Turnaround time was a critical factor for the patients coming from the North-East, West Bengal and Orissa who had to incur out-of-pocket travel and stay costs for self and attendants/relatives, in addition to the hospital charges. For them, the total cost of their trip to CMC, Vellore, was an important component of their satisfaction with CMCH and their willingness to recommend CMCH to others.

Exhibit 6.1 Christian Medical College Hospital, Vellore Medical Services, Teaching and Research*

Vision Statement: The Christian Medical College, Vellore, seeks to be a witness to the healing ministry of Christ, through excellence in education, service and research.

The Objective: The objective of the Christian Medical College, Vellore, is the establishment, maintenance and development of a Christian Medical College and Hospitals in India, where men and women shall receive

* *Source:* CMC web site.

an education of the highest grade in the art and science of medicine, nursing, or one or other of the related professions, to equip them in the spirit of Christ, for service in the relief of suffering and in the promotion of health (CMC web site).

The range of services offered by CMC includes

1. Medical services,
2. Education and training, and
3. Research

1. **Medical Services:** CMC's medical staff of 1,290 doctors and 2,481 nurses is involved in providing medical care. Almost every clinical specialty is catered for, and many departments are subdivided into units each of which may have particular expertise in specific areas as well as providing services of a more general nature. For example the Division of Surgery is further broken down into eight units specializing in Head and Neck Surgery, Endocrine Surgery, Vascular Surgery, Colorectal, and so on.

   CMC is particularly well known for certain departments such as Gasteroenterology, Neurosciences and Hematology (where it is a national leader in the treatment of rare blood disorders and bone marrow transplantation). However, it also gives high importance to less prominent specialties such as Rheumatology, Physical Medicine and Rehabilitation, Developmental Pediatrics and Palliative Care. Ophthalmology and Psychiatry departments are located on different campuses, as is the Rehabilitation Institute.

   There are 95 wards including 15 ICUs. About 76 per cent of the beds are in general wards and are subsidized to reduce the financial burden on patients. There are 39 major operation theatres and a further 18 facilities for minor procedures. An average of 125 operations is carried out each day.

   Diagnostic services are provided in house by the Radiology Department, Nuclear Medicine and the Laboratories. Radiology reporting is through a filmless digital system (PACS), enabling doctors to view X-rays and scans on any computer on the network. All laboratory test results are also available through the hospital intranet, as part of the 'clinical workstation' hospital information system.

2. **Education and Training:** Right from the beginning Ida Scudder knew that she could have little impact working on her own, and her vision was not just to treat, but also to train others. So she began teaching 'compounders' (modern day pharmacists) and nurses. The first formal nursing course was started over a hundred years ago in 1909. Medical training for women began in 1918 with a Licensed Medical Practitioner course. In 1942 the MBBS degree course was started and in 1947 the College became coeducational.

   Today CMC, Vellore, offers, in addition to MBBS and Nursing BSc and Diploma courses, 66 post graduate medical degrees, 35 Allied Health Science courses, eight further Nursing programmes and PhD programmes in various disciplines. Training is available in fields as diverse as Dialysis Therapy, Medical Records Science and Neurosurgery. In 2010 CMC was voted second best Medical College in India (perceptual) and top rank (factual) in the annual *India Today* survey and is consistently listed amongst the top colleges for MBBS.

   There are a number of distinctive features of CMC courses. All of them, including nursing, are taught by qualified, experienced faculty who also participate fully in the clinical and administrative operations of the hospital. The courses are extremely practical, with students learning skills on the job in clinical and working laboratory settings. While providing a full exposure to the very best in hospital medicine, there is also a strong emphasis on community and family medicine, and students spend time in rural community settings and small secondary hospitals in different parts of India. There is also a commitment to nurture and mentor the students to enable all round growth in social and spiritual spheres as well as intellectual.

One of CMC's key roles is to help train the skilled and caring medical professionals who are desperately needed for hospitals throughout remote and rural areas of India. The educational fees are amongst the lowest in the world for a private institution and students from economically disadvantaged backgrounds are helped still further through scholarships that can cover all fees as well as hostel accommodation and food. This ensures that no one needs to be burdened by an educational loan to study at CMC, and many can then go on to serve in deprived areas of India.

3. **Research:** Research is an integral part of the mission of CMC, having a wide and long-lasting impact on the nation's health. Over the past century, CMC has contributed significantly in generating and advancing knowledge which has improved curative and preventive medical services locally, throughout India and internationally. The main thrust is orientated towards cost effective solutions to health issues where the need is greatest, in order to optimize the use of resources. However research also improves both teaching and clinical standards through fostering a spirit of enquiry and ensuring that faculty remains up to date with the latest medical advances.

CMC is engaged in cutting edge research into the causes and treatment of diseases, and collaborates with hospitals and universities throughout the world. It is one of the leading contributors of medical research articles in India. There are numerous research programmes funded by national and international agencies as well as through internal resources. It is the home of the South Asian Cochrane Network and Centre and the internationally recognized Infectious Diseases Training and Research Centre and boasts a state of the art Stem Cell Research Centre funded as a centre of excellence by the Indian government. CMC hosts many conferences and workshops and runs courses in research methodology, epidemiology and biostatistics, and so on.

During the year 2010–11, the Christian Medical College Hospital had a total staff of almost 8,000, including over 1,290 doctors and 2,481 nurses. It handled a load of 5,000 outpatients, 2,000 inpatients, 25,000 laboratory tests, 1,500 radiology investigations and 125 surgeries daily (tables 6.1 and 6.2).

Table 6.1 Hospital Staff

Sr. No.	Staff	Strength
1	Administrative staff	726
2	Chaplains	13
3	Doctors	1,290
4	Engineering staff	269
5	House keeping staff and attendants	1,424
6	Library staff	56
7	Nurses	2,481
8	Social workers	51
9	Teaching staff (non-medical) and technical staff	1,657
Total		**7,967**

Source: CMC web site.

Table 6.2 Medical Services

Location	Beds	Inpatients	Outpatients	Births	Outreach
Main Hospital	2,140	94,675	1,505,176	11,411	–
Community Health and Development	130	10,898	86,955	3,199	123,198
Rural Unit for Health, Social Affairs	70	4,480	101,459	1,421	37,878
Schell Eye Hospital	100	6,926	94,107	–	18,801
Low Cost Effective Care Unit	48	2,080	55,095	235	675
Mental Health Centre	98	1,001	88,971	–	–
Nambikkai Nilyam	24	137	3,747	–	3,327
Rehabilitation Institute	85	658	–	–	120
Total	**2,695**	**120,855**	**1,935,510**	**16,266**	**183,999**

Source: CMC web site.

In addition to the main hospital, CMCH also provides a number of medical services such as:

Eye Hospital: CMCH's Ophthalmic Department, is equipped with all the latest equipments like Lasers, and Computerized Field Testing. It does cataract surgery with intraocular lens implantation, phaco emulsification, corneal transplantation and vitreo retinal surgery. Inpatient services are also available.

Mental Health Centre: CMCH's Department of Psychiatry runs a mental healthcare centre. This centre is also involved in the evaluation and training of children with mental retardation.

Rehabilitation Institute: The Physical Medicine and Rehabilitation Department provides long term therapy and training for physically handicapped persons to cope with activities of daily living within the limits of their disability.

Community Health and Development (CHAD): The 80-bed CHAD Hospital is a programme of the Community Health Department of Christian Medical College, Vellore. This comprehensive health programme which serves a population of almost 1 million in the rural areas of Kaniambadi is affected through the joint efforts of public health teams, socio-economic development workers and part-time community health workers. In addition, the department also provides consultancy services to a population of 1,20,000 in Anaicut block which is south-west of Vellore. Primary healthcare in both the blocks is carried out by close collaboration with the existing government services.

Rural Unit for Health and Social Affairs (RUHSA): Twenty-five kilometers north-west of Vellore in the K.V. Kuppamblock, is RUHSA. This is an integrated rural health and development project, which runs a variety of field programmes actively involving the villagers, government and banks. RUHSA provides a 60 bed base hospital, training programmes to empower the rural youth, programmes for the poorest of the poor, with over 110 local family care volunteers who live in the villages. It serves a population of over 100,000.

College of Nursing Community Health Program (CONCH): Ever since Dr Ida S. Scudder identified the need for taking healthcare to the doorstep of the community, Community Health Nursing has become an integral part of nursing, both in the education and service areas. In 1987, it was decided to establish a community health programme for a population of 45,000 in the nearby villages of Vellore and Arcot blocks under the leadership of College of Nursing. The overwhelming support from the villages and the enthusiastic cooperation from the Government and local administration gave a good start to the programme. The nursing personnel engage in regular family visits according to priority needs, home care, maternal child health clinics, treatment of minor ailments, health education, organizing school health programmes, and so on. Through this programme, the nursing students get a firsthand knowledge of the common health problems of India and gain skill in working with health personnel from Government Agencies to meet the health problems of rural India efficiently.

Exhibit 6.2 CMC Hospital, Vellore: OPD Load 2010–11

Sr. No.	OPD Services	OPD Load
1	Cardiology 1,2,3	69,916
2	Casualty	43,814
3	Clinical Immunology and Rheumatology Clinic	24,883
4	Dental 1,2	15,521
5	Dermatology 1,2	54,258
6	ENT 1,2,3	62,568
7	Endocrinology	35,581
8	Endo-diabetes	23,622
9	Gastroenterology	54,048
10	Gynecology 1,2,3,4,5	47,110
11	H.L.R.S.	19,508
12	Hematology	29,716
13	Hepatology	21,773
14	Ida Scudder Citizen's Clinic	23,419
15	Medical Oncology	12,034
16	Medicine 1,2,3	1,22,028
17	Neonatology	11,108
18	Nephrology 1,2	28,236
19	Neurology	30,417
20	Neuro Surgery	18,123
21	Obstetrics 1,2,3,4,5	66,038
22	Ortho Spinal Disorders Clinic	27,407
23	Orthopedics 1,2,3,4,5	91,500
24	PMR	13,704
25	Pediatric Casualty	20,383
26	Pediatric Ent 1,2,3	13,652
27	Pediatric Orthopedics	12,876
28	Pediatric Surgery 1,2	17,547
29	Pediatric Unit 1,2,3	60,204
30	Radiation Therapy 1,2	29,500
31	Reproductive Medicine	13,001
32	Respiratory Medicine	33,465
33	Surgery 1,2 3,4,5,6	79,544
34	Staff Student Health Service	58,449
35	Urology 1,2	48,418
1–35	Sub Total	13,33,371
All other OPD services		1,71,805
Grand Total		**15,05,176**

Source: CMC web site.

MAJESTIC HOSPITALS* CASE 6.2

The CEO of Majestic Hospitals, Mr Sanjiv Verma, was very conscious about maintaining a high quality of services. A recent feedback obtained from a few patients of the hospital highlighted the discharge process of its inpatients at the end of their stay at the hospital as a problem area. The hospital policy mentioned a two to three hour period for inpatient discharge after the consultant gave the discharge orders, but the feedback form from patients showed an average delay of five hours for discharge. The CEO therefore was keen to review the inpatient discharge process and recommend ways to improve the service level.

Majestic Hospital, Mahanagar[ii]

Majestic Hospital, Mahanagar, is a leading hospital chain in Western India. It is a multi-super speciality hospital with over 300 beds, seven major operation theatres and 80 Intensive Care Unit (ICU) beds. It has emerged as a dominant player and a premier healthcare service provider. It offers high quality medical and surgical care in a host of specialties such as Cardiology and Cardio-vascular Thoracic (CVT) surgeries, Neurology and Neuro-surgeries, Nephrology and Kidney Transplant, Emergency Care and so on. The hospital provides its services through a medical team of 70 doctors on its roll, along with more than 300 visiting consultants. The medical team is complemented by a team of about 800 paramedical and non-medical personnel. It has already started its multi-specialty tertiary care hospitals in two more metropolitan cities, and plans to expand its operations to cross the 1000-bed mark with additional state-of-the art hospitals across four more cities in Western India by 2013.

Over the years, Majestic Hospital received many awards and accolades in recognition of its pioneering achievements in Indian healthcare. It was rated the Best Hospital (2007) by IMRB[iii] and *The Week* magazine. It had performed more than 200 successful Cadaver and Renal Transplants, more than 13000 Angiographies and 4200 Angioplasties, and achieved a 99.6 per cent success rate in Cardiac bypass

---

* Reproduced with the permission of the copyright owner.

Prepared by Professor K.V. Ramani, Indian Institute of Management, Ahmedabad.

Cases of the Indian Institute of Management, Ahmedabad, are prepared as a basis for classroom discussion. They are not designed to present illustrations of either correct or incorrect handling of administrative problems.

©2010 by the Indian Institute of Management, Ahmedabad, Revised 14 May 2012.

[ii] Real name of the hospital and its location have been changed.

[iii] IMRB is one of the top 20 Market Research companies in the world.

surgeries. It was one of the few hospitals in Western India which received NABH[iv] for excellence in quality healthcare services and also NABL[v] accreditation for its high quality testing and diagnostics capabilities. Majestic Hospital's accreditation was the result of the strong emphasis laid within the organization on strengthening policies, procedures and protocols, reviewing performance through patient satisfaction surveys, conducting audits and training the staff including clinicians, nurses, management and outsourced staff. It was the extension of this thought that compelled the management to seek the help of Management Consultants to improve the discharge process of its inpatients, an area that was found lacking in terms of customer satisfaction.

Inpatient Care at Majestic Hospital

Registration: Upon arrival at the hospital, each patient registered as an inpatient and was given a unique registration number which remained her/his identification throughout life. The registration form, besides carrying personal information about the patient, also carried the name of the admitting consultant and the details of insurance coverage, if any. At the time of registration, the inpatients were given options for accommodation ranging from shared beds in economy class to suites with single bed and facility for relatives to stay with the patient. A patient file was created during the registration process.

Ward Admission: The billing department, upon receipt of patient information from the registration desk, collected the deposit as per the admission class and issued a receipt to the patient. The patient was then taken to her/his room and the patient file (created at the time of registration) updated upon admission. Once admitted in the room/bed the admission nurse gave each patient a general orientation of the hospital. The patient file was maintained at the nursing station till the patient was discharged. It contained all information about the patient (name, age, address, and so on) and patient care details such as doctor's visits and observations, medicines prescribed, services given, and so on.

Treatment: Treatment began within 30 minutes of ward admission. A unit nurse was assigned to the patient, who was responsible for all the medical care to be provided. She was responsible for maintaining the patient file. One unit nurse

---

[iv] National Accreditation Board for Hospitals and Healthcare Providers (NABH) is a constituent board of Quality Council of India, set up to establish and operate accreditation programme for healthcare organizations.

[v] National Accreditation Board for Testing and Calibration Laboratories (NABL) is an autonomous body under the aegis of Department of Science and Technology, Government of India, authorised as the sole accreditation body for Testing and Calibration laboratories in accordance with ISO/IEC 17025:2005 and ISO 15189:2007.

was assigned to five patients. The unit nurse reported to the sister-in-charge assigned for each ward. Treatment could be broadly classified under medical or surgical care.

Discharge: When the admitting consultant (Consultant doctor) was satisfied with her/his patient's progress, and felt that hospital care was not needed any more, she/he initiated the discharge process. The discharge process started with the discharge advice given by the consultant doctor to the unit nurse.

Patient discharges were classified into two categories, namely, planned discharges and unplanned discharges. Planned discharges were those where the patient was informed of discharge well in advance, at least one day before. Unplanned discharges were those where the patient was discharged the same day following the morning ward visit by the consultant. Planned discharges were more in surgical cases whereas unplanned discharges happened more in medical cases.

Once the consultant doctor advised discharge, there were a number of tasks to be performed. The unit nurse ensured that all the discharge procedures were completed before the patient left the hospital.

Figure 6.2 shows the various tasks in the discharge process.

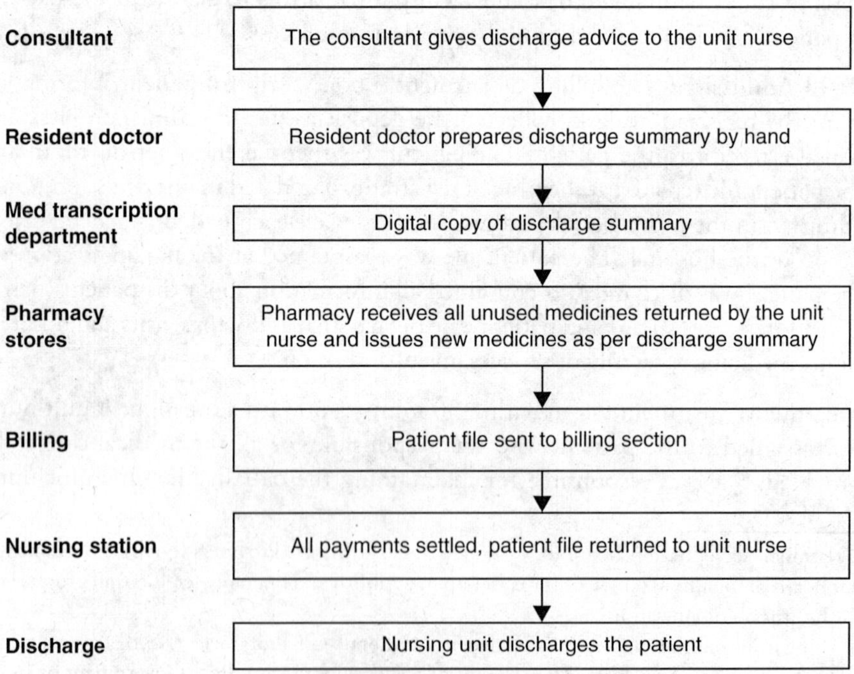

Figure 6.2 Discharge Process

Discharge Summary: Following the discharge advice by the consultants, the resident doctor prepared the discharge summary by hand and handed it over to the medical transcription department, where a digital copy of the discharge summary was made by typing it in the prescribed format. The resident doctor checked the typed discharge summary and then the final copy was printed and submitted to the consultant doctor for her/his signature. The consultant doctor signed the discharge summary after completing the morning ward visit.

Pharmacy Store: The unit nurse returned the unutilized medicines to the pharmacy store. If some medicines were prescribed to be taken after discharge, the same were requisitioned by her from the pharmacy store. The pharmacy store posted the above transactions under the patient ID, for billing purposes.

Ambulance Department: The unit nurse sent a requisition to the ambulance department for transport if required by the patient.

Billing Department: After completing the patient file, with all related information including the doctor visits and the services provided, the unit nurse sent it to the billing department. The billing department ensured that all the doctor visits and/or services mentioned in the patient file were billed and then prepared the final bill. Once the bill was ready, the patient/family members were asked to settle the bill.

The settlement of bills in the case of uninsured patients was very easy, as payment was made either in cash or through credit/debit cards by the patient's family. It was equally easy for patients who could claim reimbursement later from the insurance providers. However, in the case of patients who were insured under 'cashless service' (or from the corporate sector), the process took a little longer. The final discharge summary and the bill were sent to the insurance provider, Third Party Administrator (TPA) or the employer for authorization, to ensure receipt of the billed amount in full. If the insurance provider did not pay the full billed amount (for example, the insurance did not cover costs of certain procedures, restrictions on room charges, and so on), then the patient's family had to settle the remaining amount. Patients had to pay all non-admissible charges, not approved by insurance/corporate offices. If any additional approval was required, the process could get delayed further. Upon settlement of the bills, the billing department gave a clearance slip to the patient.

Physical Discharge: After receiving the patient file along with the clearance slip from the billing department, the unit nurse gave the discharge summary to the patient/family member, counselled the patient and handed over the prescribed medicines to patient/family members. The patient/family member acknowledged receipt of the discharge summary before the patient left the hospital.

A Patient's Experience

This was the experience of a patient at Majestic Hospital.

On the 14th August, my husband was admitted to Majestic Hospital for multiple problems related to possible renal failure, extreme weakness requiring blood transfusions, and impacted stools that called for colon cleansing. Everything was compounded by the fact that he had had a fall the day before he was hospitalized and suffered a muscle tear in the leg that had been operated on three years earlier for fracture of the neck of the femur. He could not walk.

We are covered by insurance on my son's plan as a cashless transaction. Realizing that it might take long, I informed the nursing staff to start getting the data ready three days before we were to be discharged. We were set to leave on the 24th, that is, after 10 days in the hospital.

On the 21st, I told the people at the nursing station that I had been warned of delay but that given my husband's condition I should like to be as speedy as possible. I was assured that everything was on the computer and it would be speedy.

On the 24th morning, the day we were to be discharged, I went to the billing section on the ground floor and asked when we could leave. They said, by lunchtime. I went down at 1 pm thinking it would be done and that I had given sufficient notice, but the young man at the desk said he was just putting everything together and would fax it to the insurance company as soon as he could. That fax went off at about 2 pm The hours went by with my niece and myself making several trips from the 4th floor to the ground floor, pleading with the man at the desk to ascertain why the delay. He said all that data had to be checked by a panel appointed by the insurance company and that there was no response as yet. At 4.30 pm, I called my son in Bangalore and asked him to do something at his end. He alerted his HR Department and half an hour later he told me it had been passed and that Majestic Hospital had been informed. That was 5 pm. Once that was confirmed, I had to go again to the billing section to get my deposit back, which took another half an hour.

It was 6 pm when we brought my stretcher-bound husband home. Dreading just this sort of thing, I had informed all concerned about the date of our discharge three days in advance, and been repeatedly assured that it was all being taken care of and would be prompt. While all concerned were well-meaning, the inordinate delay was very tiring, especially with a sick patient. The general explanation was that cashless transactions take longer. These questions come to my mind: Why is the computation not done each day so that, at the last moment, only the final day's medicines need to be added? Why does it take till afternoon for the whole bill to be put together and then faxed? Is there some mechanism by which the transaction between insurance company and hospital can be speeded up?

Other Administrative Procedures

The hospital had incorporated a number of operational guidelines to record the time spent in the discharge of the patient. The tools used for this purpose were the following:

Discharge Checklist: Each patient file had a discharge checklist printed on the back of the file (Exhibit 6.3). The required information was to be filled by the hospital staff, namely, the resident doctor, medical transcriptionist, unit nurse, pharmacist and the billing officer. The purpose of the checklist was to track the time taken in the discharge process by each concerned department against the norm of a total of 60 minutes decided by the hospital management.

Continuous Quality Improvement (CQI) Sheet: This sheet (Exhibit 6.4) was utilized to record the time spent in the discharge of patients who were insured by TPA, Insurance companies or their employer. This checklist had to be filled by the resident doctor, unit nurse, medical transcriptionist, billing officer, corporate medical officer and Credit Patients Dept. The purpose of this sheet was to track the time consumed at each department during the billing process, especially the time taken for the settlement of the bill.

Exhibit 6.5 gives data on inpatient discharge from medicine ward for a few days.

Exhibit 6.3 Discharge Checklist (To be filled and followed by concerned department)

	Starting/ Receiving Time	Sending/ Handover Time	Actual Time (min.) to be Filled in by MRD	Normal Time (min.)	Reason for the Delay	Name and Employee ID	Sign and Date
Discharge summary prepared by the resident doctor				10			
Computerized discharge summary				10			
Completion of file by the concerned unit nurse				10			
Pharmacy store				10			
Billing department				20			
Nursing Station				–			
Total				**60**			

Note: All the procedures should be completed within 60 minutes.

Nursing Station	**Yes**	**No**	**NA**
Whether the discharge intimation was given to			
a. Pharmacy. Please specify time __________ Hrs.	☐	☐	☐
b. Billing department. Please specify time __________ Hrs.	☐	☐	☐
1. If clearance of file took more than normal time hether the billing department was informed?	☐	☐	☐
2. Whether pending medicines were counted and returned to the pharmacy stores?	☐	☐	☐
3. Whether relative's signature was taken upon receipt of all reports, X-ray films, discharge summary, and so on?	☐	☐	☐
4. Whether the final bill was settled? (Please verify settlement of receipt)	☐	☐	☐
5. Whether Attendant, Reliever and Relative Passes were collected?	☐	☐	☐

____
Sign of Unit Nurse

EID No. __________

Pharmacy Stores	**Yes**	**No**	**NA**
1. Whether all stores related charges were posted and credit for return medicine given?	☐	☐	☐
2. If clearance of file took more than normal time, was the billing department and sister-in-charge/unit nurse informed?	☐	☐	☐
3. Whether the signature from stores for NOC (with Emp. Code) was present?	☐	☐	☐

____
Signature of Pharmacist

EID No. __________

Billing	**Yes**	**No**	**NA**
1. Whether all relevant charges were checked and posted?	☐	☐	☐
2. Whether '0' dialling was deactivated by reception and telephone bill collected?	☐	☐	☐
3. If the clearance of file took more than the time prescribed, whether the sister-in-charge/unit nurse was informed?	☐	☐	☐

4. Whether the final billing was done? ☐ ☐ ☐
5. Whether the final bill settled? ☐ ☐ ☐
6. In case of mediclaim, whether all relevant papers had been handed over? ☐ ☐ ☐

____
Signature of Billing Officer

EID No. ____________

Exhibit 6.4 Continuous Quality Improvement (CQI)

DATE: ___/___/___

TPA Discharges Form				**If Delayed for More Than the Prescribed Time, then Write Remarks**
TPA Name			**Ward Floor**	
Process	**In Time**	**Out Time**	**Sign with Code**	
Primary Nurse to Unit Secretary			Unit Secretary	
Unit Secretary to House Officer			House Officer	
House Officer to Unit Secretary			House Officer	
Unit Secretary to Billing Department			Billing	
Billing Department to CMO/DMA			CMO/DMA	
CMO/DMA to Billing Department			Billing	
Billing Department notifying the time and calling relatives			Billing	
Billing to Credit Operations			CPD	
Credit Operations to Corporate			AM Corporate (Head Corporate Billing)	

- This form has to be filled in by all TPA patients, otherwise file should not be received by Corporate.
- In case of CMO/DMA is not available, send the file to Chief Medical Administrator (CMA).

Terminology Used

TPA	Third Party Administrator
Primary Nurse	Staff Nurse
Unit Secretary	Medical Transcriptionist
House Officer	Resident Doctor
CMO	Corporate Medical Officer
DMA	Deputy Medical Administrator
Credit Operations	Credit Patient Department (CPD)
AM Corporate	Assistant Manager

Exhibit 6.5 Inpatient Discharge Data: Discharges from Medicine Department

Discharge Summary				Nursing Station		Pharmacy Department		Billing Department				Mode of Discharge
Order Given		Res. Dr Signs		Patient File Ready		Return/Buy Med		File Received		Bills Ready		
Date	Time	Date	Time	Date	Time	Date	Time	Date	Time	Date	Time	
03/08	9.00	03/08	11.00	03/08	9.10	03/08	9.50	03/08	9.45	03/08	11.00	Unplanned Cash
03/08	9.30	03/08	11.30	03/08	9.40	03/08	10.10	03/08	10.30	03/08	11.30	Unplanned Cash
03/08	10.00	04/08	12.00	03/08	Night Shift	03/08	Night Shift	04/08	13.00	04/08	18.30	Planned Cashless
03/08	10.00	03/08	11.30	03/08	10.20	03/08	10.50	03/08	11.00	03/08	12.00	Unplanned Cash
03/08	10.00	03/08	11.30	03/08	10.10	03/08	10.50	03/08	11.00	03/08	12.30	Unplanned Cash
03/08	10.30	03/08	11.30	03/08	10.40	03/08	10.50	03/08	11.45	03/08	12.30	Unplanned Cash
03/08	11.00	04/08	11.00	03/08	Night Shift	03/08	Night Shift	04/08	11.20	04/08	12.30	Planned Cashless
03/08	11.30	04/08	11.30	03/08	Night Shift	03/08	Night Shift	04/08	12.00	04/08	14.00	Planned Cash
03/08	11.30	03/08	13.00	03/08	11.40	03/08	12.10	03/08	12.30	03/08	16.00	Unplanned Cash
03/08	12.00	03/08	14.30	03/08	12.10	03/08	12.40	03/08	13.00	03/08	15.00	Unplanned Cashless
03/08	12.00	03/08	14.30	03/08	12.10	03/08	12.40	03/08	12.50	03/08	15.00	Unplanned Cash
03/08	12.30	04/08	14.00	03/08	Night Shift	03/08	Night Shift	04/08	13.00	04/08	13.00	Planned Cash
03/08	13.00	03/08	13.45	03/08	13.10	03/08	13.40	03/08	14.00	03/08	14.30	Unplanned Cashless
03/08	13.00	03/08	15.00	03/08	13.10	03/08	13.40	03/08	14.00	03/08	16.30	Unplanned Cash
04/08	11.00	04/08	14.00	04/08	11.15	04/08	11.50	04/08	12.00	04/08	14.00	Unplanned Cash
04/08	12.00	04/08	14.00	04/08	12.10	04/08	12.50	04/08	13.00	04/08	14.30	Unplanned Cash
04/08	12.30	04/08	13.30	04/08	12.40	04/08	12.50	04/08	13.40	04/08	14.30	Unplanned Cashless

04/08	12.30	04/08	14.30	04/08	12.45	04/08	12.50	04/08	13.40	04/08	15.00	Unplanned Cash
04/08	12.30	04/08	14.00	04/08	12.40	04/08	12.50	04/08	13.30	04/08	15.00	Unplanned Cash
04/08	13.00	04/08	14.00	04/08	13.10	04/08	13.50	04/08	14.00	04/08	16.00	Unplanned Cashless
04/08	15.00	04/08	16.30	04/08	15.30	04/08	15.35	04/08	16.00	04/08	17.00	Unplanned Cash
05/08	9.30	06/08	10.00	05/08	Night Shift	05/08	Night Shift	06/08	10.00	06/08	11.00	Planned Cash
05/08	11.30	06/08	11.30	05/08	Night Shift	05/08	Night Shift	06/08	11.40	06/08	12.30	Planned Cash
05/08	12.00	06/08	13.00	05/08	Night Shift	05/08	Night Shift	06/08	13.00	06/08	18.00	Planned Cashless
05/08	12.00	06/08	13.30	05/08	Night Shift	05/08	Night Shift	06/08	12.35	06/08	14.00	Planned Cash
05/08	12.00	06/08	12.30	05/08	Night Shift	05/08	Night Shift	06/08	12.30	06/08	14.00	Planned Cash
05/08	12.30	06/08	12.30	05/08	Night Shift	05/08	Night Shift	06/08	12.45	06/08	14.30	Planned Cash
06/08	10.00	06/08	11.45	06/08	10.10	06/08	10.50	06/08	11.45	06/08	15.30	Unplanned Cashless
06/08	10.00	06/08	12.00	06/08	10.10	06/08	10.50	06/08	11.00	06/08	12.00	Unplanned Cash
06/08	11.00	06/08	12.15	06/08	11.20	06/08	11.50	06/08	12.15	06/08	14.30	Unplanned Cashless
06/08	11.00	07/08	11.30	06/08	Night Shift	06/08	Night Shift	07/08	11.00	07/08	12.30	Planned Cash
06/08	11.00	06/08	12.00	06/08	11.10	06/08	11.50	06/08	11.45	06/08	12.30	Unplanned Cash
06/08	11.30	06/08	12.30	06/08	11.40	06/08	12.10	06/08	12.45	06/08	15.30	Unplanned Cashless
06/08	11.30	06/08	13.00	06/08	11.40	06/08	12.10	06/08	12.45	06/08	14.30	Unplanned Cash
06/08	12.00	06/08	13.00	06/08	12.10	06/08	12.40	06/08	13.00	06/08	14.00	Unplanned Cash
06/08	12.30	06/08	14.00	06/08	13.00	06/08	13.00	06/08	14.00	06/08	17.00	Unplanned Cashless
06/08	13.00	06/08	14.00	06/08	13.10	06/08	13.40	06/08	14.00	06/08	15.00	Unplanned Cash
06/08	13.00	06/08	14.30	06/08	13.30	06/08	13.40	06/08	14.00	06/08	15.30	Unplanned Cash

ARAM HOSPITAL (APOLLO GROUP)* CASE 6.3

Abdur Razzaque Ansari Memorial (ARAM) Weavers' Hospital was set up in 1996 in Ranchi by the Chotanagpur Regional Handloom Weavers' Cooperative Union Ltd, to fulfill the dream of Mr Ansari who dedicated his entire life to the upliftment of the weaver community. Starting as a 75 bed secondary care health facility, ARAM Hospital managed by the Apollo Hospitals Group has grown over the years into a Super Specialty hospital with 200 beds under the dynamic leadership of Mr Sayeed Ahmed Ansari and Mr Manzoor Ahmed Ansari, sons of Mr Abdur Razzaque Ansari. There was a demand for ARAM Hospital to add new super specialties, as well as to expand some of the existing super specialty units. Mr Sayeed Ansari wished to understand the utilization of the two Cath Labs, considering the huge investments already made.

In the midst of the devastating First World War which wrecked the socio-economic conditions of every nation on earth, the family of Asad Ali, a weaver, was blessed with a son Abdur Razzaque Ansari in a small town on the outskirts of Ranchi in present day Jharkhand state in 1917. Mr Ansari founded the Chotanagpur Regional Weavers' Cooperative Union Ltd in 1978, and devoted his entire life to the upliftment of the weaver community. Following his visit to Apollo hospital in Chennai for cardiac care in 1987, Mr Ansari was determined to build a small hospital for the weavers and the downtrodden tribal population of Jharkhand. Unfortunately, he died in March 1992 without fulfilling his dream.

In the board meeting of the Chotanagpur Regional Weaver's Cooperative Union (CRWCU) Ltd held on 4 May 1991, it was unanimously decided to build a hospital for the weavers and tribal community in Ranchi. In 1992, Mr Sayeed Ahmed Ansari met Dr Pratap Reddy, Chairman of Apollo Hospitals Group, for his ideas in setting up a small hospital in memory of his father, the late Abdur Razzaque Ansari. In April 1993, the Apollo Hospitals Group submitted a proposal to the CRWCU Board for setting up a 75 bed secondary care hospital. Encouraged by a generous contribution of almost ₹2 crores by the Weavers' union and a grant of ₹1.5 crores from the Central Government, the Abdur Razzaque Ansari Memorial (ARAM) Hospital was commissioned in July 1996 by the weaver's community with a Sarvdharam Puja. This is the only hospital in the country set up by a Weavers' Cooperative Society.

---

* Reproduced with the permission of the copyright owner.

Prepared by Professor K.V. Ramani of Indian Institute of Management, Ahmedabad and Dr Ambrish Tripathi of Apollo Hospitals Group, Ranchi.

Cases of the Indian Institute of Management, Ahmedabad, are prepared as a basis for classroom discussion. They are not designed to present illustrations of either correct or incorrect handling of administrative problems.

© 2011 by the Indian Institute of Management, Ahmedabad, Revised 14 May 2012.

1996 was an important year for the Hospital. The hospital started functioning in July 1996 with General Medicine, Cardiology and Dermatology departments. The hospital was elevated to a high secondary care hospital by installing a CT Scan in August 1996. Nephrology department started functioning in October 1996 with two dialysis machines.

Since then, the hospital has grown into a Super Specialty Tertiary Care Hospital with 20 clinical units and 200 beds. In the year 2010–11, the hospital handled an annual load of over 37,000 outpatients and 9,000 inpatients (Exhibit 6.6), while the investigation loads on its pathology and radiology departments were over 227,000 and 41,000 tests respectively (Exhibit 6.7). A new building with an additional 50 beds and an MRI unit became functional in July 2011.

The hospital opened a City Medical Centre in the year 2000 for the benefit of those who do not have to travel 20 kms to the main hospital. The city centre provided a wide range of services from morning to evening under one roof. The same consultants who work in the main hospital are available for consultation in the city centre as well.

In addition to the main hospital, Mr Sayeed Ahmad Ansari established a tie-up with the Bangalore based Healthcare Global Enterprises Ltd for setting up a state of the art Cancer Institute. Curie-Abdur Razzaque Ansari Cancer Institute was inaugurated by the Vice President of India in 2000. This centre provides comprehensive treatment in oncology such as Medical Oncology, Surgical Oncology and Radiation Oncology. The hospital is the first of its kind in Jharkhand and has done much to fulfill Mr Ansari's dream to stop the migration of poor weavers and the tribal population for cancer treatment to other cities in the country.

Cardiac Sciences Department

The Cardiac Sciences department at ARAM Hospital is as old as the hospital itself. It started in 1996 with one cardiologist, and one technician. The Cardiothoracic unit, Cath Lab and CCU started in April 2000. The services offered by the Cardiac Sciences Department at ARAM Hospital include a wide range of diagnostic tests and interventional procedures.[vi] The increasing demand for cardiac care services can be seen from Exhibit 6.8.

The cardiothoracic department performed its first Coronary Artery Bypass Surgery in the year 2000, completed 100 heart surgeries by June 2001, 100 Valve Replacement surgeries by July 2003, and 1000 cardiac surgeries by August 2004.

[vi] Please refer to Annexure 1 for a brief explanation of various services offered by the Cardiac Sciences Department.

Cardiology Department

The Cardiology department at ARAM Hospital started functioning in 1996. The hospital commissioned its first Cath Lab in 2000 and the second Cath Lab in 2005. Installation of the latest generation Flat Panel Cath Lab with Intra Vascular Ultrasound (IVUS) opened up a new dimension in cardiac imaging and interventions providing high level tertiary care services.

In the year 2010–11, the cardiology department performed over 2000 interventional procedures. The cardiology department had two consultants, two doctors, five nurses, two technicians and five paramedics. The Cardiology service process consisted of OPD consultations, non-invasive diagnostic tests, and interventional procedures, if required; see Exhibit 6.9 on the load for cardiology services over the last few months, for illustration.

Figure 6.3 shows the various steps a patient goes through for receiving cardiology services.

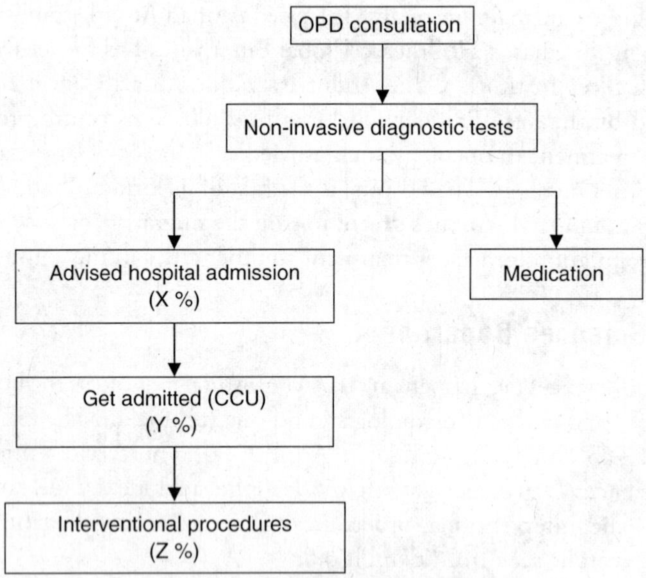

Figure 6.3 Cardiology Service Process

Consultation: OPD consultations were provided at the main hospital from 1 pm to 6 pm and at the City centre from 7 pm to 9 pm, Monday through Saturday.

Non-invasive Diagnostic Tests: Following the OPD consultation, all outpatients underwent non-invasive diagnostic tests. Non-invasive diagnostic ECHO and

ECG services were available at the City Centre, while additional non-invasive diagnostic services such as TMT, Color Doppler, Holter, and PFT were available only at the main hsopital. ICU facilities were recommended for non-invasive diagnostic procedures such as TMT, and hence available only at the main hospital.

Inpatient Admission, CCU: Based on the outcomes of the diagnostic tests, a majority of those who were advised hospital admission were admitted in the Coronary Care Unit (CCU). The pre-intervention CCU at ARAM (called CCU 1) had seven beds.

Patients who were admitted in the pre-intervention CCU underwent certain basic pathological tests. Cath Lab procedures were performed only after ensuring that all the reports of pathology lab and other investigations were OK. For example, before doing a CAG procedure, it was necessary to study the creatinine levels since the use of dye during the process could slightly increase the creatinine level. Also, a deranged kidney could be a contraindication for CAG.

It took about five minutes to prepare the patients for CAG and TPI, while it took 15 minutes to prepare a patient for PTCA, BMV, and PPI. It took another 10 minutes to shift the patient from CCU 1 to the Cath Lab.

Interventional Procedures: After all the pre-intervention procedures were completed, those patients who were required to undergo interventional procedures were moved to the Cath Lab. About 75 per cent of the inpatients underwent interventional procedures. Patients were taken into the Cath Lab for interventional procedures on a First-Cum-First Served basis (FCFS Rule), as per their time of admission. All the interventional procedures were scheduled from 1 pm to 5 pm Monday through Saturday. Emergency cases which were handled on a priority basis rarely disrupted the planned schedule of Cath Lab procedures, since ARAM Hospital had two Cath Labs.

Cath Lab interventions started with diagnostic CAG. Based on the findings from CAG, the consultant took decisions on appropriate interventions if required, and consulted the patient's relatives and/or attendants. Any interventional procedure was done only after getting consent from the patient's relatives and/or attendants. If any interventions were to be carried out, they were advised to have them done in the same sitting. Cath Lab Interventional procedures offered at the main hospital included Diagnostic Angiography (CAG), Coronary Angioplasty (PTCA), Balloon Mitral Valvotomies (BMV), and Temporary/Permanent Pacemaker Implantation (TPI/PPI). See Exhibit 6.10 on interventional procedures carried out in the month of February 2012; this exhibit gives complete data for four days on each Cath Lab procedure, namely, the name of the procedure, the cardiologist who did the procedure, the Cath Lab reference where this procedure was done, and the time taken for the procedure.

Post Intervention CCU: Following the Cath Lab interventional procedures, all patients were shifted to the Post-intervention CCU unit (CCU 2) for continuous monitoring of their health conditions. CCU 2 had eight beds. Patients who had undergone only CAG were discharged after 8 hours (Day 1). All other patients who had undergone other interventional procedures spent one day in CCU 2. Following the morning visit by the consultants next day, these patients were either discharged (Day 2) or admitted in the general ward for an additional day if required and discharged from the general wards on Day 3. Post procedure activities in Cath Lab took about 15 to 20 minutes which included shifting the patient to CCU 2 and making the Cath Lab ready to receive the next patient.

Management Concerns

ARAM Hospital administrator was wondering how to manage the Cath Lab services since the demand has been increasing over the years. He wanted to test if it would be possible to complete the current daily load of Cath Lab procedures in less amount of time, perhaps by a different rule from the current FCFS rule for scheduling the procedures. By ding so, if the throughput from the Cath Lab can be increased, would the availability of CCU beds be a constraint?

Exhibit 6.6 ARAM Hospital: Load on Outpatient and Inpatient Services

Sr. No.	Clinical Department	Year Started	Number of Outpatient Registrations					No. of Inpatient Registrations				
			2006–2007	2007–2008	2008–2009	2009–2010	2010–2011	2006–2007	2007–2008	2008–2009	2009–2010	2010–2011
1	Cardiology	1996	3,528	3,372	4,177	4,678	4,643	1,446	1,462	1,714	1,879	1,766
2	Dermatology	1996	1	397	354	347	349	11	9	4	7	7
3	General Medicine	1996	5,149	5,622	6,046	7,130	8,285	1,140	1,279	1,312	1,334	1,451
4	Nephrology	1996	1,700	1,803	1,830	2,069	2,178	617	463	478	646	839
5	Neurology	1996	2,804	2,779	3,461	3,846	4,374	388	386	515	596	647
6	Obs and Gynecology	1996	352	865	880	1,217	1,303	187	186	137	196	193
7	Orthopedics	1996	219	1,558	1,663	1,895	1,870	268	296	288	310	269
8	Pediatrics	1996	506	378	551	824	800	146	105	141	149	150
9	Psychiatry	1996	0	0	0	44	472	0	0	118	10	30
10	ENT	1996	576	742	810	799	820	103	108	90	78	71
11	General surgery	1996	46	1,189	1,441	1,549	1,537	628	621	678	666	675
12	Neurosurgery	1996	751	776	1,110	1,035	1,313	367	368	430	469	608
13	Plastic surgery	1996	280	214	302	332	334	130	106	121	121	139
14	Endocrinology	1996	433	285	159	42	10	70	36	14	7	7
15	Gastroenterology	1998	2,470	2,312	2,386	3,047	3,213	462	374	397	578	553
16	Urology	1998	1,249	1,430	1,589	1,878	1,941	367	417	374	423	464
17	Cardiac surgery	2000	585	615	722	1,338	2,174	51	56	65	92	81
18	Renal transplant	2007	56	83	98	91	84	35	36	60	35	43
19	Rheumatology	2007	0	0	454	1,648	1,928	0	0	20	149	189
20	Nuclear medicine	2008	0	180	300	242	292	0	0	0	0	0
Total			**20,705**	**24,600**	**28,333**	**34,051**	**37,920**	**6,416**	**6,308**	**6,956**	**7,745**	**8,182**

Exhibit 6.7 ARAM Hospital: Load on Investigation Services

Department	Sections	2007–08	2008–09	2009–10	2010–11
Laboratory	Bio Chemistry	102,522	114,692	128,410	142,248
	Hematology	24,364	27,341	31,109	33,436
	Immunology	19,709	21,620	24,946	27,685
	Microbiology	5,131	6,960	7,571	8,105
	Clinical Path	10,474	11,611	12,721	13,502
	Histopathology	695	841	991	1,002
	Cytology	269	430	506	625
	Body Fluid	393	494	626	626
	Total	**163,557**	**183,989**	**206,880**	**227,229**
Radiology	X Ray	19,599	22,421	21,690	23,858
	Ultrasound	8,967	10,487	11,907	13,273
	CT Scan	2,847	3,597	4,452	4,691
	BMD	86	107	70	55
	Mammography	40	79	65	65
	Total	**31,539**	**36,691**	**38,184**	**41,942**

Exhibit 6.8 ARAM Hospital: Growth of Cardiac Care Services

Procedures	Types of procedure	2007–08	2008–09	2009–10	2010–11
Non-interventional Diagnosis	ECG	7,933	8,467	10,585	10,651
	ECHO	5,013	5,553	6,643	6,499
	TMT	823	787	879	1,074
	PFT	309	297	377	343
	Total	**16,044**	**17,338**	**21,089**	**20,812**
Cardiology interventions	CAG	938	1,069	1,297	1,227
	PTCA	382	447	572	514
	BMV	118	128	111	69
	TPI	104	98	137	127
	PPI	115	122	157	132
Cardiothoracic	Device closure	5	4	2	8
	Renal/others	39	43	42	18
	CABG	84	87	73	48
	Open heart	148	206	195	92
	Closed heart	33	30	19	10

Exhibit 6.9 ARAM Hospital: Cardiology OPD and Non-invasive Diagnostic Services: Monthly Load

Services	Services	Oct 2011	Nov 2011	Dec 2011	Jan 2012	Feb 2012	Mar 2012
Main Hospital	OPD	535	506	493	471	599	575
	ECG	850	967	903	843	603	943
	ECHO	546	505	510	470	603	588
	TMT	76	58	52	65	78	106
	PFT	35	16	11	19	28	42
	Holter	10	14	10	09	17	10
City Centre	OPD	89	82	74	83	75	86
	ECG	66	55	56	56	66	60
	ECHO	94	82	84	90	80	86

Exhibit 6.10 ARAM Hospital: Cath Lab Schedule for a Few Days

Sr. No.	Date	Hospital No.	Name of Procedure	Consultant	Patient in at	Patient out	Cath Lab
1	1/2/12	305239	PTCA	Dr X	1.30 pm	2.05 pm	1
2	1/2/12	305368	CAG	Dr X	3.55 pm	4.00 pm	1
3	1/2/12	288787	BMV	Dr X	5.05 pm	5.20 pm	1
4	1/2/12	305367	CAG	Dr Y	5.45 pm	5.55 pm	1
5	1/2/12	305334	BMV	Dr Y	2.00 pm	2.15 pm	2
6	1/2/12	305333	CAG	Dr Y	3.00 pm	3.06 pm	2
7	1/2/12	305348	CAG + PTCA	Dr Y	3.20 pm	4.15 pm	2
8	1/2/12	305344	CAG + PTCA	Dr Y	4.25 pm	5.10 pm	2
9	1/2/12	305337	CAG	Dr Y	5.45 pm	5.50 pm	2
10	2/2/12	305395	CAG	Dr X	1.25 pm	1.30 pm	1
11	2/2/12	305424	CAG + PPI	Dr Y	2.40 pm	3.30 pm	1
12	2/2/12	305412	CAG + PPI	Dr X	4.25 pm	5.00 pm	1
13	2/2/12	305393	CAG	Dr X	5.40 pm	6.40 pm	1
14	2/2/12	305405	CAG	Dr X	6.40 pm	7.00 pm	1
15	2/2/12	305420	CAG	Dr X	2.35 pm	3.45 pm	2
16	2/2/12	305423	CAG	Dr Y	4.00 pm	4.20 pm	2
17	2/2/12	305440	CAG	Dr Y	4.40 pm	4.45 pm	2
18	2/2/12	303829	BMV	Dr Y	5.06 pm	5.20 pm	2
19	2/2/12	162333	CAG	Dr Y	6.15 pm	6.20 pm	2
20	3/2/12	305448	CAG	Dr Y	1.45 pm	2.00 pm	2
21	3/2/12	305465	CAG + PTCA	Dr Y	3.00 pm	3.50 pm	2
22	3/2/12	305452	CAG	Dr X	3.30 pm	3.40 pm	1
23	3/2/12	305477	CAG	Dr X	4.15 pm	4.25 pm	1
24	3/2/12	305468	CAG + PTCA	Dr Y	4.50 pm	5.45 pm	1
25	4/2/12	305335	CAG + PTCA	Dr Y	2.15 pm	4.20 pm	1
.							
.							
.							

ANNEXURE 1

A Note on Cardiac Catheterization and Coronary Artery Disease

The Human Heart

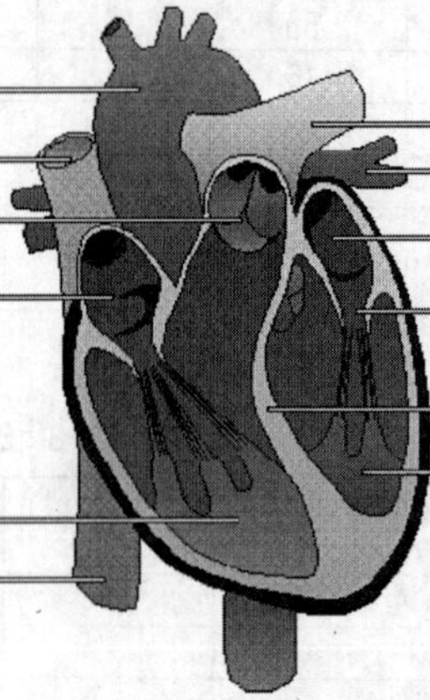

Source: http://worldinvisible.com/apologet/humbody/heart.htm.

The human heart has four chambers, two superior atria and two inferior ventricles. The atria are the receiving chambers and the ventricles are the discharging chambers. Deoxygenated blood flows through the heart in one direction, entering through the anterior *vena cava* into the *right atrium* and is pumped into the *right ventricle* before being pumped out through the *pulmonary valve* to the *pulmonary arteries* into the *lungs*. It returns from the *lungs* through the *pulmonary veins* to the *left atrium* where it is pumped through the atrioverticular *(mitral) valve* into the *left ventricle* before leaving through the *aortic valve* to the *aorta*.

Cardiac catheterization is done to:

- Check blood flow and blood pressure in the chambers of the heart.
- Check blood flow in the coronary arteries and, if you have *coronary artery disease* (CAD), determine whether surgery or another type of procedure, such as angioplasty with stenting, is needed to open the blocked blood vessels.

Cardiac catheterization is also done to:

- Check the pumping action of the heart.
- Find out if a congenital heart defect is present and how severe it is. Cardiac catheterization sometimes can also be used to help correct the defect.
- Check blood flow through the heart after surgery.

A Brief Account of Interventional Procedures Being Performed in Cardiac Care

CAG: It is a diagnostic tool in which a contrast (radio opaque dye) is being injected via catheter into the heart coronary arteries in order to investigate the condition of the heart.

PTCA: It is a therapeutic procedure by which the identified coronary artery disease is rectified by putting a wire mesh (Stent) in order to restore normal flow in the compromised/diseased artery.

BMV: It is a therapeutic procedure where a BMV Balloon is sent inside a narrowed (stenosed) valve and inflated at the origin to bring the valve to its normal size.

TPI: It is a life saving procedure where a temporary pacing lead is introduced by the venous route to the right ventricle of heart and connected to external temporary pacemaker to provide the desired electrical support.

PPI: A permanent pacemaker is implanted in order to get rid of the temporary pacemaker. In this process, the lead placed in right ventricle of the heart is connected to a battery (Permanent pacemaker) to provide required electrical impulse as when required by the body.

Device Closure: Device closure is usually the domain of pediatric patients and done by pediatric interventional cardiologist.

Coronary Artery Bypass Grafting (CABG): If the CAG investigation reveals clogged arteries, the patient is advised to undergo Coronary Artery Bypass Grafting Surgery. Here, the patient is either put on Heart Lung machine (on Pump) or without putting him on pump (off Pump/Beating Heart Surgery). The blocked arteries are bypassed by putting venous/arterial grafts taken from hands/legs.

Open Heart Surgery (OHS): In this surgery, all patients are to put Heart Lung machine (on Pump) and the surgery includes Mitral Valve Replacement (MVR), Aortic Valve replacement (AVR), Double Valve Replacement (DVR), Atrial Septal Defect (ASD), Ventricular Septal Defect (VSD), Tetralogy of Fallot (TOF), Left/Right Atrium Myxoma and so on.

Closed Heart Surgery (CHS): Closed heart surgery implies that the 'heart lung machine' or 'bypass' machine is not used and the heart is visualized but not cut open.

A Brief Account of Non-invasive Diagnostic Tests

ECG (Electrocardiogram): This is the most basic test. It involves taping electrical leads onto your legs, arms and chest to take readings of the electrical activity of your heart. These are prined out onto a piece of paper for the doctor to examine.

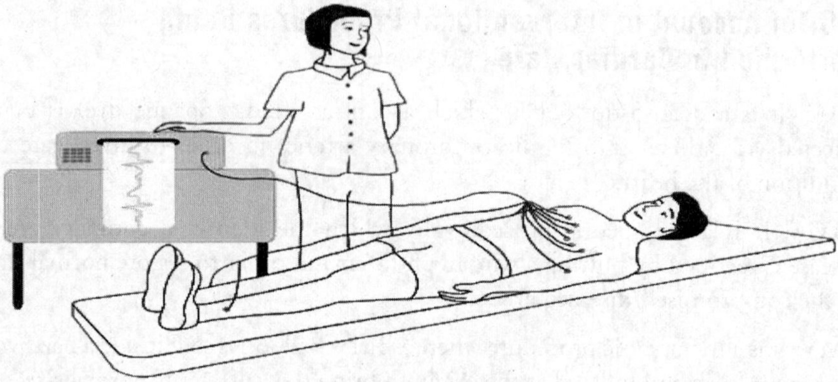

Echocardiogram: The operator puts some clear gel on your chest and then places an ultrasound probe on it. The probe sends ultrasound beams into your body and their reflections are detected and used to generate images of the heart. You can see different parts of your heart on a screen as the probe is moved around on your chest. The test is similar to the ultrasound scan that is used to examine a pregnant woman's unborn baby. It is completely painless.

This test is useful for people whose ECG shows changes which may have damaged the heart—for example a previous heart attack that you may not have even been aware of. An echocardiogram can also detect inheritable conditions such as cardiomyopathy and mitral valve prolapse.

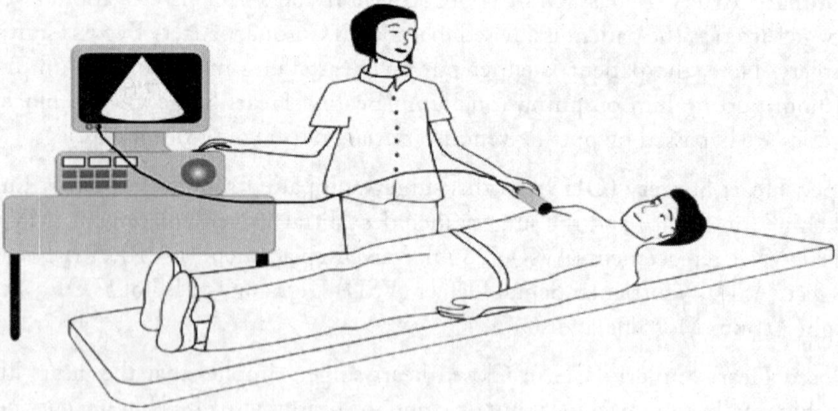

Exercise Test (Tread Mill Test): Electrical leads from the ECG machine are taped to your body and you are monitored while you exercise either on an exercise bike or treadmill. If you are having a 'cardiopulmonary exercise test', your doctor will ask you to breathe in and out of a special piece of equipment while you are doing the exercise, in order to monitor how efficiently your body uses oxygen.

This test is the same as the ECG, but is recorded before, during and after a period of time spent exercising on a treadmill or an exercise bike. This allows the doctor to examine any changes in the electrical patterns that occur with exercise, and analyse any abnormalities.

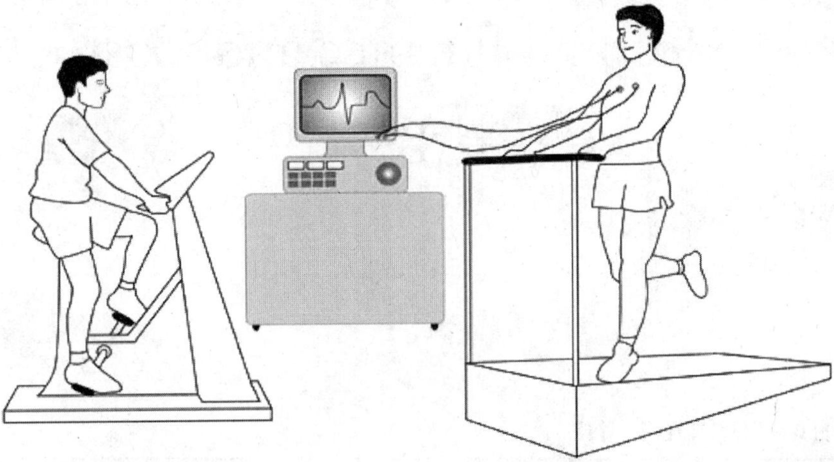

Holter: The Holter monitor is attached by 4 or 6 electrical leads to your body. It monitors your heart's electrical activity over a period of time. You wear the device on a belt round your waist. Four or six ECG leads from the device are taped to your chest. The device records the electrical activity of your heart for 24 to 48 hours, or for up to seven days if a digital one is used. The doctor can then analyse the electrical activity and rhythm of your heart to find out if you have any arrhythmias.

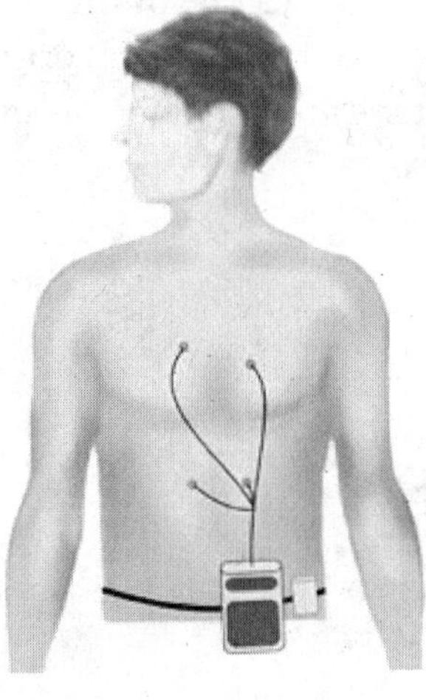

Source: http://www.sads.org.uk/cardiac_tests.htm.

chapter 7

Hospital Finance and Cost Management

CHAPTER OUTLINE

CHAPTER OBJECTIVE

The main objective of this chapter is to apply the concepts of finance and cost management (discussed in Chapter 4) to two large hospitals through real-life case studies.

APOLLO HOSPITALS*

CASE 7.1

Vision 20.6: A Blueprint for Smarter Healthcare

Annual Report 2010–2011

Exhibit 7.1 Balance Sheet as at 31st March 2011

(₹ in million)

	Schedule	31.03.2011		31.03.2010	
I. Sources of Funds					
1. Shareholders' Funds					
(a) Share capital	A	623.55		617.85	
(b) Preferential issue of equity share warrants		685.07		–	
(Refer clause 12 of Schedule 'J')					
(c) Reserves and Surplus	B	16,413.03	17,721.65	14,799.93	15,417.78
2. Loan Funds					
(a) Secured loans	C	5,496.07		4,714.30	
(b) Unsecured loans	D	1,914.04	7,410.11	2,185.57	6,899.87
3. Deferred Tax Liability*			1,071.06		751.46
*Refer clause 18 of Schedule 'J'					
Total			**26,202.82**		**23,069.11**
II. Application of Funds					
1. Fixed Assets	F				
(a) Gross block		14,444.95		12,555.11	
(b) Less: Depreciation		3,987.44		3,314.74	
(c) Net block		10,457.51		9,240.37	
(d) Capital work in progress		3,523.96		2,734.12	
			13,981.47		11,974.49
2. Investments	G		6,241.12		4,897.88
3. Current Assets, Loans and Advances	H				
(a) Inventories		1,505.21		1,343.44	
(b) Sundry debtors		2,696.43		2,055.34	
(c) Cash and bank balances		1,413.76		2,855.58	
(d) Loans and advances		5,714.98		5,170.72	
		11,330.38		11,425.08	

(Continued)

* Reproduced with the permission of the copyright owner.

Exhibit 7.1 (*Continued*)

			(₹ in million)		
	Schedule	**31.03.2011**		**31.03.2010**	
Less: Current Liabilities and Provisions	E				
(a) Liabilities		2,658.07		2,629.84	
(b) Provisions		2,692.08		2,598.62	
		5,350.15		5,228.46	
Net Current Assets			5,980.23		6,196.62
4. Miscellaneous Expenditure (to the extent not written off or adjusted)	I		–		0.12
Total			**26,202.82**		**23,069.11**

Schedules 'A' to 'I' and notes in Schedule 'J' form part of this Balance Sheet

As per our report annexed

For and on behalf of the Board of Directors

For M/s S. Viswanathan
Chartered Accountants
Firm Registration No.: 004770S

V.C. Krishnan
Partner
(Membership No: 022167)
17, Bishop Wallers Avenue (West)
Mylapore, Chennai 600 004

Place: Chennai
Date: 24 May 2011

Krishnan Akhileswaran
Chief Financial Officer

S.M. Krishnan
General Manager - Project Finance and Company Secretary

Dr Prathap C. Reddy
Executive Chairman

Preetha Reddy
Managing Director

Suneeta Reddy
Executive Director – Finance

Exhibit 7.2 Profit and Loss Account for the Year Ended 31st March 2011

(₹ in million)

	Schedule	31.03.2011	31.03.2010
Income			
(a) Income from Healthcare Services		23,319.62	18,257.79
(b) Other income	I	213.70	329.66
Total		**23,533.32**	**18,587.45**
Expenditure			
(a) Operative expenses	II	12,788.04	9,944.64
(b) Payments to and provisions for employees	III	3,572.00	2,863.81
(c) Administration and other expenses	IV	3,186.86	2,633.37
(d) Financial expenses	V	587.32	377.47
(e) Preliminary and other expenses incl. public issue		–	0.18
(f) Deferred revenue expenditure (Refer clause 37 of Schedule 'J')		3.28	3.27
Total		**20,137.50**	**15,822.74**
Profit Before Depreciation and Tax		3,395.82	2,764.72
Less: Depreciation		702.58	543.06
Profit Before Tax		2,693.24	2,221.65
Less: Provision for taxation		570.00	577.12
Add: Excess provision of earlier years written back		13.55	–
Less: Deferred tax		319.61	124.89
Profit After Tax		1,817.18	1,519.64
Surplus in Profit and Loss Account brought forward		1,474.07	1,208.76
Amount available for appropriations		3,291.25	2,728.40
Dividend		467.67	432.49
Dividend tax payable		75.86	71.83
Transfer to debenture redemption reserve		100.00	–
Transfer to general reserve		1,000.00	750.00
Balance of Profit in Profit and Loss Account		1,647.72	1,474.07
Total		**3,291.25**	**2,728.40**
Earnings Per Share (Refer clause 30 of Schedule 'J'))			
Basic Earnings Per Share of face value ₹5 (2009–10: ₹5) each		14.66	12.31
Diluted Earnings Per Share of face value ₹5 (2009–10: ₹5) each		14.24	12.26
Schedules 'I' to 'V' and notes in Schedule 'J' form part of this Profit and Loss Account			

(*Continued*)

Exhibit 7.2 (*Continued*)

As per our report annexed

For and on behalf of the Board of Directors

For M/s S. Viswanathan
Chartered Accountants
Firm Registration No.: 004770S

V.C. Krishnan
Partner
(Membership No: 022167)
17, Bishop Wallers Avenue (West)
Mylapore, Chennai 600 004

Place: Chennai
Date: 24 May 2011

Krishnan Akhileswaran
Chief Financial Officer

S.M. Krishnan
General Manager – Project Finance and Company Secretary

Dr Prathap C. Reddy
Executive Chairman

Preetha Reddy
Managing Director

Suneeta Reddy
Executive Director – Finance

Exhibit 7.3 Schedules to Balance Sheet

				(₹ in million)
		31.03.2011		31.03.2010
SCHEDULE (A)				
Share Capital				
Authorized				
200,000,000 Equity Shares of ₹ 5 each (2009–10: 150,000,000 Equity Shares of ₹ 5 each)	1,000.00		750.00	
1,000,000 Preference Shares of ₹ 100 each (2009–10: 1,000,00 Preference Shares of ₹ 100 each)	100.00	1,100.00	100.00	850.00
Issued				
a) 125,243,728 Equity Shares of ₹ 5 each (2009–10: 124,102,736 Equity Shares of ₹ 5 each)		626.22		620.51
Subscribed and Paid up*				
b) 124,710,710 Equity Shares of ₹ 5 each fully paid up (2009–10: 123,569,718 Equity Shares of ₹ 5 each fully paid up)		623.55		617.85

* (a) Includes 1,836,596 Equity shares of ₹ 5 each fully paid up allotted on conversion of first 2 years interest on debentures, 20% on the face value of debentures and 41,624,462 Equity shares of ₹ 5 each fully paid up allotted to the shareholders of amalgamated companies for consideration other than cash

(b) Includes 4,159,860 Equity shares of ₹ 5 each fully paid up allotted on preferential basis during the year 2004–05

(c) Includes 3,062,800 (2009:10 9,326,000) underlying Equity shares of ₹ 5 each fully paid up, representing Global Depository Receipts issued during the year 2005–06 (Refer Clause 13 of Schedule 'J')

(d) Includes 2,079,930 Equity shares of ₹ 5 each fully paid up allotted during the year 2006–07 on conversion of Equity share warrants issued on preferential basis during the year 2005–06

(e) Includes 14,094,238 Equity shares of ₹ 5 each fully paid up were allotted to Apax Mauritius FDI One Limited during the year 2007–08 on preferential basis

(f) Includes 3,100,000 Equity shares of ₹ 5 each fully paid up allotted during the year 2008–09 on conversion of Equity share warrants issued on preferential basis during the year 2006–07

(g) Includes 3,098,314 Equity shares of ₹ 5 each fully paid up allotted during the year 2009–10 on conversion of Equity share warrants issued on preferential basis during the year 2007–08

(h) Includes 1,140,992 Equity shares of ₹ 5 each fully paid up allotted during the year 2010–11 on conversion of FCCBs amounting US $ 7,500,000 issued to International Finance Corporation (IFC), Washington.

Equity shares of face value of ₹ 10 each subdivided into two shares of ₹ 5 each on 3 September 2010. The number of equity shares allotted prior to 3 September 2010 are adjusted to face value of ₹ 5 per share.

(*Continued*)

Exhibit 7.3 (*Continued*)

				(₹ in million)
		31.03.2011		**31.03.2010**
SCHEDULE (B)				
Reserves and Surplus				
A. Capital Reserve				
(1) Capital reserve				
(2) Profit on forfeited shares		17.85		17.85
B. Capital Redemption Reserve		0.41		0.41
C. Securities Premium Account		60.02		60.02
Balance as per last Balance sheet	10,490.73		9,735.22	
Add: Premium received during the year[#]	339.45		–	
Add: Premium received from Promoters' issue	–	10,830.18	755.51	10,490.73
D. General Reserve				
Balance as per last balance sheet	2,749.03		1,999.03	
Add: Transfer during the year	1,000.00		750.00	
		3,749.03		2,749.03
E. Other Reserves				
Investment allowance reserve		7.63		7.63
Foreign exchange fluctuation reserve		0.19		0.19
Debenture redemption reserve		100.00		–
Profit and Loss Account		1,647.72		1,474.07
Total		**16,413.03**		**14,799.93**

[#]Refer Clause 8 of Schedule 'J'

SCHEDULE (C)				
Secured Loans				
A. Non-convertible Debentures				
(i) 10.3% Debentures		1,000.00		–
B. Loans and Advances from Banks				
(i) Cash credit		12.26		–
(ii) Indian Bank	609.52		952.38	
(iii) Bank of India	761.90		904.76	
(iv) Canara Bank	1,503.60	2,875.02	2,160.00	4,017.14
C. Other Loans and Advances				
IFC loan (External Commercial Borrowings)		1,608.79		697.16
Total		**5,496.07**		**4,714.30**

Refer clause 7 of Schedule 'J' for details and security.
Amount repayable within one year ₹642.12 million
(Previous year ₹642.12 million) excluding Cash Credit.

SCHEDULE (D)				
Unsecured Loans		579.16		507.52
(i) Fixed deposits				
(ii) Short term loans and advances HDFC		1,000.00		1,000.00
(iii) Other loans and advances				
Foreign currency convertible bonds		334.88		678.05
Total		**1,914.04**		**2,185.57**

Exhibit 7.3 (*Continued*)

				(₹ in million)
	31.03.2011		31.03.2010	
SCHEDULE (E)				
Current Liabilities and Provisions				
A. Current Liabilities				
1. Acceptances		358.40		302.35
2. Sundry Creditors*				
(i) Total outstanding dues of micro enterprises and small enterprises	48.76		153.26	
(ii) Total outstanding dues of creditors other than micro enterprises and small enterprises	1,635.48		1,627.81	
(a) For goods	1,109.04		968.24	
(b) For expenses	201.13		448.71	
(c) For capital goods	125.43		171.90	
(d) For others	248.63	1,684.24	192.21	1,781.07
3. Advances				
(a) Inpatient deposits	100.99		97.79	
(b) Rent	48.68		35.26	
(c) Others	1.59	151.26	13.60	146.66
4. Investor Education and Production Fund shall be credited by the following (Not due)				
(a) Unclaimed dividend		18.28		16.36
(b) Unclaimed deposits		–		3.15
5. Other Liabilities				
(a) Tax deducted at source	86.51		77.73	
(b) Retention money on capital contracts	0.96		1.38	
(c) Outstanding expenses	291.91	379.38	254.16	333.27
6. Interest accrued but not due		66.51		46.98
		2,658.07		2,629.84
B) Provisions				
7. For Taxation	2,083.90		2,050.95	
8. For Dividend				
(i) Equity shares	467.67		432.49	
9. Bonus	140.51		115.18	
		2,692.08		2,598.62
Total of Current Liabilities and Provisions		**5,350.15**		**5,228.46**

*Refer Clause 35 of Schedule 'J'

(*Continued*)

Exhibit 7.3 (*Continued*)

SCHEDULE (F)
Fixed Assets (₹ in million)

Sr. No.	Name of the Assets	Gross Block				Depreciation/Amortization				Net Block	
		As at 01.04.2010	Additions	Deletions	As at 31.03.2011	As at 01.04.2010	For the year		As at 31.03.2011	As at 31.03.2011	As at 31.03.2010
							Additions	Deletions			
	Tangible Assets										
1	Land	1,082.00	9.58	–	1,091.57	–	–	–	–	1,091.57	1,082.00
2	Buildings	2,568.84	382.92	13.37	2,938.40	261.19	38.60	0.22	299.57	2,638.83	2,307.65
3	Leasehold Building*	363.25	77.91	105.23	335.93	70.99	44.25	0.98	114.25	221.68	292.27
4	Medical Equipment and Surgical Instruments	5,057.24	904.15	39.75	5,921.63	1,845.24	349.62	16.52	2,178.34	3,743.30	3,212.00
5	Electrical Installations and Generators	875.12	139.37	4.76	1,009.73	257.10	36.82	2.86	291.06	718.67	618.01
6	Airconditioning Plant and Airconditioners	347.28	94.08	6.98	434.37	92.06	26.40	0.44	118.02	316.35	255.22
7	Office Equipment	660.53	134.90	3.67	791.76	303.82	83.08	1.06	385.84	405.92	356.71
8	Furniture and Fixtures	1,269.29	247.66	39.73	1,477.22	355.96	93.05	4.22	444.79	1,032.43	913.33
9	Fire Fighting Equipment	32.73	1.27	–	34.00	4.76	0.81	–	5.58	28.42	27.97
10	Boilers	1.87	–	–	1.87	1.00	–	–	1.00	0.87	0.87
11	Kitchen Equipment	26.04	6.31	–	32.35	8.56	0.21	–	8.77	23.58	17.47
12	Refrigerators	27.80	3.33	0.31	30.82	6.09	0.94	0.06	6.97	23.85	21.71
13	Vehicles	215.65	90.16	8.07	297.73	82.18	20.94	3.53	99.59	198.15	133.47
14	Wind Electric Generator	26.85	–	–	26.85	25.57	1.28	–	26.85	–	1.28
	Intangible Assets										
15	Computer Software	0.63	20.09	–	20.72	0.22	6.59	–	6.81	13.90	0.41
	Total	**12,555.11**	**2,111.71**	**221.87**	**14,444.95**	**3,314.74**	**702.58**	**29.88**	**3,987.44**	**10,457.51**	**9,240.37**
	Previous year	**9,406.67**	**3,220.39**	**71.95**	**12,555.11**	**2,779.92**	**543.06**	**8.24**	**3,314.74**	**9,240.37**	
	Capital work-in-Progress (Includes capital advances)**									3,523.96	2,734.12
	Capital Work-in-Progress (Previous year)									2,734.12	

* Refer clause 1 (D) (v) in Schedule 'J'.

** Refer clause 1 (F) (b) in Schedule 'J'.

Exhibit 7.3 (*Continued*)

				(₹ in million)
	31.03.2011		31.03.2010	
SCHEDULE (H)				
Current Assets, Loans and Advances				
A. Current Assets				
1. Inventories (at cost)**				
(i) Medicines	1,231.57		1,059.83	
(ii) Stores, spares	49.36		60.93	
(iii) Lab materials	24.72		23.95	
(iv) Surgical instruments	127.26		125.45	
(v) Other consumables	72.30	1,505.21	73.28	1,343.44
(As taken, certified, and valued by management)				
**Refer clause 1(B) of Schedule 'J'				
2. Sundry Debtors				
Refer clause 22 of Schedule 'J'				
(a) Debtors outstanding for a period exceeding six months	915.31		417.86	
Less: Provision for bad debts	24.95	890.36	13.49	404.38
(b) Other debts		1,806.07		1,650.96
3. Cash and Bank Balances				
(a) Cash balance on hand	47.39		33.29	
(b) Bank balance				
(i) With scheduled banks				
(a) Current account	969.45		1,715.51	
(b) On deposit account	396.92	1,413.76	1,106.78	2,855.58
Refer clause 7(G) in schedule 'J'				
B. Loans and Advances				
4. Loans				
(i) To Subsidiary				
(a) Imperial Hospital and Research Centre Ltd		234.00		214.00
C/f		5,849.40		6,468.36
B/f		5,849.40		6,468.36
5. Advances				
Subsidiaries				
(a) Unique Home Healthcare Limited	–		0.05	
(b) Imperial Hospital and Research Centre Ltd	62.80		35.99	
(c) AB Medical Center Limited	–		1.47	
(d) Samudra Healthcare Enterprises Ltd	28.89		14.72	
(e) Apollo Hospitals (UK) Limited	0.86		0.32	
(f) Pinakini Hospitals Limited	25.18		9.66	
(g) Apollo Health and Lifestyle Limited	4.47		0.97	
(h) Apollo Cosmetic Surgical Centre Pvt. Ltd	4.69		–	
(i) Alliance Dental Care Private Limited	6.60		1.58	

(*Continued*)

Exhibit 7.3 (*Continued*)

	(₹ in million)			
	31.03.2011		31.03.2010	
Others				
(a) For capital items	175.92		202.37	
(b) To suppliers	380.94		124.32	
(c) Other advances	1,362.59		1,336.36	
(d) Staff advances	33.61	2,086.56	37.97	1,765.78
6. Advance tax		1,579.28		1,750.64
7. Deposits				
(a) With government	56.38		50.54	
(b) With others	652.52	708.90	580.16	630.70
8. Prepaid Expenses		79.70		64.03
9. Rent Receivables		2.48		4.33
10. Service Charges Receivables		–		2.83
11. Tax Deducted at Source		919.48		689.52
12. Interest Receivable		93.48		40.18
13. Franchise Fees Receivable		11.10		6.57
14. Royalty Receivable		–		2.14
Total of Current Assets, Loans and Advances (A + B)		**11,330.38**		**11,425.08**
SCHEDULE (I)				
Miscellaneous Expenditure				
(To the extent not written off or adjusted)				
(a) Deferred Revenue Expenditure		–		0.12
Total		**Nil**		**0.12**

Exhibit 7.4 Schedules to Profit and Loss Account

	(₹ in million)	
	31.03.2011	31.03.2010
SCHEDULE - (I)		
Other Income		
(a) Interest earned (TDS ₹11.08 million: 2009–10 ₹11.55 million)	110.89	115.47
(b) Dividend		
(i) From current investment	18.57	94.34
(ii) From long term investment	30.79	25.81
(c) Income from Treasury operations	11.77	31.35
(d) Profit on sale of investment	0.03	62.09
Current Investment		
(e) Profit on sale of asset	0.13	0.60
(f) Foreign exchange gain	41.52	–
Total	**213.70**	**329.66**

Exhibit 7.4 (*Continued*)

		31.03.2011		31.03.2010
				(₹ in million)
SCHEDULE - (II)				
Operative Expenses				
Materials Consumed				
(a) Opening stock	1,343.44		1,065.57	
ADD:				
Purchases	12,425.33		9,763.52	
Customs duty	0.31		1.39	
Freight charges	11.85		17.32	
	13,780.93		10,847.81	
LESS: Closing stock	1,505.21	12,275.73	1,343.44	9,504.37
(b) Power and fuel		378.60		302.29
(c) House keeping expenses		88.93		99.30
(d) Water charges		44.79		38.68
Total		**12,788.04**		**9,944.64**
SCHEDULE - (III)				
Payments to and Provisions for Employees				
(a) Salaries and wages		2,992.83		2,376.73
(b) Contribution to provident fund		149.44		132.29
(c) Employee state insurance		20.11		16.22
(d) Employee benefits		79.56		57.56
(e) Staff welfare expenses		177.33		155.47
(f) Staff education and training		12.22		10.37
(g) Bonus		140.51		115.18
Total		**3,572.00**		**2,863.81**
SCHEDULE - (IV)				
Administrative and Other Expenses				
(a) Rent		834.53		703.41
(b) Rates and taxes		53.12		49.56
(c) Printing and stationery		149.71		159.43
(d) Postage and telegram		24.55		23.30
(e) Insurance		31.17		28.86
(f) Directors sitting fees		2.06		1.64
(g) Advertisement, publicity and marketing		379.15		236.55
(h) Travelling and conveyance		208.79		165.11

(*Continued*)

Exhibit 7.4 (*Continued*)

				(₹ in million)
		31.03.2011		**31.03.2010**
(i) Subscriptions		9.08		7.95
(j) Security charges		65.43		49.66
(k) Legal and professional fees		222.58		149.49
(l) Continuing medical education and hospitality expenses		9.24		11.22
(m) Hiring charges		36.42		27.57
(n) Seminar expenses		4.19		2.33
(o) Telephone expenses		73.95		67.59
(p) Books and periodicals		7.35		6.93
(q) Miscellaneous expenses		71.81		69.06
(r) Bad debts written off		54.75		82.46
(s) Donations		13.62		4.05
(t) Provision for bad debts		14.24		7.89
(u) Repairs and maintenance				
(i) Equipment	198.15		199.76	
(ii) Building	114.25		125.94	
(iii) Vehicles	28.18		18.23	
(iv) Office maintenance and others	162.48	503.07	106.82	450.75
(v) Loss on sale of assets		31.59		20.09
(w) Royalty paid		1.26		1.56
(x) Outsourcing expenses		383.55		306.49
(y) Loss on sale of current investment		1.66		0.43
Total		**3,186.86**		**2,633.37**
SCHEDULE - (V)				
Financial Expenses				
(a) Interest on				
(i) Fixed loans	453.06		305.28	
(ii) Fixed deposits	51.14		29.79	
(iii) Debentures	14.96	519.16	–	335.07
(b) Bank charges		30.85		25.10
(c) Brokerage and commission		1.43		2.26
(d) Foreign exchange loss		35.88		15.05
Total		**587.32**		**377.47**

Exhibit 7.5 Cash Flow Statement for the Year Ended 31st March 2011

				(₹ in million)
		31.03.2011		**31.03.2010**
A. Cash Flow from operating activities				
Net profit before tax and extraordinary items		2,693.24		2,221.65
Adjustment for:				
Depreciation	702.58		543.06	
Loss on sale of sale of investment	1.66		0.43	
Profit on sale of asset	(0.13)		(0.60)	
Profit on sale of investment	(0.03)		(62.09)	
Loss on sale of asset	31.54		20.09	
interest paid	551.44		362.42	
Misc. Exp. written off	3.27		3.44	
Foreign exchange gain/loss	(5.64)		(7.15)	
Interest received	(110.89)		(115.47)	
Dividend received	(49.36)		(120.16)	
Income from Treasury operations	(11.77)		(31.35)	
Provision for bad debts	14.24		7.89	
Bad debts written off	54.75	1,181.71	82.46	682.98
Operating profit before working capital changes		3,874.95		2,904.64
Adjustment for:				
Trade or other receivables	(710.09)		(538.34)	
Inventories	(161.76)		(255.02)	
Trade payables	(40.77)		1,048.45	
Others	(357.56)	(1,270.18)	(628.05)	(372.96)
Cash generated from operations		2,604.77		2,531.68
Foreign exchange loss/gain		5.64		7.15
Taxes paid		(657.96)		(846.44)
Adjustments for Misc. Exp. written off		(3.15)		(3.10)
Net cash from operating activities		1,949.30		1,689.28
B. Cash flow from investing activities				
Purchase of fixed assets (Including capital work in progress)[#]		(2,901.55)		(3,581.87)
Sale of fixed assets		160.53		44.22
Purchase of investments		(3,641.83)		(881.18)
Investment in subsidiaries and joint ventures and associates		(243.92)		(2,280.47)

(Continued)

Exhibit 7.5 (*Continued*)

		(₹ in million)
	31.03.2011	**31.03.2010**
Sale of investments	2,540.87	4,618.24
Interest received	57.60	79.14
Dividend received	49.36	120.16
Cash flow before extraordinary item		
Net cash used in investing activities	(3,978.94)	(1,881.77)
C. Cash flow from financing activities		
Proceeds from issue of equity shares	–	
Proceeds from issue of securities premium	–	679.96
Proceeds from issue of equity share warrants	685.07	–
Proceeds from long term borrowings	1,911.62	1,375.20
Proceeds from short term borrowings	83.90	1,378.23
Repayment of finance/lease liabilities	(1,140.14)	(311.75)
Interest paid	(531.92)	(363.41)
Income from Treasurary operations	11.77	31.35
Dividend paid	432.49	(401.60)
D. Net cash from financing activities	587.82	2,401.92
Net increase in cash and cash equivalents (A + B + C)	(1,441.82)	2,209.42
Cash and cash equivalents (opening balance)	2,855.58	646.16
Cash and cash equivalents (Closing balance)	1,413.76	2,855.58
Component of cash and cash equivalents		
Cash on hand	47.39	33.29
Balance with banks		
1) Available with the company for day to day operations	1,348.09	2,802.78
2) Amount available in unclaimed dividend and unclaimed deposit payment accounts	18.28	19.51

Notes:

1. Previous year figures have been regrouped wherever necessary.
2. Figures in bracket represent outflow.

Purchase of Fixed Assets includes and Interest paid excludes ₹154,42 million (previous year – ₹198.68 million) of interest capitalized.

Exhibit 7.5 (*Continued*)

As per our report annexed		For and on behalf of the Board of Directors
For M/s S. Viswanathan Chartered Accountants Firm Registration No.: 004770S	**Krishnan Akhileswaran** Chief Financial Officer	**Dr Prathap C. Reddy** Executive Chairman
	S.M. Krishnan General Manager – Project Finance and Company Secretary	**Preetha Reddy** Managing Director
V.C.Krishnan Partner (Membership No: 022167) 17, Bishop Wallers Avenue (West) CIT Colony, Mylapore, Chennai 600 004		**Suneeta Reddy** Executive Director – Finance
Place: Chennai Date: 24 May 2011		

AUDITORS' CERTIFICATE

We have examined the attached Cash Flow Statement of Apollo Hospitals Enterprise Limited for the year ended 31 March 2011. The statement has been prepared by the company in accordance with the requirements of Clause 32 of the listing agreement with the Stock Exchanges and is based on and in agreement with corresponding Profit and Loss Account and the Balance Sheet of the company covered by our report of 24 May 2011 to the members of the company.

For M/s S. Viswanathan
Chartered Accountants
Firm Registration No.: 004770S

Place: Chennai
Date: 24 May 2011

V.C. Krishnan
Partner
Membership No.: 022167

Exhibit 7.6 Five Years Standalone Financial Performance at a Glance

(₹ in million)

Year Ended	31st Mar 11	31st Mar 10	31st Mar 09	31st Mar 08	31st Mar 07
Balance Sheet					
Sources					
Share capital	623.55	617.85	602.35	586.85	516.38
Preferential issue of equity share warrants	685.07	–	–	–	–
Reserve and surplus	16,413.02	14,799.93	13,106.20	11,793.51	7,016.90
Networth	17,721.64	15,417.66	13,708.11	12,377.30	7,525.48
Loans	7,410.10	6,899.86	4,494.82	3,056.35	1,441.80
Capital employed	25,131.74	22,317.52	18,202.93	15,433.65	8,967.28
Deferred tax liability	1,071.06	751.45	626.56	589.70	570.64
Applications					
Gross block	17,968.91	15,289.23	11,779.31	8,300.10	6,435.85
Accumulated depreciation	3,987.44	3,314.74	2,779.92	2,348.32	1,982.88
Net block	13,981.47	11,974.49	8,999.39	5,951.78	4,452.97
Investments	6,241.12	4,897.88	6,292.80	7,060.11	3,229.60
Current Assets, Loans and Advances					
Inventory	1,505.21	1,343.43	1,088.42	790.89	551.95
Debtors	2,696.43	2,055.34	1,607.35	1,261.59	978.92
Cash and bank	1,413.76	2,855.58	646.16	1,045.57	644.03
Loans and advances	5,714.98	5,170.72	3,693.22	2,721.10	1,847.08
(A)	11,330.38	11,425.07	7,035.16	5,819.15	4,021.98
Current Liabilities and Provisions					
Creditors	1,684.24	1,781.07	750.05	725.74	557.64
Other liabilities	973.83	839.95	776.96	677.20	696.94
Provisions	2,692.08	2,607.44	1,970.85	1,404.75	912.05
(B)	5,350.15	5,228.46	3,497.86	2,807.69	2,166.63
Net Current Assets (A – B)	5,980.23	6,196.61	3,537.30	3,011.46	1,855.35
Miscellaneous Expenditure	–	0.12	0.45	3.07	7.80
Key Indicators					
OPM%	16.93	16.90	16.38	17.54	16.71
NPM%	7.72	8.18	7.98	8.85	11.12
Collection growth %	26.61	25.56	28.72	27.85	25.10
OP growth (%)	30.16	29.72	20.27	14.15	21.82
Earnings Per Share (₹) (Basic)* Equity shares of face value of ₹5 each	14.66	12.31	9.90	9.31	9.82
ROI (PBIT/AV.CE)%	13.83	12.83	11.33	13.52	14.95
RONW %	10.97	10.43	9.09	10.22	9.84
Employee cost to collections %	15.18	15.40	14.93	14.65	14.21
Debt/Equity ratio	0.42	0.44	0.33	0.25	0.19

Exhibit 7.6 *(Continued)*

(₹ in million)

Year Ended	31st Mar 11		31st Mar 10		31st Mar 09		31st Mar 08		31st Mar 07	
		%		%		%		%		%
Profit and Loss Account										
Income	23,533.32		18,587.45		14,803.50		11,500.66		8,995.15	
Operative expenses	12,788.04	54.34	9,944.64	53.50	8,096.51	54.69	6,207.33	53.97	4,901.83	54.49
Salaries and wages	3,572.00	15.18	2,863.81	15.41	2,210.51	14.93	1,684.82	14.65	1,278.70	14.21
Administrative expenses	3,186.86	13.54	2,633.37	14.17	2,065.74	13.95	1,582.37	13.76	1,297.76	14.43
Other expenses	3.27	0.01	3.43	0.02	5.81	0.04	8.72	0.08	13.68	0.15
Operating profit	3,983.14	16.93	3,145.63	16.92	2,424.94	16.38	2,017.41	17.54	1,503.48	16.71
Financial expenses	587.32	2.50	377.47	2.03	223.16	1.51	198.98	1.73	164.24	1.83
Depreciation	702.58	2.99	543.06	2.92	439.20	2.97	367.46	3.19	308.01	3.42
Provision for loss on investment					–	–	–	–	–	–
Extraordinary items			–	–	40.19	0.27	–	–	325.07	3.61
PBT	2,693.24	11.44	2,221.65	11.95	1,722.39	11.63	1,450.98	12.62	1,356.30	15.08
Tax - Current	570.00	2.42	577.12	3.10	479.79	3.24	381.12	3.31	288.16	3.20
Previous	(13.55)	(0.06)	–	–	–	–	13.27	0.12	33.48	0.37
Deferred	319.61	1.36	124.89	0.67	36.86	0.25	19.06	0.17	20.44	0.23
Fringe benefit tax			–	–	25.04	0.17	20.07	0.17	13.52	0.15
PAT	1,817.18	7.72	1,519.63	8.18	1,180.69	7.97	1,017.45	8.85	1,000.70	11.12
Dividend	467.67		432.49		401.60	–	352.11	–	258.18	–

CITY MUNICIPAL HOSPITAL[i,*] CASE 7.2

The head of the general surgery department at City Municipal Hospital was not happy with the current system of charging all major surgeries uniformly, since each type of surgery consumes different amounts of each surgical resource. He was wondering if it would be possible to get a handle on the costing of surgical procedures and thereby determine an appropriate pricing of surgical procedures. He has recently attended a one week course on Hospital Management conducted by a leading Institute of Management, where one of the professors mentioned Activity Based Costing as an alternative to traditional costing methodology.

The OT complex at the City Municipal Hospital worked as an independent unit, situated in a separate building with its own furniture, equipment and instruments. The three operating rooms in the OT complex for general surgery worked from 9.00 am to 5.00 pm Monday through Saturday. It had its own staff of surgeons, resident surgeons, anesthetists, resident anesthetists, and interns supported by nurses, technicians and attendants. It drew its requirement of consumables and disposables from the hospital medical stores every month.

The municipal hospital system grouped all the surgical procedures into two categories, namely, minor and major surgeries. Minor procedures included dressings, suturing, biopsies, and so on and accounted for almost fifty per cent of the total number of surgeries. Major surgeries covered all other procedures ranging from simple appendectomy to radical procedures such as pancreatechtomy.

The municipal hospital's policy was to charge a fixed price for all major surgeries, even though the wide range of major surgeries varied significantly in the consumption of hospital resources. A fixed price for all major procedures consciously ignored the distortions in the costing of surgical procedures arising from uneven consumption of resources.

Activity Based Costing

The above situation presented an ideal opportunity to explore the possibility of applying Activity Based Costing to get a better handle on the costing of surgical

---

* Reproduced with the permission of the copyright owner.

Prepared by Prof. K.V. Ramani, Indian Institute of Management, Ahmedabad and Dr Tushar Lakhia, Professor of Surgery, NHL Medical College, Ahmedabad.

Cases of the Indian Institute of Management, Ahmedabad, are prepared as a basis for classroom discussion. They are not designed to present illustrations of either correct or incorrect handling of administrative problems.

© 2009 by the Indian Institute of Management, Ahmedabad.

[i] This case study is based on the M.Phil Dissertation titled 'Costing of Surgical Operations Theatre Services' at Sheth LG Hospital, Ahmedabad, by Dr Lakhia TS under the supervision of Professors Rajesh Agarwal and K.V. Ramani of the Indian Institute of Management, Ahmedabad.

procedures. This required data on OT activities, resources used for surgical procedures and a detailed analysis of cost allocation based on cost drivers.

OT Activities

OT activities consisted of the following:

- OT complex preparation
- Pre-operative patient care
- Pre-operative preparation of patients
- Anesthesia
- Surgery
- Post operative patient care

Cost Drivers (Level 1)

In order to estimate the activity costs, Dr Tushar Lakhia, who has been performing surgeries for more than 20 years in the City Hospital OT complex, undertook a detailed data collection on all the procedures done for three months (Exhibit 7.7). The OT complex at the City Municipal Hospital performed about 200–250 surgeries every month. Major surgeries were performed in the morning hours (9.00 am to 1.00 pm) in all the three OTs. Minor procedures were done in the afternoon hours from 2.30 pm to 5 pm in two OTs. A total of 626 procedures were done during the study period of three months. OT costs for our three month study are given in Exhibit 7.8.

Pre- and post-operative care activities took about one hour during each shift in each OT/day. The pre-operative preparation of patients took an additional hour per shift per OT per day. Anesthesia and surgical procedures took about three hours in the morning shift and an hour and a half in the afternoon shift per OT per day.

Using the duration of each activity as the activity cost driver, OT costs were allotted to the above OT activities.

Cost Drivers (Level 2)

Identifying the cost drivers for allocating OT activity costs to OT procedures was not so easy. Each surgical procedure consumed different amounts of OT resources: staff, materials, and instruments. Staff costs were fixed, materials costs were variable, while the cost of instruments and equipment had to be estimated from their purchase costs and depreciation.

Staff Costs: OT had its own staff, staff costs were fixed irrespective of the nature of surgery.

Material Costs: The City Municipal Hospital followed the system of tray accounting to account for the consumption of materials. Based on the OT schedule for each day, the stores supervisor prepared two trays of materials for each surgery – an anesthesia material tray and a surgical material tray. Additional trays were prepared based on requirements. Each tray was prepared as per the needs of the surgeon and anesthetist; for example, anesthesia materials depended on the type of anesthesia given – local, spinal, general, and so on. Items were taken out of these trays during surgery, and the unused items in their respective trays were returned to the OT stores after surgery. The difference between the materials issued and materials returned was taken as the materials consumed and the cost of materials computed.

Dr Tushar Lakhia was wondering how to identify the utilization of resources by each activity for each procedure. In other words, what would be the level 2 cost drivers?

Exhibit 7.7 OT Data

Date: ....

OT Number: ....

OT Complex: Open time ....

OT Complex: Closed time ....

Procedure: Name, description: ....

Activities	Pre-op care patients: Start Time	
	Pre-op care patients: End Time	
	Pre-op preparation patients: Start Time	
	Pre-op preparation patients: End Time	
	Anesthesia: Start Time	
	Surgery: Start Time	
	Surgery: End Time	
	Anesthesia: End Time	
	Post Op Care patient: Start Time	
	Post Op Care patient: End Time	
Resources	Anesthetist: Name	
	Resident Anesthetist: Name	
	Surgeon: Name	
	Resident Surgeon: Name	
	Number of Support Staff	
	Materials used: Anesthesia	
	Materials used: Surgical	
	Materials used: Others (linen, gowns,...)	
	Instruments/Equipment: Sets	

Exhibit 7.8 OT Expenses Collected for Our Study (All Surgeries in Three Months)

Sr. No.	Expense Head	Activities Causally Related	Expenses in ₹
E1	Building	A1 to A6	97,416
E2	Furniture and fixtures	A1 to A6	3,895
E3	Electricity	A1 to A6	19,440
E4	Salary of support staff	A1 to A6	371,131
E5	Overheads of support departments	A1 to A6	83,780
E6	Linen, gowns, and so on laundry	A2 to A6	23,900
E7	Instruments and equipments	A3 to A6	34,970
E8	Central sterilization and supply department	A3 to A6	56,375
E9	OT Stores	A3 to A6	368,383
E10	Salary of surgeons and anesthetists	A3 to A6	409,762
Total			**1,469,052**

chapter 8

Hospital Human Resource Management

CHAPTER OUTLINE

CHAPTER OBJECTIVE

The main objective of this chapter is to apply the concepts of human resource management (discussed in detail in Chapter 4) to live case studies on three large hospitals.

CMC HOSPITAL, VELLORE (B)* CASE 8.1

The increasing load on doctors whose responsibilities included teaching and research in addition to patient care had been a matter of great concern to Dr Suranjan Bhattacharji, the Director of Christian Medical College (CMC) Hospital, Vellore. Post graduate teaching load was expected to go up following a decision by the Medical Council of India (MCI) to double the number of annual post graduate admissions from the academic year 2012–13. Under graduate teaching load would also increase as CMC has decided to increase its annual intake from 60 to 100 students for its MBBS programme from 2012–13. Dr Bhattacharji, therefore, wanted to explore the possibility of generating a formal schedule of activities for his doctors, which would also provide some flexibility and autonomy in their work schedule, without any compromise on service quality.

Dr Ida Scudder founded the Christian Medical College Hospital, Vellore, after she returned to India following her graduation from Cornell University Medical College, USA. The medical school which she established in 1918 as a medical college for women with a Licensed Medical Practitioner course became a full-fledged medical college offering MBBS degree for men and women in 1947.

By 2011, CMC had become a centre of excellence in medical and health education, with over 150 different post graduate courses in medical, nursing, and allied health disciplines in which nearly 2,000 students were enrolled. The CMC Hospital with a dedicated staff of over 8,000 which included 1,290 doctors and 2,480 nurses was involved in

(i) patient care,
(ii) teaching and training, and
(iii) research activities.

During the year 2010–11, the hospital handled a daily load of 5,000 outpatients, 2,000 inpatients, 25,000 laboratory tests, 1,500 radiology investigations, and 125 surgeries. In the same year, its teaching and training activities produced 60 MBBS doctors, 99 post graduate medical degree and diploma holders,

---

* Reproduced with the permission of the copyright owner.

Prepared by Professor K.V. Ramani, Indian Institute of Management, Ahmedabad and Dr Anand Zachariah, Christian Medical College, Vellore.

Cases of the Indian Institute of Management, Ahmedabad, are prepared as a basis for class discussion. They are not designed to present illustrations of either correct or incorrect handling of administrative problems.

© 2012 by the Indian Institute of Management, Ahmedabad.

240 nurses, and 243 allied medical and health professionals. Its research efforts led to 230 publications in academic journals, 270 internal research proposals, 108 external proposals and total internal research funds of ₹82.36 million.

Medical Council of India

Medical Council of India (MCI), the regulatory body for medical education in India, had laid down minimum standard requirements for medical colleges offering MBBS-Under Graduate (UG) programme, and Post Graduate (PG) degree/diploma programmes. UG Programme guidelines were for a given number of annual admissions. Non-clinical teaching in the first 18–24 months of the MBBS curriculum focused on Anatomy, Physiology, Biochemistry, Sociology, and Community Health. Clinical teaching which began in the second year focused on ENT, Ophthalmology, Community Health[i], Medicine, Surgery, Obstetrics and Gynecology, Pediatrics, Orthopedics, Dermatology, Psychiatry, Anesthesia, and Radiology.

As per MCI guidelines, each medical college was organized into clinical and non-clinical departments (see Exhibit 8.1 for the number of Doctors in Clinical Departments and Exhibit 8.2 for the number of Doctors in Non-Clinical Departments). Each clinical department was further divided into 'Units' for administrative convenience. The number of beds per unit and the minimum staff strength per unit for offering UG and PG programmes as per MCI guidelines are given in Annexure 1 and Annexure 2 respectively.

CMC admitted 60 students annually for its MBBS programme from a total of about 12,000 applications from all over India. In addition to the MBBS course, CMC admitted a total of 153 students per year for its various post graduate medical degree, diploma, and Fellowship programmes.

Each clinical department in CMC was given a certain amount of resources (beds, staff, equipment and so on) and was expected to

(i) provide patient care (outpatient and inpatient care) and outreach services,
(ii) offer teaching under graduate MBBS programme and post graduate diploma and degree programmes MD/MS, DM/M.Ch., and
(iii) excel in research contributions through publications in international journals.

---

[i] Community Health training occurred in three phases in the pre-clinical, clinical phase, and during the internship.

Department of General Medicine

The department of general medicine was one of the busiest departments at the hospital. It had a staff composition of 24 faculty, 32 post graduate students, and about 100 nurses. As a teaching hospital, its doctors were called Professors, Associate Professors, Assistant Professors, Registrars, Senior Residents, and Junior Residents, and Interns. Professors and Associate Professors were also known as Senior Consultants, while Assistant Professors were known as Junior consultants. PG students were called Registrars and Junior residents. Senior residents were those who had just completed PG training in the previous three years and were not yet full teaching faculty.

The weekly activities of a doctor in the general medicine department included the following:

1. OPD Consultation

Each unit had two OPD days from 8.00 am to 5.00 pm. The total OPD load was around 300–350 general patients and 100–150 private patients per day.

2. Inpatient Care

Split Rounds: Each unit had 40 general beds and 10–15 private patients. Each unit was divided into three teams, each of which looked after their male, female and private patients separately. Each team had one consultant, one or more PG registrars and one or more interns. Each team did morning and evening rounds every day. The consultant conducted the morning rounds while the PG registrar did the evening rounds. These rounds were known as split rounds, as the unit was split into three teams.

Grand Round: In grand rounds, the entire unit visited all its patients as a single team. Grand rounds offered excellent opportunities for the MBBS students to review many more cases and thereby add immense value to teaching and decision making in relation to complex cases.

Ward Work: Ward work included patients who were admitted for investigations, seriously ill patients in emergency, Intensive Care Unit (ICU) or semi-ICU. Interns, PGs and faculty took care of the patient on hour-to-hour and day-to-day basis from admission to discharge along with other team members (nurses, physiotherapist and so on). Various procedures and other ward work were also part of inpatient care. The registrars along with their interns ensured that their patients' medical needs were well taken care of, and proper documentations were maintained. Usually, ward work and procedures reached their peak after the grand and split rounds, when fresh investigations and/or medicines were ordered. During the initial admission the focus was on history, examination, and ordering investigations. In the middle phase, focus was on further investigation, assessing the progress of treatment, and on-going analysis of the problem. At the end, ward activities focused on preparation of the discharge summary, explaining the disease and treatment to the patient and family, followed by planning for discharge.

3. Outreach Services

Units had outreach activities such as clinic in secondary care hospitals or linkage to mission hospitals including telemedicine link, visits to mission hospitals, faculty exchange, joint projects and so on. This was highly encouraged in CMC so as to expose the students to the health care needs of the rural population.

4. Teaching

UG Teaching: UG teaching involved formal classroom teaching as well as bedside teaching during OPD consultation and ward visits (Split rounds and Grand rounds). Under graduate clinics were conducted every day in the morning, Monday through Saturday. Formal classroom theoretical lectures were usually scheduled in the afternoons.

PG Teaching: PG teaching also involved formal classroom teaching and bed-side teachings. Formal classroom theoretical lectures were scheduled only in the afternoons. PG students also took part in academic meetings, such as journal clubs, seminars, clinical meeting presentations, and so on.

5. Academic Meetings

Academic meetings included journal club, seminar, special sessions, and death audit. Journal club met once a week usually in the morning, where a journal article was presented by a PG student and discussed jointly by the entire unit. Weekly seminars were held every week where a PG student made a detailed presentation on a particular topic. Clinical meetings were held once a week, where PGs presented interesting cases. Usually cases of four to six patients were presented. This was a forum for much debate and discussion. Once in a month Clinico-pathologic conferences were held, where a faculty presented a chosen and complex case prepared by another unit. The faculty was not aware of the diagnosis and had to make a final diagnosis and investigation plan. This was a popular and challenging teaching exercise.

6. Death Audit

All death cases over the previous one month were discussed in detail focussing on lessons, errors both of omission and commission. The reports were sent to the Medical Superintendent's office.

7. Research

Research was an essential component of a faculty member's work. Faculty members had to undergo research methodology and research ethics workshop. Faculty also supervised PG thesis (two per Professor and one per Associate Professor). Each unit had special areas of clinical work (example Infectious Disease and Clinical Toxicology for Medicine I, Clinical Epidemiology for Medicine II). The research in these units focussed on these areas and thereby helped in improving the quality of patient care. Recent studies from CMC showed that the most common cause of epilepsy in India was CNS parasitic disease (neurocysticercosis). Follow up studies of patients receiving anti-retroviral therapy on the publicly funded ART programme at CMC showed high rates of compliance and survival. Each faculty member presented papers at one to two research conferences every year.

8. External Examiners

Every year, about three to four faculty members were external examiners in theory and practical examinations in UG and PG courses. This was considered a part of teaching activity.

9. Administration

The unit head was in-charge of all the unit clinical activities, such as (OPD, inpatient, emergency), teaching activities (UG and PG), research, faculty development, financial aspects, and office work. The Head of Department coordinated across all the units in relation to clinical work, training, and research.

Exhibit 8.3 gives the teaching staff composition of each medicine unit for UG and PG teaching. Load on MBBS teaching is given in Exhibit 8.4. During half day postings, total duration of classroom teaching was six hours (one hour per day for six days), and clinical teaching was 12 hours (two hours per day for six days). During whole day postings, total duration of classroom teaching was 12 hours (two hours per day for six days) and clinical teaching was 22 hours (four hours per day for five days, and two hours on Saturdays).

As far as PG teaching was concerned, each unit had 12 MD students, four students in each year of the PG programme.

Exhibit 8.5 provides estimates of the total weekly load on teaching, research and patient care for a General Medicine consultant/staff.

Conclusion

Dr Bhattacharji said,

> We have a new module on out-reach services. This is in addition to the traditional modules on Teaching, Clinical work, and Research. We are placing more emphasis on out-reach services so that faculty will not be inward looking, instead they will constantly be aware of the need of the real *Bharath* (India) and respond to it. We send our staff and students to rural areas and require them to be involved in the community. Our real purpose is to serve those who cannot come to us! It was this that compelled Dr Ida to start roadside clinics ....

Dr Bhattacharji needed a rough schedule to capture the current workload on the medicine department faculty on patient care, teaching, research and so on.

Exhibit 8.1 Number of Doctors in Clinical Departments

Department	No. of Faculty
Accident and Emergency Services	02
Anesthesiology	42
Cardio vascular and Thoracic Surgery	09
Clinical Hematology	08
Clinical Immunology and Rheumatology	07
Cardiology	18
Community Medicine	15
Dental Surgery	10
Dermatology, Venerology and Leprosy	09
Development Pediatrics	09
Distance Education	03
Endocrine Surgery	04
Endocrinology	06
Family Medicine	10
Genitor-urinary Surgery	14
General Medicine	34
Geriatrics	04
General Surgery	24
Hand and Leprosy Reconstructive Surgery	05
Hepatology	05
Hepato Pancreato Billary Surgery	05
Medical Gastroenterology	08
Medical Genetics	02
Medical Oncology	03
Neonatology	11
Nephrology	09
Neurology	
Neurosurgery	13
Obstetrics and Gynecology	23
Ophthalmology	21
OTO – Rhino – Laryngology, Speech and Hearing	31
Pediatric Surgery	09
Pediatrics	32
Palliative Care Unit	04
Physical Medicine and Rehabilitation	15
Plastic Surgery and Reconstructive Surgery	04
Psychiatry	34
Pulmonary Medicine	10
Radiation Therapy	17
Radio-diagnosis	35
Reproductive Medicine	05
Vascular Surgery	04
Total	**533**

Source: Hospital Records.

Exhibit 8.2 Number of Doctors in Non-clinical Departments

Non-clinical Departments	No. of Faculty
Anatomy	08
Biochemistry	05
Clinical Biochemistry	10
Bioengineering	01
Biostatistics	09
Cytogenetics Unit	01
Forensic Medicine	06
Microbiology	14
Nuclear Medicine	04
Pathology	29
Pharmacology and Clinical Pharmacology	09
Physiology	09
Transfusion Medicine and Immunohematology	11
Virology	06
Total	**122**

Source: Hospital Records.

Exhibit 8.3 Teaching Staff Composition for UG and PG Teaching (Department of General Medicine)

Doctors	Unit 1		Unit 2		Unit 3		Unit 4		Total
Professors	3		1		2		1		7
Associate Professors	1		2		2		2		7
Assistant Professors	3		3		3		3		12
Tutor/Registrars									
Senior Residents	1		1		1		1		4
Junior Residents	6		6		6		6		24
Any Others (Interns??) and so on	5		5		5		5		20
Total									

Doctors teaching counted in both UG and PG.

Source: Hospital Records.

Exhibit 8.4 MBBS Teaching Load for a Medicine Unit

Unit	Year	Teaching Load per Week		
		Classroom Teaching Hrs/Week	Bed Side Teaching Hrs/Week	Total Teaching Hrs/Week
Unit 1	Year 2 (10 weeks)	6	12	
	Year 3 (4 weeks whole day)	6	22	
	Year 4 (6 weeks whole day and 4 weeks half day)	12	Whole day-22 Half day-12	
	Year 4 +			

Source: Hospital Records.

Exhibit 8.5 Estimated Weekly Work Load of a Doctor in Department of General Medicine

Main Activity	Activities	Prof. Hrs/Week	Assc. Prof. Hrs/Week	Asst. Prof. Hrs/ Week	....	....
OPD	Consultation which includes UG teach bedside PG teach bedside	15	15	15		
IPD (Grand Round)	Consultation which includes UG teach bedside PG teach bedside	5	5	5		
IPD (Split Round)	Consultation which includes UG teach bedside PG teach bedside	12	12	12		
Out-reach		Variable		11		
Formal Classroom Teaching	UG teaching PG teaching Non Formal (Dist Edu)	4	4	4		
Other Academic Activities	Journal Club (PG) Seminar (PG) Regular Staff Meet (PG) Special Staff Meet (PG) Death Audit	4	4	4		
Quality Circles		1	1	1		
External Exam duties		Variable				
Research		4	4	4		
Admin.		4	2	2		
Other Activities	1 2 3					

Note: Activities such as out-reach services, external exam duties do not happen every week. Work load on such activities are therefore mentioned as 'Variable'.
Source: Hospital Records.

ANNEXURE 1

Under Graduate Medical Education

Minimum Standard Requirements for Medical Colleges for 100 Admissions Annually

(Regulations 1999, Amended up to November 2010, Medical Council of India)

Teaching Hospital

Requirement of Beds and Units: Clinical Departments in the Hospital

The number of beds required for 100 admissions annually is 500.

They may be distributed for the purposes of clinical teaching as under, namely:

(i) **Medicine and Allied Specialities**

No. of beds and units required	Beds/units
1. General Medicine	120/4
2. Pediatrics	60/2
3. Tuberculosis and Respiratory Diseases	20/1
4. Dermatology, Venerealogy and Leprosy	10/1
5. Psychiatry	10/1
Total	220

(ii) **Surgery and Allied Specialities**

No. of beds and units required	Beds/units
1. General surgery	120/4
2. Department of Orthopedics	60/2
3. Department of Ophthalmology	20/1
4. Oto-Rhinolaryngology	20/1
Total	220

(iii) **Obstetrics and Gynecology**

No. of beds and units required	Beds/units
1. Obstetrics	30
2. Gynecology	30
Total	60/2

(iv) **Grand Total** **500**

Staff Requirements: Clinical Departments in the Hospital: The minimum staff complement of each unit shall consist of the following:

Professor/Reader	1
Lecturer	1
Senior Resident/Tutor/Registrar	1
Junior Residents	3 to 4

Department of General Medicine: The Number of units, beds and staff for each department shall be as follows:

(a) **General Medicine**

No. of units/beds:	4/120
Staff strength required	
Professor	1
Associate Professor/Reader	3
Assistant Professor/Lecturer	4
Tutor/Registrar/Senior Resident*	6**
Junior Residents	12

*With three years resident experience.

(b) **Tuberculosis and Respiratory Diseases**

No. of units/beds:	4/120
Staff strength required	
Professor	1
Associate Professor/Reader	
Assistant Professor/Lecturer	1
Tutor/Registrar/Senior Resident*	2**
Junior Residents	3

*With three years resident experience.

(c) **Dermatology Venereology and Leprosy**

No. of Units/beds:	1/10
Professor	1
Associate Professor/Reader	
Assistant Professor/Lecturer	1
Tutor/Registrar/Senior Resident*	2**
Junior Residents	3

*With three years resident experience.

(d) **Psychiatry**

Number of Units/beds:	1/10
Professor	1
Associate Professor/Reader	
Assistant Professor/Lecturer	1
Tutor/Registrar/Senior Resident*	2**
Junior Residents	3

*With three years resident experience.

Source: www.mciindia.org.

ANNEXURE 2

Post Graduate Medical Education Regulations, 2000

(Amended up to February 2012, Medical Council of India)

General Conditions to Be Observed by Post Graduate Teaching Institutions

Post graduate Medical Education in broad specialities shall be of three years duration in the case of Degree course and two years in the case of Diploma course after MBBS and in the case of super specialities the duration shall be of three years after MD/MS with the exceptions wherever indicated.

Period of Training

The period of training for the award of various post graduate degrees or diplomas shall be as follows:

(a) **Doctor of Medicine (MD)/Master of Surgery (MS):** The period of training for obtaining these degrees shall be three completed years including the period of examination.

Provided that in the case of students possessing a recognized two-year post graduate diploma course in the same subject, the period of training, including the period of examination, shall be two year.

(b) **Doctor of Medicine (DM)/Master Chirurgiae (M.Ch.):** The period of training for obtaining these degrees shall be three completed years including the examination period.

(c) **Diplomas:** The period of training for obtaining a post graduate diploma shall be two completed years including the examination period.

(d) **Ph.D. (Doctor of Philosophy):** The period of training for Ph.D. shall be two years for candidates who possess MD/MS/PG/ diploma in three years for candidates with M.Sc. (medical subjects).

Staff: Faculty

A clinical department or its unit training candidates for Broad or Super Specialities, shall have a minimum of three fulltime faculty members belonging to the concerned disciplines of whom one shall be a Professor, one Associate Professor/ Reader and one Assistant Professor/Lecturer, possessing requisite qualification and teaching experience prescribed by the Medical Council of India.

Provided that the second or subsequent unit may be headed by an Associate Professor along with two Assistant Professors/Lecturers. Of these faculty members only those who possess a total of eight years teaching experience, of which at least five years teaching experience is as Assistant Professor gained after obtaining post graduate degree, shall be recognized as post graduate teachers.

A guide for the Ph.D. degree shall have not less than fifteen years teaching and research experience after obtaining his post graduate qualification and shall also have not less than 10 years post graduate teaching experience as a faculty member.

Bed Strength in Clinical Departments

A Department to be recognized for training of post graduate students, shall have at least 60 (Sixty) beds each of General Medicine, General Surgery, Obstetrics and Gynecology and 30(thirty) beds each for others specialities for Degree and Diploma courses, and 20 (twenty) beds each in case of Super Specialty courses.

Explanation: A unit shall consist of not less than 30 and more than 40 beds for Degree/Diploma courses and not less than 20 and more than 30 beds for Super Specialty courses respectively.

Number of Post Graduate Students to Be Admitted

The ratio of recognized post graduate teacher to the number of students to be admitted for the degree course where diploma is not prescribed shall be 1:2 for a Professor and 1:1 for other cadres in each unit per year subject to a maximum of 4 PG seats for the degree per unit per academic year provided 10 teaching beds are added to the prescribed bed-strength of 30 for the unit for broad specialities.

Source: http://www.mciindia.org.

AMC HOSPITALS* CASE 8.2

In 2001, the Ahmedabad Municipal Corporation (AMC) increased the number of fresh admissions for its Bachelor of Medicine, Bachelor of Surgery (MBBS) programme by 50 seats. This prompted the Dean of the NHL Medical College (under the administrative control of AMC) to reorganize the clinical departments in each of the three hospitals affiliated to NHL Medical College. As a result, certain clinical departments were asked to reduce the number of clinical units so as to comply with the Medical Council of India (MCI) norms on staffing. The hospital superintendents were concerned about the impact of reducing the number of clinical units on patient care. The Ahmedabad Municipal Commissioner was looking for a solution to resolve the dilemma between teaching and patient care arising from the increased intake of students for the MBBS programme.

The AMC administered three large general hospitals, namely: VS Hospital, SCL Hospital, and LG Hospital for providing tertiary healthcare services. These hospitals were attached to the NHL Medical College for MBBS and the KM School of Post Graduate Medicine and Research[ii].

NHL Medical College

The VS Hospital, established in 1931 with 120 beds, was the oldest municipal hospital in Ahmedabad. Over the last 80 years, it had grown into a large hospital with more than 1,200 beds offering many specialty and super-specialty services. It also served as a teaching hospital for graduate and post graduate studies. It housed the NHL Medical College for MBBS programme and the KM Institute for Post Graduate (PG) education. The LG hospital established in 1954 with 60 beds, and the SCL hospital established in 1958 as a maternity home had both transformed gradually into large general hospitals offering many specialty services. In 1965, both LG and SCL hospitals came under the NHL Medical College.

---

* Reproduced with the permission of the copyright owner.

Prepared by Professor K.V. Ramani, Indian Institute of Management, Ahmedabad and Dr Tushar Lakhia, Professor of Surgery, NHL Medical College.

Cases of the Indian Institute of Management, Ahmedabad, are prepared as a basis for class discussion. They are not designed to present illustrations of either correct or incorrect handling of administrative problems.

© 2003 by the Indian Institute of Management, Ahmedabad, Revised June 2012.

[ii] On registration of the Ahmedabad Medical Education Trust in 2008, the above medical education institutions have been brought under the administrative control of the Ahmedabad Medical Education Trust.

As teaching hospitals, VS, SCL, and LG hospitals were bound by the norms laid down by the Medical Council of India (MCI) regarding the staffing of hospital departments and resources for teaching and patient care. These norms were based on the number of annual student admissions for MBBS and MD courses (Annexure 1):

- **Minimum number of beds:** 500 beds for 100 annual admissions to MBBS, and 750 beds for 150 admissions to MBBS.
- **Patient care:** A maximum of 30 beds per clinical unit.
- **Number of consultants:** Each clinical unit to have at least two consultants for under graduate teaching, and three consultants for post graduate teaching.

So far AMC had been admitting 100 students into its MBBS programme every year with 1,000 beds at VS hospital, 450 beds at LG hospital, and 470 beds at SCL hospital. Exhibit 8.6 gives the number of beds in each clinical department and the number of clinical units in each department. Each clinical unit had two or three consultants and two PG students. Consultants were either full-time or part-time honorary. Honorary consultants were required to be available only in forenoons, while full-time consultants were present in the hospitals from 9 am to 5 pm on Mondays through Fridays, and from 9 am to 1 pm on Saturdays.

Reorganization of Clinical Departments

The additional 50 seats for MBBS were to be offered as paid seats with a certain number of seats reserved for NRI students on payment in US dollars. With the increased number of seats, the AMC hospitals had to comply with MCI norms. Also, the new MCI norms did not allow part-time honorary consultants in teaching hospitals.

The dean of NHL Medical College had to reorganize the clinical departments in each hospital in order to comply with the new MCI norms. He re-designated all part-time honorary consultants as full-time honorary consultants and hired new consultants to para-clinical departments such as pathology, physiology, PSM department, and so on to comply with the MCI norms. He also reduced the number of clinical units in each department so that each unit had three consultants to meet MCI norms. By reducing the number of clinical units there was no need to hire new consultants to the clinical departments. This step was taken to ensure that AMC did not face any additional financial burden. For illustration, the department of general surgery at LG hospital had 90 beds. It had six consultants (two fulltime and four honorary), four PGs, and two resident doctors. Before the reorganization, these consultants were allocated to three clinical units with 30 beds per unit. The reorganization of the clinical departments by the dean in order to comply with MCI norms, resulted in the general surgery department working with only two clinical units, each unit having three consultants. The reorganized set-up of each clinical department in each hospital is given in Exhibit 8.7.

The hospital superintendents of VS, SCL, and LG hospitals were worried about the impact of these organizational changes on patient care.

Exhibit 8.6 Number of Beds and Clinical Units: Before Reorganization

Clinical Department	VS		LG		SCL	
	No. of Beds	No. of Clinical Units	No. of Beds	No. of Clinical Units	No. of Beds	No. of Clinical Units
Medicine	180	6	90	3	90	3
Surgery	180	6	90	3	75	3
Gynec.	192	6	91	3	109	3
Pediatric	90	3	60	2	70	2
Ortho.	108	3	30	1	30	1
Eye	–	–	–	–	30	1
ENT	30	1	30	1	30	1
Total		**25**		**13**		**14**

Exhibit 8.7 Number of Beds and Clinical Units: After Reorganization

Clinical Department	VS		LG		SCL	
	No. of Beds	No. of Clinical Units	No. of Beds	No. of Clinical Units	No. of Beds	No. of Clinical Units
Medicine	180	4	90	2	90	2
Surgery	180	4	90	2	75	2
Gynec.	192	–	91	2	109	2
Pediatric	90	2	60	1	70	1
Ortho.	108	3	30	–	30	1
Eye	–	–	–	–	30	1
ENT	30	1	30	–	30	–
Total		**14**		**7**		**9**

ANNEXURE 1

Minimum Standard Requirements for Medical Colleges for 150 Admissions Annually

(Regulations 1999, Medical Council of India)

B. Teaching Hospital

B.1 General Remarks

B.1.1: All the teaching hospitals shall be under the academic, administrative and disciplinary control of the Dean/Principal of the medical college or medical institution.

B.1.9: *Clinical Departments in the Hospital: Requirement of Beds and Units:* The number of beds required for 150 admissions annually is 750. They may be distributed for the purposes of clinical teaching as under, namely:

(i) **Medicine and Allied Specialities**

No. of beds and units required	Beds/units
1. General Medicine	180/6
2. Pediatrics	90/3
3. Tuberculosis and Respiratory Diseases	30/1
4. Dermatology, Venerealogy and Leprosy	15/1
5. Psychiatry	15/1
Total	330 beds

Note:

1. There shall be well equipped and updated Intensive Care Unit (ICU), Intensive Coronary Care Unit (I.C.C.U.) Intensive Care Pediatric beds and preferably Intensive care in Tuberculosis and Respiratory Diseases.
2. Wherever possible, the facilities available in larger tuberculosis and chest diseases hospitals, infectious diseases hospitals and mental hospitals may be utilized for training in these specialities. However, if these hospitals are not under the total administrative control of the Medical College, the required beds in these specialities shall have to be provided in the attached teaching hospital itself.

(ii) **Surgery and Allied Specialities**

No. of beds and units required	Beds/units
1. General surgery	180/6
2. Department of Orthopedics	90/3
3. Department of Ophthalmology	30/1
4. Oto-Rhinolaryngology	30/1
Total	330 beds

Note: There shall be well-equipped and updated intensive Care Burn Unit and Surgical post operative critical care Unit.

(iii) **Obstetrics and Gynecology**

No. of beds and units required	Beds/units
1. Obstetrics	50
2. Gynecology	32
3. Postpartum	08
Total	90/3

(iv) **Grand Total** **750**

Note:

1. In case a super specialty is developed, it shall necessitate creation of extra beds. Along with additional staff over and above the minimum requirement stated here in above in accordance with the provisions of the post graduate Medical Education Regulations, 1971.
2. The teaching hospital may provide additional beds in any specialty depending upon their patients load.

Schedule-II: Staff Requirements

- Emphasis in medical education being on practical instruction and demonstration in small groups. The number of teachers must be as per provisions of this Schedule adequate to enable such instruction to be imparted effectively.
- The teaching staff of all departments of medical college shall be full-time.
- These regulations cover the minimum requirements of under graduate medical education.
- Additional teaching staff will be required in institutions where post graduate education is also imparted. Additional teaching staff will also be required where the work load involved in emergency care patient care, clinical laboratory work/field work is heavy or of a specialized nature.

- To ensure the exposure of under graduate students to experienced teachers, it is essential to provide adequate number of higher posts (Professors/ Readers) in every department of teaching.
- In department of anatomy, Physiology, Biochemistry, Pharmacology and Microbiology, non-medical teachers may be appointed to the extent of 30 per cent of the total number of posts in the department. A non-medical approved medical M.Sc. qualification shall be a sufficient qualification for appointment as lecturer in the subject concerned but for promotion to higher teaching post a candidate must require Ph.D. degree qualification or equivalent qualification. However, in the department of Biochemistry, non-medical teachers may be appointed to the extent of 50 per cent of the total number of posts in the department. In view of the paucity of teachers in non-clinical departments, relaxation upto the Head of the department may be given to non-medical persons in case a suitable medical teacher in the particular non-clinical specialty is not available for the said appointment in said department. However, all such appointments will be made only with the prior approval of the Medical Council of India. However, a non-medical person cannot be appointed as Director/Principal/Dean/Medical Superintendent or equivalent of an institution in any case. In the department of Community medicine, Statistician cum Lecturer in Statistics should possess M.A./M.Sc. qualification in that particular subject from a recognized university. These requirements are as per the Teacher Eligibility Qualification Regulations.
- Teacher in higher specialities like Cardiology, neurology, Neuro-Surgery shall not be counted against the complement of teachers required for under graduate medical education.

Department-wise Staff Requirements: Clinical Departments

1. General

   (i) Each department shall have a Head of the Department of the rank of full time Professor who shall have overall control of the Department.

   (ii) The Staffing pattern of the departments shall be organized on the basis of units.

   (iii) A unit shall have not more than 30 beds in its charge. However, in departments of Tuberculosis and respiratory diseases, Dermatology, Veneralogy and Leprosy, Psychiatry, Ophthalmology and ENT one unit shall be of MCI sanctioned strength for that specialty even if the total number of beds is less than 30.

(iv) The minimum staff complement of each unit shall consist of the following, namely:

(a)	Professor/Reader	1
(b)	Lecturer	1
(c)	Senior Resident/Tutor/Registrar	1
(d)	Junior Residents	3 to 4

In addition to the above staff, additional Senior Residents and Junior Residents shall be provided according to the load in Burn Ward ICU, emergency, ICCU, Nursery, Labour Room and in other critical/intensive care unit/units for providing services round the clock.

2. Department of General Medicine

The Number of units, beds and staff for each department shall be as follows:

(a) *General Medicine*

No. of units/beds: 6/180

Staff strength required

Professor	1
Reader	5
Lecturer	6
Tutor/Registrar/Senior Resident*	6
Junior Residents	18

*With three years resident experience.

3. Department of Pediatrics

No. of units/beds: 3/90

Staff strength required

Professor	1
Reader	3
Lecturer	2
Tutor/Registrar/Senior Resident*	3
Junior Residents	9

*With three years resident experience.

4. Department of General Surgery

No. of units/beds:	6/180
Staff strength required	
Professor	1
Reader	5
Lecturer	6
Tutor/Registrar/Senior Resident*	6
Junior Residents	18

*With three years resident experience.

5. Department of Orthopedics

No. of units/beds:	3/90
Staff strength required	
Professor	1
Reader	2
Lecturer	3
Tutor/Registrar/Senior Resident*	3
Junior Residents	9

*With three years resident experience.

6. Department of Obstetrics and Gynecology

No. of units/beds:	3/90
Staff strength required	
Professor	1
Reader	2
Lecturer	3
Tutor/Registrar/Senior Resident*	3
Junior Residents	9

*With three years resident experience.

Source: MCI web site.

BANGALORE BAPTIST HOSPITAL (A)* CASE 8.3

"By God's grace our hospital has grown from an 80 bed secondary care centre to a multi super specialty hospital over the years. We have been awarded the 'Excellence in Teaching' by the National Board. Our mission is to care for the marginalized and to this end we reach out to those in need through outreach programmes such as palliative care, community health, as well as address vulnerable groups like HIV/AIDS, mental health, and geriatric care. In response to the critical need for palliative care services in the city of Bangalore, the Palliative Care Division was started in January 1995 in partnership with the Wake Forest University Baptist Medical Center, North Carolina, USA." With these words, Dr Alexander Thomas, CEO Bangalore Baptist Hospital (Bangalore) initiated the discussions on case development.

Bangalore Baptist Hospital

Dr Jasper McPhail, the first Southern Baptist missionary appointed in India started the Bangalore Baptist Hospital Project, when he acquired fourteen acres of land in Hebbal, north Bangalore in the late 60s. The construction began in 1971, and on 15 January 1973, Bangalore Baptist Hospital (BBH) opened its doors to serve the community. The Governing Board of BBH consists of six members from the Christian Medical College, Vellore (CMC, Vellore), and steers the organization with policies from time to time.

BBH began as an 80-bed general hospital. Over the years, it grew into a large multi super specialty hospital, with 300 beds and 1000 staff. In the year 2011–12, the hospital handled 238,000 outpatients, 17,000 inpatients, 4,600 surgeries and 2,600 childbirths. BBH was accredited by the National Accreditation Board of Laboratories in April 2011 and the National Accreditation Board of Hospitals in July 2011. In the same year, BBH received the Best Teaching Award for its Diplomate of the National Board (DNB) Programme (Exhibit 8.8).

---

* Reproduced with the permission of the copyright owner.

Prepared by Professor K.V. Ramani, Indian Institute of Management, Ahmedabad, Professor Nagesh Rao, Director, Mudra Institute of Communication, Ahmedabad and Dr Ravi Livingston of Bangalore Baptist Hospital.

Cases of the Indian Institute of Management, Ahmedabad, are prepared as a basis for class discussion. They are not designed to present illustrations of either correct or incorrect handling of administrative problems.

© 2012 by the Indian Institute of Management, Ahmedabad.

The Palliative Care Unit

Palliative care addresses the problems of the incurable and terminally ill patients. It moves the emphasis to 'caring' when all hope of 'curing' has been lost. Key elements of palliative care include symptom and pain control, special nursing, specific palliative care round the clock, as well as psychological and emotional support for the patient and the family (Annexure 1).

The Palliative Care Unit at BBH was started in partnership with the Wake Forest University Baptist Medical Center (WFUBMC), Winston Salem, North Carolina, USA in January 1995, following the return of Dr Stanley Macaden after completion of his Fellowship in Palliative Care. The objective of setting up a palliative care unit was to fulfill the need of caring for persons with terminal or chronic illnesses. Most patients had an undignified and painful death. Patients and families had nowhere to go to fulfill their physical, emotional and spiritual needs. The Palliative Care unit was designed to improve the quality of life and ultimately facilitate peaceful death.

The Palliative care service at BBH was integrated with clinical departments. For example, a patient with breast cancer was initially evaluated by an oncologist and a surgeon. If the disease recurred and all possible treatments were vetted, the patient continued to be under the clinical department, but assisted by the palliative care team. As the disease progressed, the palliative care team took complete charge of such patients and continued to provide the necessary care at home. Bereavement visits and counseling were provided at the family's request. While cancer patients made up the largest number in palliative care, there were some geriatric and chronic patients as well.

Home care services started in April 1998 as a majority of patients preferred to stay at home with their families. BBH started providing palliative radiotherapy services, an important aspect of palliative care, with the setting up of 'The Edward G. Shaw Radiotherapy Unit' in January 2010.

Activities of the Palliative Care Unit

The Palliative Care Unit performed two sets of major activities, Patient Care and Training, and some other related activities.

Patient Care: The Palliative Care Unit team had one doctor, three nurses (called sisters) and a pastor cum counselor. Dr Ravi Livingston, head of the Palliative care unit, and his team were a devoted, passionate, committed and self-reflective group as reflected in the words and feelings of patients. It is summed up by one of the notes of a patient, 'They take care of us when all others have given up. They feel our sorrow, soothe our pain, and are there whenever we need them. They are, I think, angels on Earth.'

The team divided their work; the doctor and a sister took inpatient rounds along with the chaplain/counselor to address spiritual and psychological needs. The second sister cleared the previous day's bills (cash payment to the business office), pharmacy purchases, exchange of sterile dressing and so on. The third sister organized bags (drugs, chart and so on), made phone enquiries about patients and also planned their visits for the day. The team visited four to seven patients every day, Monday through Friday. One senior nurse stayed in the office to see new ward referrals, OPD referrals, dispense morphine and update all the registers. By 2004, the unit had served more than 2,500 patients (Cancer 74.8 per cent; Chronic medical disease 22.5 per cent and geriatric 2.6 per cent), made more than 8400 home visits and conducted about 3600 Palliative-Oncology Clinics. More than 94 per cent of deaths were peaceful and at home.

Training: BBH was the regional center for Indian Association of Palliative Care (IAPC). This course is meant for qualified (only allopathic) doctors and nurses. Hands-on training is an integral part of this course.

Other Activities: Other activities of the unit included supplying alfa air beds, wheel chair, and so on, handling emergency admission at BBH, bereavement visits, death certification, organ donation, embalming and so on.

Home Visits: A Typical Day for the Palliative Care Team

Mrs D'Souza: It was 10 am on a Tuesday morning. Dr Ravi from the Bangalore Baptist Hospital and his palliative care team—Sister Vinayashree, Sister Ruby and Pastor K.K. Abraham—reached their first patient's home. Mrs D'Souza was a 71 year-old patient with cancer of the cervix that had spread to her lungs. She lived with her two daughters, son and her daughter-in-law. Dr Ravi was greeted by Mrs D'Souza's daughter-in-law. As Mrs D'Souza was resting, Dr Ravi checked in with the family first. One of the daughters asked if there was any chance that her mother could be cured. Dr Ravi remained calm and silent and the daughter started crying. Sister Ruby sat next to the daughter and stroked her back. It soon became clear that the son and one of the daughters were having difficulty accepting their mother's prognosis while the other daughter and the daughter-in-law were able to understand the situation.

The family also had difficulty accepting the rapid decline in Mrs D'Souza's health. A week ago, she had been walking and talking. Now, she was mostly bedridden and not speaking much. She was in a lot of pain and cried through the night. Dr Ravi explained that it was time to think of morphine to relieve Mrs D'Souza's pain. The family reacted quite strongly, wondering if morphine was addictive and if their mother would be conscious. The doctor explained that morphine was not addictive and that Mrs D'Souza would still be able to sit up and talk. The doctor explained that the cancer could progress irrespective of treatment with palliative drugs or morphine.

Mrs D'Souza was upset initially, and refused to talk with Dr Ravi and the team, because she was forcefully taken to the hospital by her children. She felt that the doctor had not briefed her properly before conducting the pelvic examination. But her children assured the visiting BBH team that the doctor was gentle, kind and gave adequate time before the examination and also explained the procedures prior to it in detail.

Dr Ravi spent about fifteen minutes with Mrs D'Souza, mostly reassuring her and making sure she was not in pain. Mrs D'Souza had only two requests: to be independent and to die pain free.

Dr Ravi and his team got into their car to continue their day of home visits. They had committed to three more visits before the end of the day.

Mr Sriram: Mr Sriram, a 74 year old male had been diagnosed with locally advanced cholangio-carcinoma (cancer of bile ducts), and referred to BBH for further symptom management. The patient's son Sunder had briefed Dr Ravi about the history, diagnosis, and prognosis of his father, and pleaded with them not to tell his father about the advanced stage of cancer. The BBH palliative care team visited Mr Sriram's home. They were Kannada Brahmins, very well educated, from an upper middle-class family. As soon as the team parked in front of the house, Sunder came out and greeted the team, followed by the daughter-in-law a little later.

Sunder: Doctor, don't tell anything to my father. Just tell him that he will be alright in few days.

Dr Ravi: It may not be wise to say that considering his disease status. He can also deteriorate.

Sunder: Tell him that he will get better. He would be depressed if you reveal the truth.

Dr Ravi: Even if you don't tell him the truth, he would be pondering about his deteriorating health and would not trust the doctor or his family. He can become frustrated or sleepless.

Sunder: At least, not now.

With this background, the team went into the house. Mr Sriram was lying on a couch in the living room, in deep sleep. His wife and other relatives were sitting around. With their permission, Dr Ravi gently woke him up and introduced the BBH team to him. Sriram was not very comfortable, Dr Ravi started the conversation slowly.

Dr Ravi: Sir, how are you feeling today?

Sriram: I am feeling very tired, not able to walk to the toilet.

Dr Ravi: Are you feeling bad about it?

Sriram: Yes. There was no improvement at all with the treatment at the hospital. I went to the hospital walking and was brought out in a wheel chair.

Dr Ravi: Did the doctors tell your diagnosis? (Family members became very anxious at this question).

Sriram: They said that something was wrong with my liver.

Dr Ravi: Did they assure you of getting better?

Sriram: I don't know what they said. They were discussing with my family.

Dr Ravi: Do you want to know what it is? Or shall I discuss with your doctor and let you know?

The patient accepted by nodding his head.

Dr Ravi: Since we have come home, we will give you simple medications for your problems. Can you tell me all your problems?

Sriram: Very tired, unable to walk and I am finding it difficult to pass stools.

Dr Ravi: Do you have any pain, nausea, vomiting, and loss of appetite, itching or any other symptoms?

Sriram: There is no appetite but other than that I don't have any other symptoms.

Dr Ravi: Okay sir, take rest. I will prescribe simple medications. You can take them if you have any complaints. Do you want us to visit you, again?

Sriram: Okay.

Dr Ravi: In our next visit, do you want us to tell you about the disease?

Sriram: Yes, tell me.

Dr Ravi: The news could be good or bad, would you still like to know or do you want us to tell your family?

Sriram: (After hesitation) tell me.

After this conversation, Dr Ravi explained to the family members about the stage of the disease (Mr Sriram was deeply jaundiced, having flaps in the hand which predicted that he might slip in to coma, anytime), the possible complications, the necessity to tell the truth and handling emergencies. 'Life is not in our hands now. How long he will live or if he can get better and go back to normal activity or not – only God has control over his life.' Several family members started crying. The BBH team left after clarifying their doubts.

During the next visit a week later, the BBH team noticed that Mr Sriram's condition had deteriorated further. He was not in a condition to talk. The BBH team discussed and prepared the family about 'end of life care issues' and taught them how to administer subcutaneous injections for predictable distressing symptoms. Mr Sriram passed away peacefully at home few days later.

Mr Raja: Mr Raja, a 40 year old male, software engineer with his own business establishment, was diagnosed with locally advanced stomach cancer. He was a Tamil Brahmin, recently married, and staying in his own villa in a gated community. He had an elder sister, Lalitha and a brother Raghu, both married and settled independently in Bangalore. His parents had come down from Tamil Nadu to be with them.

The BBH team introduced themselves to Raja and his family, who were seated in the living room. Dr Ravi asked the family about their expectations. Lalitha replied that Raja would get better and get back to his old normal self. Raja smiled and asked the doctor to sit next to him.

Raja: Doctor, tell me, what is my condition now?

Dr Ravi: What did the oncologist tell you?

Raja: Doctor said that he has done everything, there is not much option. But, doctor, I have done whatever he had told me, whether it is investigation, CT scan or treatment on time, how then did the disease recur?

Dr Ravi: The tumor, sadly, is a high grade tumor. Though it responded well initially to chemotherapy, now the tumor is growing faster than what medicines can do. We cannot continue chemotherapy now, as it may cause more side effects. The benefit of treatment could be outweighed by the risks.

Raja: What is the remedy now? Doctor, I never smoked or had a drink till date. Though I traveled all over the world, I have continued to be a vegetarian. I used to go to gym and keep myself fit.

Lalitha: Doctor, he was disciplined in following the diet and exercised regularly. He used to have a perfect 'v' shaped body. Why should he suffer with this disease? His friends, in the corporate, used to drink, smoke and eat all junk food, but they are quite healthy.

Dr Ravi: Yes. I know .... it is difficult and frustrating .... (unable to finish)

Raja: How long am I going to live? How far has the disease progressed now?

Dr Ravi: I am seeing you for the first time, so I may not be able to answer your first question. Probably, after one or two visits, I might be able to make some assessments. Regarding, the second question, the possibilities are: there can be progressive weakness, leading to a bedridden state, (patient and family were intently listening, so I continued) loss of appetite and increasing pain. These can be controlled very effectively by medications. We will be teaching your caretaker how to manage these symptoms, if at all they occur.

Dr Ravi: Is it worrying you?

Raja: Yes. Everything is over now. My dream, married life. I planned and built this home, my dream house … (Silence …)

The patient was trying to control his tears. Dr Ravi went to him and gently touched his shoulder. The mother and the daughter invited us outside Raja's room to talk.

Lalitha: I don't want my brother to suffer. What about 'Euthanasia'? Will you allow him to die without pain?

Dr Ravi: I am sorry, it is not possible.

Lalitha: Why not?

Dr Ravi: It is against the law in our country.

Lalitha: You mean to say that cancer can kill him, but he can't choose to end his life?

Dr Ravi: Yes. As a doctor, I only have the right to treat him or in a situation like this to keep him comfortable.

Lalitha: But, what if we all agree for mercy killing and demand it?

Dr Ravi: Sorry, it is not legal in our country.

Lalitha: This is absolute rubbish (she became very agitated and angry). I will approach the higher authorities and policy makers to debate on this issue.

Finally the family agreed to go along with our plan. We taught the family how to manage the symptoms and left. Two days later the patient was brought to the casualty and admitted in the special private ward where he passed away.

Mr Chikappa: A 55 yr old male, Mr Chikappa, agriculturist by profession, from a village near Bangalore was referred by the department of surgery and oncology at BBH. He had been diagnosed in 2008 with stomach cancer and had undergone surgery and chemotherapy at Victoria Hospital. His wife worked in the fields for daily wages and was the sole bread winner. Chikappa had two elder daughters and a son. The first daughter was married and had a supportive son-in-law. The second daughter did her schooling, but stopped taking care of her father. His youngest son was in high school.

The palliative care team went to visit him at home. Chikappa and his second daughter were standing outside to receive the team. He had been bed ridden in the hospital and the BBH team was thrilled to see him walking about.

Dr Ravi: How are you feeling today?

Chikappa: Symptoms are better now. The medications you prescribed are working well.

The BBH team discussed his symptoms, family, income and other general issues. Dr Ravi had a mixed feeling, happy and also apprehensive, about the patient being better as he did not want them to mistake it for a cure.

Dr Ravi: Tell us briefly about your illness.

The patient told them his past and present medical history. He knew that he had a tumor in the stomach and was being treated for it. He was not fully aware of the possibility of recurrence. At least, he thought that he had been cured, like last time.

Dr Ravi What did the doctors at BBH tell you?

Chikappa: They said that your team (palliative care) will be visiting us at home.

Dr Ravi : What about further treatment at the hospital?

Chikappa: They said that your team will do everything at home.

Dr Ravi : Did they tell anything about the disease?

Chikappa: No. (Dr Ravi was not sure whether he was told and was in denial or wanted a new opinion).

Dr Ravi: Okay, I can explain to you, if you want.

Chikappa: Tell me.

Dr Ravi: What if the news is not good?

Chikappa: What to do? We have to face the truth.

Dr Ravi You got the symptoms due to recurrence of the disease.

Chikappa: I thought that the tumor was removed and treated.

Dr Ravi: Investigation shows that disease has become worse. That is the reason you had these symptoms. (Dr Ravi stopped and looked at the patient and his daughter. The Nurse had to console the daughter as she was moved to tears.) Are you feeling bad?

Chikappa: I didn't expect this … anyway nothing is in my hands now. God will look after everything. I thought of getting my daughter married and my son educated. Instead of me helping the family, I will be troubling them.

Dr Ravi: It is everybody's duty to help you. We can come home and take care of your symptoms. We can give the medications free ……. Even now, since you can walk around, you can arrange for your daughter's wedding.

Chikappa: She is not interested. She wants to study further.

Daughter: I want to achieve something in my life time.

Dr Ravi: If you are interested in nursing, you can join BBH Nursing School. Education, food and lodging everything can be sponsored. After completing the course, you have to honour a bond to serve BBH for a period of 2–3 years. You will get a decent salary and gain rich experience. (Nurses were continuing the discussion with her and explaining the benefits.)

Chikappa: Please come regularly and see me. I don't want to suffer. Nothing is in my hands, nothing. HE will look in to the needs.

Both father and daughter waved us good bye. The BBH team was astonished at their capacity to come to terms with this news. One weekend, the patient became very sick and the symptoms became uncontrollable (subcutaneous route not started yet), got admitted under surgery, and was diagnosed with outlet obstruction. Chikappa died after four days in the hospital. His daughter joined the BBH nursing school.

The Challenges

In April 2012, Dr Ravi decided to relocate to serve another missionary hospital. After considerable discussions, the BBH management moved its palliative care unit to the Community Health Department, following the highly successful model of North Kerala where palliative care services are managed by community networks (Annexure 1). The Community Health Department at BBH headed by Dr Gift Norman has been doing excellent work and impacting the communities (Annexure 2). Though much thought went into this decision, Dr Alex wanted to analyze the implications of this organizational change on the quality of palliative care services.

Exhibit 8.8 DNB Programme Award to BBH

No. NBE/AWARD/2012/...5013....

National Board of Examinations
New Delhi

NBE Award for Excellence in Teaching
DNB Programme (Accredited Hospital)

is presented to

Bangalore Baptist Hospital, Bengaluru

in recognition of the
outstanding contributions of the hospital
for successfully running DNB Programme.
This award is presented at the ceremony
held on February 1st, 2012
at New Delhi

Dr. Bipin Batra
Executive Director

Dr. K. Srinath Reddy
President

ANNEXURE 1

A Note on Palliative Care

The World Health Organization defines palliative care as an approach that improves the quality of life of patients and their families facing the problem associated with life-threatening illness, through the prevention and relief of suffering by means of early identification and impeccable assessment and treatment of pain and other problems, physical, psychological and spiritual.

Palliative care addresses the problems of the incurable and terminally ill patients. It moves the emphasis to 'caring' when all hope of 'curing' has been lost. Key elements of palliative care include symptom and pain control, special nursing, specific palliative care round the clock, as well as psychological and emotional support for the patient and the family.

The origin of palliative care services in India can be traced back to the National Cancer Control Programme of the Government of India in 1975 which was subsequently modified in 1984 to make pain relief one of the basic services to be delivered at the PHC level. The Medical Council of India recognized Palliative Medicine as a medical specialty only in 2011[iii], even though palliative care has been developing in India since the mid-1980s. Palliative care needs understanding, a certain degree of medical skill, and most importantly, compassion and psychological support. The philosophy is to value life until death, and to give the dying the dignity of breathing their last in surroundings of their choice. Despite palliative care services being in existence over 30 years, our national coverage remains under 20 per cent[iv]. There is no national policy for palliative care. The Government of Kerala is probably the only state government in India to declare a Palliative Care Policy in 2008[v]. The palliative care policy of the Government of Kerala recommends the inclusion of palliative care in each Primary Health Centre (PHC).

The state of Kerala alone has almost 65 per cent of all palliative care units in India, and spread throughout the state. The Palliative care movement in Kerala started with the establishment of the Pain and Palliative Care Society (PPCS)

[iii] Pallium India Newsletter, January 2011: *http://palliumindia.org/newsletetr/.*

[iv] Libby Sallnow, Suresh Kumar, Mathews Numpeli: 'Home based palliative Care in Kerala, India: the Neighborhood Network in Palliative Care', Invited review, Progress in Palliative Care, 2010, Vol 18, No. 1, pp 14–17.

[v] G.O (P) No. 109/2008/Health and Family Welfare Department, Thirivananthapuram, April 15, 2008.

at Kozhikode in 1993[vi], followed by the Palliative Care Society, Trissur, in 1997[vii]. Recently, there has been a move in Kerala to establish community-led Neighborhood Network in Palliative Care (NNPC) units. Well trained NNPC volunteers are formed into groups of 10–15 community volunteers who would work along with the professional healthcare team in providing home based palliative care services[viii]. Kerala's initiative in starting the Neighborhood Network Palliative Care (NNPC) units is very laudable.

> NNPC is an attempt to develop a sustainable 'community led' service capable of offering long term care and palliative care to the needy in the developing world. In this programme, volunteers in the local community are trained to identify problems of the chronically ill in their area and to intervene effectively with active support from a network of trained professionals. Essentially, NNPC aims to empower the local communities to look after the chronically ill and dying patients in that community. Almost 80 per cent of NNPC programme funds are mobilized locally through donations within the community.
>
> [Suresh Kumar 2005].

ANNEXURE 2

Community Health Department[ix]
Bangalore Baptist Hospital

Poverty, ignorance, food insecurity, poor living conditions, poor access to information and healthcare are major problems faced by most rural communities. 40 per cent of families who belong to the lower socio-economic strata are the most affected. The rural and urban poor are both wading through a myriad of health and socio-economic challenges that the Government programmes alone may not be able to meet.

[vi] Anil Paleri, Mathews Numpeli: 'The evolution of palliative care programmes in north Kerala', Indian Journal of Palliative Care, June 2005, Vol 11, pp 15–18.

[vii] Dr Rajagopal was then Professor of Anesthesiology, Medical College, Kozhikode. Currently he is the Chairman of Pallium India, Thiruvananthapuram.

[viii] Suresh Kumar, Mathews Numpeli: 'Neighbourhood network in palliative care', Indian Journal of Palliative Care, June 2005, Vol 11, pp 6–9.

[ix] Note prepared by Dr Norman Gift, Head of the Community Health Department, Bangalore Baptist Hospital, exclusively for this case study.

The Community Health Department (CHD) of Bangalore Baptist Hospital has come alongside the existing efforts of the government and private organizations to alleviate the effects of poor access to affordable quality healthcare, health information and barriers to social and economic development. The work of CHD focuses on the poor and the marginalized communities living in the rural and urban districts of Bangalore. The main strategies of the department include health promotion and disease prevention, strengthening government programs, improving access to primary healthcare services and community development.

Since 2010 CHD has initiated a consolidated effort through several programmes to address these issues in the rural and urban areas namely: three Primary Health Center areas of 50 villages in Devanahalli Taluk, covering a population of approximately 35,000. The urban area of coverage includes government defined geographical areas under the Revised National Tuberculosis Control Programme (RNTCP), National Leprosy Eradication Programme (NLEP) and an urban slum of DJ Halli (Ward 47). The programmes are serving individuals of all age groups particularly the children, women and the elderly.

Mother Teresa Hospital (MTH) the rural hospital is located in Kannamangalapalya in Devanahalli Taluk. MTH is the base hospital offering mainly primary care services as well as speciality services as per the needs of the community. Need based speciality clinics are in medicine, psychiatry, ophthalmology, orthopedics and others. The hospital has an average outpatient attendance of 300 every month. Other health services like mobile clinics and projects are also coordinated from MTH in the region. Early morning and evening mobile clinics reach out to 20 villages twice every month with an average total attendance of 600 a month. Camps, awareness programmes and follow-up of referrals for quality care are a regular feature of the programme. In order to address the changing health needs of Devanahalli, which have to do with the rapid urbanisation of the region with the Bangalore International Airport now stationed at Devanahalli, CHD is working on developing special health projects. These include a rural cardiovascular disease prevention model with field assistants as outreach workers, 'Restore—a de-addiction programme with the support of Alcoholics Anonymous' and 'Empower—a community based rehabilitation programme for persons with disability.

The urban slums of DJ halli have regular evening clinics and health worker assistance. Health promotion through IEC activities has benefitted the many SHGs, schools and so on. The needs of the community are learnt to be prevention of CVD, Obstetric services, education of hygienic living conditions and accessing available health services. To respond to the same, CHD is soon to work from an urban health centre in DJ halli.

Community development activities of CHD are vocational training (tailoring course, beautician course, training of the disabled for BPOs), strengthening of SHGs, strengthening of youth groups, income generation programmes and formation of health committee meetings.

CHD has engaged the Dip. NB Family Medicine students to draw from the enriching experience of programmes initiated by the Department. They receive adequate exposure from a range of activities of CHD like strategic planning sessions, awareness programmes, clinical exposure in the community, review meetings and above all impact them with the important perspective as viewing Family Medicine as a key contributor in the field of medical science. CHD also engages in the academic sessions and periodic appraisals. There is a constant effort to track best practices and innovative approaches to solve community related health issues. Thereby, stepping up the research element is the need of the hour. The department has worked keenly with the DNB students to identify relevant and appropriate research topics for their thesis. The students will be able to glean from the processes and programmes of CHD to enhance their research acumen.

The goal to provide the quality services at low costs for the marginalized populations is achieved through the CH team of 25, which ranges from Community Health Workers to doctors. The approaches and experiences of CHD are consistently reviewed to improve operations in order to develop models that can serve larger populations.

chapter 9

Hospital Materials Management

CHAPTER OUTLINE

CHAPTER OBJECTIVE

The main objective of this chapter is to apply the concepts of materials management (discussed in detail in Chapter 4) to live case studies on two large hospitals.

MPS HOSPITAL*

CASE 9.1

In February 2003, Dr Pankaj Shah, was appointed as the new Director of Gujarat Cancer Research Society, also known as MP Shah (MPS) Cancer Hospital. Having served as deputy director at MPS Hospital for a number of years, Dr Pankaj Shah was aware of the challenges facing the hospital. While the input costs for healthcare services were increasing over the years, financial support from the Government had not increased in the same proportion. Any shortfall in financial support from the Government put enormous constraints on variable expenses for patient care towards purchases of hospital supplies such as medicines and drugs, lab chemicals, X-ray films, and so on. A common complaint from Clinical Heads was the frequent shortfalls of certain critical items and long waiting periods for receipt of several regular items from stores. Dr Shah was worried about the adverse impact of the archaic purchase management systems on the quality of patient care.

MPS Cancer Hospital

The idea to create a Cancer Centre in Gujarat was conceived in 1960 by His Excellency, the then Governor of Gujarat Shri Mehdi Nawab Jung. The Chief Minister of the State Dr Jivraj Mehta blessed this activity by providing land in the Civil Hospital campus. A generous donation of UK £ 55,000 by the MP Shah Charitable Trust, London paved the way towards the foundation of MP Shah Cancer Hospital, and the hospital started functioning from 1966. To accelerate the development of MP Shah Cancer Hospital, the Gujarat Cancer and Research Institute (GCRI) was established in 1972 under a tri-partite agreement between the Gujarat Cancer Society, Government of Gujarat, and GCRI. Under this agreement, the state government agreed to provide 100 per cent grant-in-aid to institute's all recurring expenses, and to finance future developments as and when required.

By 2003 MPS Hospital had grown to a comprehensive cancer center with 650 beds and all modern diagnostic and treatment facilities. It was recognized by the Government of India as a Regional Cancer Centre. Certain important statistics of the hospital are given in Exhibit 9.1.

---

* Reproduced with the permission of the copyright owner.

Prepared by Professor K.V. Ramani, Indian Institute of Management, and Mr Narendrabhai Chawda, Chief Administrative Officer, Gujarat Cancer Research Institute, Ahmedabad.

Cases of the Indian Institute of Management, Ahmedabad, are prepared as a basis for class discussion. They are not designed to present illustrations of either correct or incorrect handling of administrative problems.

© 2004 by the Indian Institute of Management, Ahmedabad, Revised June 2012.

When Dr Shah took over as the director, the organizational structure was very centralized, with the Director taking almost all the decisions, even though he was assisted by a Deputy Director and an Administrative Officer.

The administrative officer was responsible for the routine day-to-day administration. However, the role of the Deputy Director was unclear; heads of departments reported to the director for all their requirements, bypassing the deputy director. After a series of consultations, the hospital adopted a new organizational structure. All the activities were grouped under three departments, namely, Medical, Surgical, and Research. Each of these departments was headed by a deputy director with clear responsibilities.

Dr Shah then took up the issues on hospital supplies. He asked each of his deputy directors to prepare detailed notes regarding the problems they faced with the central stores. Many heads of clinical departments reported the unsatisfactory levels of support from the administration, especially from Stores and Purchase. A common complaint from the clinical departmental heads was the frequent shortfalls of certain critical items and long waiting periods for receipt of several regular items from stores.

MPS Cancer Hospital dealt with about 2,000 items, classified into 11 groups, namely medicines and drugs, laboratories, X-ray units, surgical department, anesthetics, rehabilitation, lamps, linen, stationery, printing, and petty items. About 260 vendors supplied these items worth rupees six crores to the hospital every year.

Every year the hospital floated tenders in the month of March asking quotations for each item for its annual requirements, for the period June 1 to May 31. All the quotations received were tabulated manually and the vendors were selected on lowest price (L1 price) basis for each item quoted. This entire process took about three months. Once the vendors were selected, the purchase officer placed purchase orders (POs) with them as and when required.

MPS hospital had about 30 user departments. Each department raised an indent at the beginning of every month, based on subjective assessment of its monthly requirements. No proper registers were maintained by the user departments to monitor their consumption of items. As a result, each user department raised ad-hoc indents throughout the month, over and above the monthly indent raised at the beginning of the month.

More than 1,200 POs were placed every year. The PO quantity was decided by the purchase officer based on subjective assessment of the quantity on hand and quantity indented. In addition to regular purchases, emergency purchases as well as purchases of new medicines and drugs were common, mainly due to changes in the treatment protocol. The purchase department was also responsible for all the follow up actions with the vendors, checking/inspecting all the items received from the vendors, and approving the bills for payment.

The finance department, upon receiving the payment approvals, made the payments to the vendors. The hospital enjoyed a three-month credit period for all its purchases.

Dr Shah who had recently attended a one week program on hospital management, was keen to apply some of the learning from the program to improve the working of the purchase department. He invited one of the professors of the hospital management program to his hospital and discussed the issues in detail. Dr Shah gave the professor certain important statistics (Exhibit 9.2) and the income and expenditure statement for a few years (Exhibit 9.3). The administrative officer was put on job to provide additional data on the working of the stores and purchase departments along with certain details of expenditures (exhibits 9.4, 9.5, and 9.6) and some data on purchase of hospital supplies (Exhibit 9.7).

Dr Pankaj Shah is keenly awaiting the professor's report.

Exhibit 9.1 The Gujarat Cancer and Research Institute: General Statistics (Year 2006–2011)

No.	Item	Year 2006	Year 2007	Year 2008	Year 2009	Year 2010	Year 2011
1	Total new cases registered (cancer and Non-cancer)	20,381	21,488	22,684	24,482	25,115	25,905
	Adult cases				23,362	24,012	24,821
	Pediatric cases				1,120	1,103	1,084
2	Total number of outdoor patients visited	2,06,503	2,12,813	2,22,899	2,32,634	2,49,650	2,73,667
3	New admission during the year	20,027	20,187	20,794	21,026	21,781	20,855
4	Inpatient days	1,80,578	1,83,481	1,74,599	1,99,489	2,32,511	2,21,164
5	Average inpatient stay	9.02	9.09	8.4	9.48	10.7	10.6
6	Strength of beds	650	650	650	650	650	650
7	Death during the year	1,008	1,041	1,227	1,265	1,186	1,332
8	Hematological investigation	6,32,159	7,21,675	7,58,305	6,39,691	6,38,360	7,04,076
9	Biochemical investigations	4,25,638	4,72,793	5,14,781	5,40,366	6,19,688	6,25,148
10	Bacteriology investigation including seriology	7,006	7,341	8,204	70,278	78,795	13,374
11	Cytological investigation	12,899	12,438	16,923	16,249	16,932	16,794
12	Histological exam.	71,923	79,729	83,144	81,771	81,134	80,925
13	Bone marrow exam.	3,234	3,290	4,020	4,008	4,023	3,722
14	Biopsy procedures (Other than Endoscopies and B.M.Bx.)	3,632	3,472	4,551	5,249	7,113	8,298
15	Total B.T. given to the patients	13,875	14,409	13,338	13,657	12,649	13,431
16	Total plasma/PRP given to the patients	10,433	9,667	8,845	8,944	15,279	14,195
17	Imaging and radiological investigation						
(i)	MMR Ba. Swallow and other X-rays	48,060	44,564	46,844	55,883	53,227	50,589
(ii)	Ultrasound exam.	15,391	15,037	17,340	17,321	17,699	19,217
(iii)	CT Scan investigation	6,739	8,816	9,906	11,577	12,495	12,546
(iv)	MRI	1,138	1,684	2,131	2,665	2,767	2,984
(v)	Memograms	2,446	2,742	2,927	3,618	3,493	3,536

(vi)	OPG			3,756	2,810	3,414	3,216
(vii)	Colour Doppler			2,019	625	655	761
18	Radiation treatment						
(i)	Brachy therapy	1,387	1,162	1,189	865	953	820
(ii)	Cobalt teletherapy	1,710	2,033	2,223	2,287	1,512	1,257
(iii)	Linear accelerator	4,229	3,997	4,421	5,040	4,920	4,859
(iv)	BHABHATRON						1,793
(v)	Mould prepared for planning	1,962	1,865	2,059	2,213	2,699	2,280
(vi)	Simulator treatment planning	6,322	5,662	6,797	7,139	7,805	7,938
19	Surgical operations						
(i)	Major	3,289	3,472	3,729	3,776	4,322	4,138
(ii)	Minor	9,358	10,433	10,459	11,424	11,036	10,030
(iii)	I.V.T.C	3,219	3,266	3,687	3,344	4,142	5,007
20	Neurosurgical operation	529	491	513	628	558	498
21	Nuclear medicine (isotope)						
(i)	PET CT SCAN						459
(ii)	ISOTOP SCAN	1,616	2,100	2,718	3,122	3,207	2,693
(iii)	IODINE THERAPY			136	133	132	84
22	RIA investigations	14,923	17,368	20,176	27,516	30,449	33,027
23	Immunochemistry	2,418	2,872	3,583	4,161	5,114	5,649
24	Biochemical investigations (Research wing)	1,796	1,966	2,372	1,342	469	438
25	Cell biology division (Research wing)	1,187	1,487	1,615	2,006	2,437	1,988
26	Physiotherapy treatment	18,275	18,838	18,906	18,686	15,911	18,650
27	Total number of chemotherapeutic procedures	22,836	25,818	29,178	33,756	38,248	41,985
28	Bone marrow transplants	–	–	–	24	29	29
29	ECG	5,766	6,822	8,742	9,895	12,563	14,382

Source: GCRI web site.

Exhibit 9.2 MPS Cancer Hospital: Important Statistics

Sr. No.	Item	2002–03	2001–02	2000–01
1	Number of beds	550	550	550
2	Outpatient visits	1,63,485	1,65,000	1,66,552
3	Inpatient admissions	13,923	13,673	16,164
4	Average length of stay (Days)	9.5	9	8
5	Lab investigations	6,88,838	6,93,493	6,34,152
6	Radiology investigations	74,221	70,717	81,472
7	RIA investigations	14,142	11,845	11,063
8	Radiation treatment	12,228	18,070	10,214
9	Surgical operations – Major	2,738	2,944	2,877
	Minor/IVTC	11,503	11,675	10,339
10	Neurological operations	559	380	248
11	Nuclear medicines	2,022	2,145	2,652
12	Bone marrow transplants	6	17	5
13	Chemotherapy procedures	15,997	14,772	13,763
14	Physiotherapy treatment	16,238	16,562	15,837

Exhibit 9.3 MPS Cancer Hospital: Income and Expenditure Statement

	2002–03	2001–02	2000–01
Income			
Grants	20,72,05,700	18,96,05,577	18,73,39,938
Hospital fees	3,90,27,925	3,94,29,820	4,32,17,467
Other income	12,64,645	15,09,199	6,72,271
Excess of expenditure over income transferred to balance sheet	1,10,15,440	1,82,83,964	2,40,95,891
Total Income	**25,85,13,710**	**24,88,28,560**	**25,53,25,567**
Expenditure			
Establishment expenses	13,88,41,501	13,19,41,420	13,22,54,518
Hospital expenses	6,61,87,363	6,42,29,403	6,76,78,516
Other operating expenses	3,27,25,257	2,97,25,984	2,92,74,677
Expenditure on projects	51,682	57,789	1,15,172
Depreciation	2,07,07,907	2,28,73,964	2,60,02,684
Total Expenditure	**25,85,13,710**	**24,88,28,560**	**25,53,25,567**

Exhibit 9.4 MPS Cancer Hospital: Establishment Expenses

Particulars	Year Ending 31-3-2002	Year Ending 31-3-2001	Year Ending 31-3-2000
Salary	11,75,94,319	11,75,71,391	10,93,55,092
Pension	2,42,154	1,38,996	1,38,996
Contributory PF	91,30,966	71,37,610	71,90,896
Group gratuity and LIC premium	34,48,664	49,77,782	46,65,240
Staff welfare expenses	1,06,962	1,51,068	2,65,066
Sub Total	13,05,23,065	12,99,76,847	12,16,15,290
Computer expenses	97,730	4,21,831	2,32,364
Stationery and printing	7,22,972	12,43,911	14,63,695
Postage and telegrams	41,588	51,393	1,00,917
Telephone expenses	3,72,628	3,82,376	4,64,051
Advance charges	1,83,437	1,78,160	1,55,547
Total	**13,19,41,420**	**13,22,54,518**	**12,40,31,864**

Exhibit 9.5 MPS Cancer Hospital: Hospital Supplies

Particulars	Year Ending 31-3-2002	Year Ending 31-3-2001	Year Ending 31-3-2000
Drugs, medicines and chemicals	2,71,51,005	2,75,29,648	1,92,98,648
Laboratory materials and chemicals	1,35,26,980	1,48,68,222	1,57,75,504
X-ray contingencies	1,04,45,905	88,67,020	95,73,279
Diet to patients	29,88,765	28,54,593	26,00,983
Research and development expenses	22,48,709	15,27,212	27,55,958
Linen and bedding	4,75,356	11,81,715	6,56,906
Surgical and physiotherapy materials	54,02,350	86,98,222	76,98,154
Ambulance car contingencies	3,16,088	2,83,217	3,45,565
Hospital contingencies	16,74,245	18,68,667	19,24,428
Other expenses	42,39,042	36,79,096	50,25,951
Grand Total Hospital Expenses	**6,42,29,403**	**6,76,78,516**	**6,06,29,425**

Exhibit 9.6 MPS Cancer Hospital: Other Operating Expenses

Particulars	Year Ending 31-3-2002	Year Ending 31-3-2001	Year Ending 31-3-2000	Year Ending 31-3-1999
Electricity charges	1,39,77,026	1,27,18,350	1,15,68,398	1,13,35,957
Insurance premium	5,23,335	4,86,484	7,85,717	7,61,453
Building repairs	20,84,669	17,60,764	22,23,089	17,69,552
Equipment repairs and maintenance	65,37,333	69,02,987	55,26,913	43,04,326
Rates and taxes	1,35,696	1,448	–	40,607
Subscriptions	16,10,960	27,91,536	35,15,979	23,90,723
Security services	13,07,079	10,55,288	–	–
Professional charges	4,84,021	8,27,226	17,81,405	20,05,661
Books and publications	1,48,013	1,42,670	1,85,130	77,517
Cancer awareness and conference	52,501	71,482	79,028	9,63,545
Travelling and conveyance	4,47,716	1,73,528	8,69,460	5,53,836
Loss on sale of fixed assets	–	45,273	–	–
Membership fees	27,250	3,500	3,000	–
Audit fees	44,100	42,000	26,250	24,000
General expenses	8,57,614	5,71,773	9,03,233	9,78,010
Interest to bank	14,88,671	16,80,368	15,78,990	15,44,051
Total	**2,97,25,984**	**2,92,74,677**	**2,90,46,592**	**2,67,49,238**

Exhibit 9.7 MPS Cancer Hospital: Existing Purchase System

Major Group	No. of Items	No. of Suppliers	No. of POs
Drugs and medicines	291	72	404
Lab	708	67	359
X-ray	103	19	44
Surgical	361	34	173
Anesthesia	067	12	30
Rehabilitation	049	9	10
Lamps	021	13	9
Linen	55	8	27
Stationery	146	17	95
Printing	163	10	77
Petty Items	142	04	52
Total	**2,097**	**265**	**1,280**

MP TRUST HOSPITAL*

CASE 9.2

Our hospital is an internationally reputed centre for kidney care. Of late, our business is facing competition from many urologists and nephrologists, who are opening their clinics nearby and offer the same services at much lower charges, since they do not have the overheads of an Institution like ours. Our lab facilities are excellent and we can extend them to patients from general practitioners, but what exists in the market in terms of remunerating the general practitioners cannot be done by a hospital like ours. Our operating profit is showing a decline since a few years. How can we attract more business to our hospital and manage our hospital resources more efficiently and effectively?

General Manager – Administration, MP Trust Hospital

MP Trust Hospital

The MP Trust Hospital (MPTH) was set up in 1978 to provide special care for kidney-related ailments. The hospital performed its first kidney transplant operation in 1980. The MP Trust Society for Research in Nephro-Urology was formed in 1984, while the Diploma Programme in Nephrology and Urology was started in 1993. MPTH was one of its kind in Asia-the first hospital in India devoted entirely to Nephrology and Urology. MPTH was awarded the ISO-9001: 2008 certificate for quality management system. An organizational chart of MPTH is given in Exhibit 9.8.

By the year 2000, MPTH had performed more than 800 kidney transplant operations. The hospital had also treated 8,000 kidney stone cases, 4,000 cases of trans-urethral resection of prostate, and conducted 40,000 dialysis procedures.

Medical Services

The Outpatient Department (OPD) provided facilities to examine six patients at a time with an Emergency Cubicle equipped to examine and treat critically ill patients. Personal consultations were arranged with consultant Urologists and

---

* Reproduced with the permission of the copyright owner.

Prepared by Professor K.V. Ramani, Indian Institute of Management, Ahmedabad.

Cases of the Indian Institute of Management, Ahmedabad, are prepared as a basis for class discussion. They are not designed to present illustrations of either correct or incorrect handling of administrative problems.

© 1998 by the Indian Institute of Management, Ahmedabad, Revised June 2012.

Nephrologists by prior appointment. The OPD department completed all the procedures of consultation, investigation, and diagnosis the same day.

For inpatient care, the hospital had a centrally air-conditioned facility with a capacity of 140 beds. The hospital offered five types of accommodations; general ward, semi-special room, special rooms, special rooms with kitchen, and deluxe rooms. More than 60 per cent of the inpatients were discharged within a week. The Dialysis department handled about 30 dialysis procedures every day and was the busiest department in the hospital. These medical services were well supported by the hospital's well equipped clinical laboratory and radiology departments. Exhibit 9.9 gives the load on medical services for a few years.

Support Services

The general manager was in charge of all support services and coordinated all the activities in the hospital.

The Administrative section provided support services under the following departments. The stores department supplied medical, surgical, and general items to the user departments. The purchase department looked after purchases for the general stores; the hospital pharmacy took care of the medical requirements of the patients, while the canteen department looked after the dietary requirements of the patients. The Personnel, Accounts, and Maintenance departments managed the staffing, financial, and maintenance requirements for running the hospital.

The stores department was responsible for the supply of all items (medical, surgical, and general) to the various user departments in the hospital such as Operation Theater (OT), new Intensive Care Unit (ICU), old ICU, dialysis, transplant ward, and so on. Each of these user departments sent a monthly indent to the stores. Upon checking the stock status, the stores-in-charge prepared a consolidated statement of requirements for each item (medical, surgical, general, and so on) and sent this statement to the purchase department. The stores department dealt with almost 1,200 items, out of which 300–350 were stocked items and the remaining 800–850 items passed through the stores directly to the user indenting departments.

At the beginning of every financial year, purchase department requested vendors to submit quotations to meet its annual requirements. Those with the lowest quotations were selected. The purchase department maintained a 90-day credit period with its suppliers. There were about 200 suppliers supplying items to MPTH in any given year. Every month, the department prepared consolidated POs orders for outside and local purchases, and initiated the purchase procedures.

The hospital started its Pharmacy department in July 1993. The Pharmacy was responsible for supply of medicines to the patients (from the hospital and outside) and not to any department in the hospital. A computer-based information system supported the pharmacy staff in monitoring and planning the purchase and sales of medicines.

Management Concerns

Majority of the beds were in the general ward and hence the management could not increase charges for patient care. Any amount of additional facilities introduced in the special rooms did not increase the occupancy in the special room category.

Over a period of time, an increasing number of Urologists and Nephrologists started practicing in nearby places offering their services at lower rates. They could do so since their overhead expenses were very little, unlike MPTH. The diagnostic facilities in the hospital like the laboratory and X-ray department were not used to the maximum. To increase the capacity utilization of these departments, the hospital could accept patients from outside, but even the inflow of such patients from outside was not much. This was because MPTH did not follow the unethical practice of remunerating the general physicians for recommending their patients to the hospital.

The hospital had been investing extensively to keep up with the developments in medical technology. On an average, per year, the hospital incurred capital expenditure of over rupees one crore. This amount had to come in the form of donations. The institution had an exemption certificate, making donations 100 per cent free from Income Tax.

Exhibit 9.10 gives the activity report. Monthly purchases for the hospital varied between rupees six to seven lakhs as can be seen in Exhibit 9.11. The hospital expenses towards inputs like personnel, consumables, and power kept increasing year after year, but charges for patient care remained the same. Exhibit 9.12 provides the financial details at a glance, while Exhibit 9.13 and Exhibit 9.14 give the income and expense statements respectively.

The hospital management was faced with the challenge of improving the hospital's business performance.

Exhibit 9.8 MPTH Organizational Chart

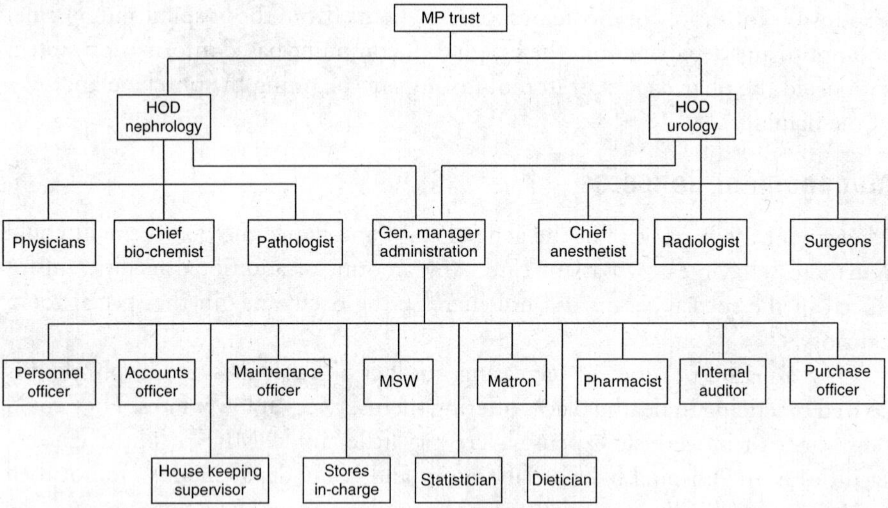

Exhibit 9.9 MPTH Medical Service Activities

Year	OPD Patients		Inpatients		No. of Dialysis Patients	No. of Surgery	No. of Lab Tests	No. of X-rays	No. of Sonography
	Nephro	Uro	Nephro	Uro					
1990	7,976	7,901	718	1,184	331	2,433	1,52,220	9,986	6,303
1991	7,867	8,136	802	1,207	427	2,562	1,57,175	10,896	6,956
1992	8,009	8,640	846	1,167	440	2,596	1,63,470	12,013	7,348
1993	8,395	9,038	861	1,285	533	2,636	1,71,721	11,316	7,056
1994	8,832	9,434	1,010	1,340	524	2,748	2,01,774	13,771	7,386
1995	8,696	11,284	1,650	2,448	1,317	3,006	2,15,569	16,007	8,247
1996	8,977	11,171	1,701	2,403	1,882	3,447	2,22,984	22,784	7,716

Exhibit 9.10 MPTH Activity Report: 1997–98

₹ in lacs

Sr. No.	Name of Activity	Avg./Mth. 1994–95	Avg./Mth. 1995–96	Avg./Mth. 1996–97	Avg./Mth. 1997–98 (Apr–Nov)	Total 1997–98 (Apr–Nov)	% Variation
1	OPD Nephro (new cases)	158	161	166	163	1,300	–3.92
2	OPD Nephro (follow up)	576	585	620	662	5,299	8.63
3	OPD Uro (new cases)	262	318	288	294	2,349	–7.07
4	OPD Uro (follow up)	522	650	688	609	4,871	–11.81
5	OPD Anr (new cases)	–	–	17	16	127	–23.72
6	OPD Anr (follow up)	–	–	30	35	277	–2.04
7	Adm. Nephro (new cases)	84	80	83	73	581	–12.03
8	Adm. Nephro (follow up)	52	58	60	54	432	–11.65
9	Adm. Uro (new cases)	112	137	128	110	876	–12.83
10	Adm. Uro (follow up)	62	77	76	73	582	–4.59
11	Adm. Anr (new cases)	–	–	0	2	18	–
12	Adm. Anr (follow up)	–	–	0	1	6	–
13	X-rays	1,123	1,875	1,943	1,811	14,486	–6.63
14	Laboratory tests	16,814	18,196	19,740	18,633	1,49,065	–3.08
15	Ultrasonography	618	667	571	611	4,891	3.91
. . .							
22	**Occupancy:**						
	(a) General ward (N + U)76	102	106	104	58	461	–44.46
	(i) General ward (N) – 28	–	–	–	67	67	–
	(ii) General ward (U) – 48	–	–	–	41	41	–
	(b) Semi-special rooms 14	51	65	47	14	108	–71.17
	(c) Special and delux rooms 11	49	52	49	49	391	–0.42
	(i) Special rooms-06	–	–	–	60	478	–
	(ii) Delux rooms 3, 4 and 5 – 03	–	–	–	21	169	–
	(iii) Super delux rooms 1 and 2 – 02	–	–	–	58	467	–
	(d) Transplant ward 12	–	–	–	33	33	–
	(e) New I.C.U.06	–	–	–	95	95	–
	(f) Post-op. ward 08	–	–	–	54	54	–
	Overall occupancy 127	–	–	–	36	36	–

Exhibit 9.11 MPTH Stores and Purchase Departments

₹ in lacs

Category	1990–91	1991–92	1992–93	1993–94	1994–95	1995–96	1996–97
A. Medical Items							
Opening balance	0.91	2.36	1.31	1.88	0.48	3.80	0.70
Purchase	4.32	4.44	6.71	6.42	5.57	7.09	7.78
Consumption	2.87	5.42	6.14	7.82	2.25	10.19	7.60
B. Surgical Items							
Opening balance	5.16	6.12	12.82	10.23	11.82	8.46	13.78
Purchase	14.06	20.34	22.35	27.94	29.82	44.93	38.49
Consumption	13.09	13.65	24.95	26.35	33.18	39.61	33.30
C. General Items							
Opening balance	0.08	0.03	0.13	0.61	0.05	0.15	0.12
Purchase	0.52	0.51	0.57	0.19	0.99	1.82	1.81
Consumption	0.57	0.41	0.48	0.75	0.90	1.84	1.80
D. Other Items							
Dialysis	6.11	8.00	6.32	6.54	9.56	7.67	13.16
Anesthetic	1.04	1.93	1.10	0.71	1.01	0.70	0.45
Laboratory	3.70	5.03	10.80	9.72	10.74	12.71	24.74
X-Ray	3.49	3.79	6.30	6.44	4.73	5.99	3.63
Blood transfusion	0.61	0.89	0.74	0.05	0.01	0.01	0.04
A/C: Elect.	7.30	9.68	10.10	11.94	13.48	13.56	14.76
A/C: Plant maint.	1.18	1.14	1.61	2.18	1.21	2.00	3.16
Oxygen	0.71	0.71	1.46	1.60	2.02	2.34	3.13
E. (A + B + C + D)	40.68	50.75	70.02	74.11	79.10	96.62	105.76

Exhibit 9.12 MPTH Financial Details

								₹ in lacs
Sr. No.	**Particulars**	**1990–91**	**1991–92**	**1992–93**	**1993–94**	**1994–95**	**1995–96**	**1996–97**
1	Opening balance	49.90	36.89	50.99	27.29	69.16	137.65	106.68
2	Revenue income	189.35	282.94	305.06	335.84	366.07	457.47	473.32
3	Donations	91.91	75.41	3.69	93.36	60.48	38.03	75.53
4	Income from other sources	0.48	1.70	0.42	2.36	3.14	4.01	1.90
5	Interest received – Bank	0.01	0.40	0.36	0.35	0.90	1.25	0.49
	Interest received – Corpus	–	–	–	2.81	18.28	24.22	36.71
6	Loans availed from financial institutions	–	6.75	20.98	26.57	23.56	24.33	25.00
	Total (1)	331.65	404.09	381.50	488.58	541.59	686.96	719.63
7	Revenue expenses (Inclusive of Interest)	175.05	264.58	295.60	316.50	327.92	411.92	446.16
8	Capital expenses	31.17	24.52	29.16	75.32	43.71	123.37	62.69
9	Loans repaid to financial institutions	88.54	64.00	29.45	27.60	32.31	44.99	29.00
	Total (2)	294.76	353.10	354.21	419.42	403.94	580.28	537.85
10	Closing balance (1) –(2)	36.89	50.99	27.29	69.16	137.65	106.68	181.78

Exhibit 9.13 MPTH Income Statement: 1997–98

							₹ in lacs
Sr. No.	**Fees**	**Avg./Mth. 1994–95**	**Avg./Mth. 1995–96**	**Avg./Mth. 1996–97**	**Avg./Mth. 1997–98 (Apr–Nov)**	**Total 1997–98 (Apr–Nov)**	**% Variation**
1	Consulting	0.49	0.52	0.54	0.73	5.87	35.67
2	X-ray	1.47	1.81	2.33	2.92	23.33	24.98
3	Laboratory	5.28	5.67	7.06	7.74	61.88	9.54
4	Stay	2.29	2.62	3.02	3.57	28.52	17.88
5	Operation	7.55	8.92	9.48	8.79	70.31	–7.32
6	Kidney transplant	3.77	2.39	2.65	2.79	22.30	5.35
7	Theatre (Other charges)	3.06	3.41	4.94	4.61	36.86	–6.67
8	Anesthetic	0.44	0.48	0.57	0.76	6.09	33.16
9	Dialysis	2.11	2.80	3.99	4.36	34.87	9.11
10	E.C.G.	0.13	0.13	0.16	0.16	1.30	–0.51
11	Urodynamic	0.34	0.45	0.70	0.71	5.65	1.50
12	Miscellaneous	1.02	1.07	0.99	0.89	7.13	–9.59
13	Special consultation	0.09	0.11	0.14	0.13	1.06	–5.92
14	Stone clinic	2.47	3.56	2.85	2.34	18.71	–17.76
15	Kidney care clinic	–	–	0.00	0.00	0.00	–100.00
16	Andrology fees	–	–	0.02	0.01	0.09	–28.95
17	Surcharge	0.00	4.19	0.00	0.00	0.00	–
	Total income	30.50	38.12	39.45	40.50	323.97	2.67
	Freeship	1.08	1.56	2.20	1.83	14.65	–16.70
	Net income	29.42	36.56	37.25	38.67	309.32	3.81
	Total expense	26.24	32.84	34.98	38.11	304.91	8.95
	Surplus/Deficit	3.18	3.72	2.26	0.55	4.41	–75.65
Other Income							
1	Rent	0.01	0.01	0.01	0.00	0.03	–43.75
2	Interest (Bank)	0.08	0.03	0.04	0.03	0.21	–35.71
3	Interest (Corpus)	1.52	2.21	3.06	3.08	24.65	0.72
4	Insurance claims	0.15	0.29	0.48	0.00	0.00	–100.00
5	Patient bill recover	0.02	0.02	0.01	0.02	0.18	68.75
6	Disposal of scraps	0.07	0.03	0.07	0.05	0.36	–39.33
	Total other income	1.86	2.59	3.68	3.18	25.43	–13.50

Exhibit 9.14 MPTH Expense Statement: 1997–98

							₹ in lacs
Sr. No.	**Particulars**	**Avg./Mth. 1994–95**	**Avg./Mth. 1995–96**	**Avg./Mth. 1996–97**	**Avg./Mth. 1997–98 (Apr–Nov)**	**Total 1997–98 (Apr–Nov)**	**% Variation**
1	Salary and wages	8.78	10.32	11.98	14.50	115.98	21.01
2	Laboratory	1.72	2.06	2.67	2.83	22.61	5.92
3	Surgical	2.74	4.00	3.37	2.77	22.18	–17.77
4	X-ray	0.59	0.63	0.54	0.51	4.07	–6.51
5	Dialysis	1.11	1.12	1.48	1.30	10.39	–12.25
6	Medicines	0.46	0.59	0.62	0.86	6.91	39.69
7	Electric	1.67	1.80	2.13	2.73	21.84	28.27
8	Maintenance	1.38	3.28	1.98	2.68	21.40	34.99
9	Medical professional	1.26	1.73	1.80	1.58	12.60	–12.46
10	Con. conv. expenses	0.34	0.38	0.50	0.48	3.85	–3.59
11	Honorarium	0.51	0.64	1.00	0.93	7.40	–7.27
12	Interest	1.41	1.29	1.07	0.99	7.91	–7.59
13	Stationery	0.40	0.62	0.53	0.46	3.67	–13.71
14	Post and telephones	0.45	0.63	0.62	0.76	6.09	23.28
15	Staff welfare and guest	0.05	0.12	0.12	0.11	0.85	–13.27
16	Travelling	0.21	0.33	0.35	0.49	3.93	42.05
17	Computer	–	0.46	0.47	0.65	5.21	39.06
18	Clothes and dress	–	0.29	0.37	0.39	3.14	5.84
19	Cleaning and washing	–	0.15	0.18	0.17	1.34	–5.19
20	Veema premium	–	0.52	0.26	0.30	2.37	12.86
21	Slide and conference	–	0.51	0.61	0.11	0.85	–82.63
22	Indoor patient food	–	–	–	0.86	6.88	
23	ESWL equipment repairs	0.35	0.00	0.32	0.10	0.81	–67.90
24	ESWL service charge	0.35	0.00	0.39	0.30	2.40	–22.35
25	Other	2.48	1.36	1.69	1.20	10.23	–24.45
	Total Expense	23.7	32.84	34.98	88.11	304.91	8.95
	Capital Expense	3.64	10.28	5.22	13.00	104.00	148.84

chapter 10

Hospital MIS

CHAPTER OUTLINE

CHAPTER OBJECTIVE

The main objective of this chapter is to apply the concepts (discussed in Chapter 5) of design and development of a hospital MIS to a large hospital, a hospital's clinical lab and a standalone clinical lab.

SJ HOSPITAL* CASE 10.1

In the last meeting of the board of directors, the chairman of SJ Hospital emphasized the need to develop a comprehensive hospital information system in order to help hospital authorities manage their resources efficiently and effectively. In his words:

> *It is our endeavor to leverage on Information Technology to provide us a competitive edge as we believe that it will play a differentiating factor between successful medical organizations and the not-successful ones. In the long run we should plan to collaborate with other reputed hospitals and diagnostic centers world-wide for patient referrals and consultation through a computer network.*

SJ Hospital

SJ Hospital, established in 1975 with 50 beds, has grown into a large hospital with 1200 beds. In 2007, the hospital had 24 full- fledged departments to provide specialty and super specialty services, including state-of-the-art diagnostic facilities to ensure the delivery of holistic patient care. Its diagnostic facilities included C.T. Scan, Radio-therapy and fully-equipped laboratory facilities with Pathology, Biochemistry, Microbiology, Histopathology labs and a Blood Bank. The diagnostic laboratories had been granted accreditation with the ISO 15189:2003 standards by the National Accreditation Board for Laboratories (NABL) of the Department of Science and Technology.

The hospital handled an OPD load of 500,000 outpatients and 46,000 inpatients, in the year 2007 (January to December). This meant an average load of 1,400 OPD patients and 130 inpatients per day. At the time of registration for outpatient services, minimal information was sought from the patient. The computer printed a registration slip in duplicate. One copy was retained by the patient for his/her records, while the other copy was to be produced for availing of hospital services (Exhibit 10.1). Billing for outpatient and inpatient services (exhibits 10.2 and 10.3 respectively) were subsequently computerized. The computer system also provided all the details of each service under each category; for illustration, see Exhibit 10.4 for complete details of diagnostic services for inpatient billing.

---

* Reproduced with the permission of the copyright owner.

Prepared by Professor K.V. Ramani, Indian Institute of Management.

Cases of the Indian Institute of Management, Ahmedabad are prepared as a basis for class discussion. Cases are not designed to present illustrations of either correct or incorrect handling of administrative problems.

© 2001 by the Indian Institute of Management, Ahmedabad, Revised July 2012.

Over the last few years, the hospital had experienced a steady increase in the number of OPD and inpatient cases. The increasing load on hospital services was a concern for the management in terms of the hospital's ability to continue providing quality services to patients.

In a recent seminar on Hospital Management Information Systems (HMIS), the chairman heard a speaker emphasize the need for identifying meaningful performance indicators in the design and development of MIS. The speaker also highlighted the data contained in the OPD and inpatient billing to derive several performance indicators. Performance indicators would throw some light on the effective and efficient management of hospital departments for delivering hospital services.

Effective performance is an indicator of output quality and quantity.

Efficient performance is an indicator of the utilization of input resources to output.

Together, effectiveness and efficiency reflect an optimal utilization of resources in the delivery of goods and/or services.

One of the current performance indicators used by the hospital was the Average Length of Stay (ALOS) for the hospital as a whole. The ALOS for the hospital as a whole was an average of all the hospital departments; some departments like orthopedics required a higher ALOS for patent recovery, while some other departments such as medicine required only a few days of hospital stay. An estimate of ALOS for each department was essential to assess the performance of the hospital.

The chairman wanted to know if the current data base on billing would suffice to assess the performance of individual departments. He wanted the hospital director to make a presentation to the hospital board on a comprehensive HMIS to address issues such as

- Identify critical areas for developing Hospital MIS.
- Elaborate on the importance of Performance Indicators in the design of HMIS.
- Suggest a few Performance Indicators to estimate hospital efficiency and effectiveness.
- Discuss data required to estimate these indicators.
- Demonstrate the computations involved in estimating a few performance indicators.
- Outline the steps required to ensure data collection.
- Identify the frequency of reporting.
- Design HMIS reports to reflect hospital performance.

The chairman was also interested to hear the director's assessments regarding the preparedness of the hospital for implementing the proposed Hospital MIS.

Exhibit 10.1 OPD Registration Slip

Date 21/06/2007	Date 21/06/07
Time ________	Time ________
Hospital Number: ________	Hospital Number: ________
New/Repeat ________	New/Repeat ________
Clinic: Medicine 1	Clinic: Medicine 1
Name and Address:	Name and Address:
________	________
________	________
________	________
Age ________ Sex ________	Age ________ Sex ________
Registration Fee: ₹50.00	Registration Fee: ₹50.00
Net Payable: ₹50.00 (₹Fifty only)	Net Payable: ₹50.00 (₹Fifty only)
Valid Until: ________	Valid Until: ________

Exhibit 10.2 Outpatient Billing

Cash Bill No.051236

O.P. No.: 1457476 Patient Name: ________ Time: 11:57:23

Sr. No.	Service/Material	Amount (₹)
1	00274 00274 E.C.G.	80.00
2	10208 10208 Urine Routine Analysis	55.00
3	10604 10604 FBS/PPBS/RBS	35.00
4	00236 00236 Disposable Needle and Syringe	5.00
5	10609 10609 Urea and Creatine	110.00
	Gross	**285.00**

Exhibit 10.3 Inpatient Billing

Patient Classification: Individual/Institution   Bill No.: D 025205   Date: 05-07-2007

Name of Patient: **********   O.P. No.: 1454926   I.P. No.: 519368

From: 28-06-2007   To: 05-07-2007   Ward/Room: ______________

	Name of Service/Supply	Amount (₹)
000	Bed charges	1,400.00
004	Professional and treatment charges	875.00
006	Operation	1,585.00
007	Anesthesia	530.00
008	Operation theatre	3,865.00
009	Anesthetics	282.00
010	O.T. materials	535.50
014	Pharmacy materials	1,564.50
016	**Laboratory Investigations**	**1,050.00**
018	Radiology investigations	**
027	Telephone calls	**
028	E.C.G.	**
037	Ultrasound	**
057	Computerized stress test	**
058	Echocardiography	**
078	Surgeon's visiting fee	**
079	Cross consultation fee	**
	. . .	
	Total Dues	**16,367.50**

Exhibit 10.4 Laboratory Investigations

Date	Test ID	Test Name	No:	Amount (₹)
29-06-07	1005	Complete Blood Count (HB, TC, DC, ESR)	1	100.00
29-06-07	10023	Prothrombin Time (PT)	1	120.00
29-06-07	10101	Activated Partial Thromboplastin (APTT)	1	225.00
29-06-07	10208	Urine Routine Analysis	1	65.00
29-06-07	10575	Creatinine	1	75.00
29-06-07	10604	FBS/PPBS/RBS	1	45.00
30-06-07	10573	Complete Liped Profile (Cholesterol, Trigl, HDL)	1	420.00
Total Lab Investigation				**1,050.00**

MAHANAGAR HOSPITAL* CASE 10.2

Dr Satish Kumar, Director, Pathology Laboratory, at Mahanagar Hospital was reviewing the annual report of his lab performance prepared by the hospital's quality control department. This report was prepared at the request of Dr Satish himself, in anticipation of a proposed visit by an NABL team, following the accreditation of his lab three years ago. Dr Satish was a little worried about some of the observations in the report on pre-analytical activities and the possible consequences on the turnaround time for report generation and patients' health. With increasing dependence on clinical lab test reports by the hospital physicians, the reliability of laboratory testing and reporting was very critical.

Investigations play a very important role in medical diagnosis. Laboratory results are estimated to affect sixty to seventy per cent of the most important decisions in patient care.

Pathology Lab at Mahanagar Hospital

The organization of the Mahanagar[i] Hospital lab department is given in Exhibit 10.5 along with the staff strength in each analytical section in the lab. The increasing load for pathology investigations (Exhibit 10.6) and the hospital management's commitment to quality services led to NABL accreditation (National Accreditation Board for Testing and Calibration Laboratories) in the year 2009.

Worksheet Preparation: Pathology lab services in Mahanagar Hospital started with the physicians ordering certain investigations/tests on their patients and communicating the same to their nursing units for onward transmission to the pathology laboratory.

Mary Joseph, the receptionist in the Pathology Laboratory at Mahanagar Hospital for over three years, received an IP Request Slip (Exhibit 10.7) from the nursing station for Mrs Parvathy Menon admitted in the gynecology department. Each request for investigation carried a Request Number, commonly referred to

---

* Reproduced with the permission of the copyright owner.

Prepared by Professor K.V. Ramani, Dr Poonam Trivedi, Research Assistant and Dr Imran Malek, Research Assistant, Indian Institute of Management, Ahmedabad as a basis for classroom discussion. Cases are not designed to present illustrations of correct or incorrect handling of administrative problems.

Cases of the Indian Institute of Management, Ahmedabad are prepared as a basis for classroom discussion. They are not designed to present illustrations of either correct or incorrect handling of administrative problems.

©2010 by the Indian Institute of Management, Ahmedabad, Revised 22 May 2012.

[i] Real names of the hospital and the lab director changed.

as Encounter Number, which gave a unique ID for each sample collection from patients.

Upon receipt of the Investigation Request Slip, Mary entered the inpatient ID on her computer screen and the Health Management System (HMS) generated Worksheets for sample collection. Separate worksheets were prepared for tests to be done in each section of the lab, namely, Biochemistry, Hematology sections and so on, since each section laid its own requirements for sample collection (Exhibit 10.8). For example, blood samples submitted to the hematology section were often different from blood samples submitted to biochemistry section. The HMS also recorded the charges for investigations in the patient database. Mary stapled the sectional worksheets with the request slip on top and dropped them in the IPD Inbox for collection by the phlebotomists.

While Mary was preparing the worksheet for Parvathy Menon, she received a telephone call from the Emergency Department nurse for sample collection. Requests for sample collection from Emergency Department were usually verbal requests to save time. Ahmed Khan, a phlebotomist was soon on his way to the emergency department.

The computer printer in Mary's cabin was continuously busy printing request slips for investigations from nursing stations on all the eight floors of the hospital, as Mary was answering a telephone call from a patient's relative. Mary took out the request slip which required samples to be collected from Viral Patel shifted to the Medical Intensive Care Unit 15 minutes ago. Mary prepared the sectional worksheets for Viral and marked them URGENT, while she continued to be on the telephone. As per the lab protocol, phlebotomists were expected to pick up urgent requests immediately, even if normal requests had arrived earlier and their worksheets were lying in the IPD Inbox.

Mary then noticed several outpatients queuing up in front of her cabin, each outpatient holding a Requisition Slip (Exhibit 10.9) which listed all the investigations ordered by the consultant. She collected the requisition slip from the first outpatient in the queue, entered the details in her computer, generated a unique encounter number in sectional worksheets and the OPD Cash Memo (Exhibit 10.10). She received the payment in cash, signed in the cash memo to acknowledge receipt of payment, returned it along with the worksheets, and asked him to wait to be called in for sample collection. She then attended to the second outpatient in the queue as the outpatient queue was building up, while the request slips for inpatients were also waiting for her attention.

Sample Collection: Ravi Kumar, a young and energetic phlebotomist working in the Mahanagar Hospital lab for almost one year, picked up the IP request slip from the IPD inbox (8:50 am) along with the worksheets for Parvathy. He went to his cabin, entered the encounter number in his computer and generated a unique barcode (8:51 am). The HMS printed out multiple copies of the barcode on self adhesive labels for pasting on each sample container. In addition to barcode labels for each lab section where the sample will be analyzed, there was also a Dispatch barcode label[ii]. Ravi then picked his phlebotomy box known as Red box (Exhibit 10.11) and took the elevator to the third floor (8:52).

Ravi identified Parvathy easily as the worksheet gave all the patient details, such as name, ID, sex, age, room number, bed number and so on. He was also able to identify the vein and prepare the site for venipuncture easily. He opened his red box and took out all the necessary materials.

Wearing gloves (8:54), he collected blood from Parvathy's arm (8:57) into a special tube having EDTA, an anti-coagulant, for hematology section. He pasted the barcode label on each sample, kept the samples in his red box along with the used materials (capped needles, gloves and so on), and went back to his cabin in the ground floor (9:00). In his cabin, he prepared a slide for Complete Blood Count (CBC) examination (9:02) and cleaned the blood stains on his table. He then disposed off all used items: burnt the used needles, threw them in the one per cent sodium hypochloride solution, and also disposed off the needle cap, gloves, syringes and so on in the appropriate colored waste bins (9:04). After giving the samples to the respective section for analysis, Ravi returned to his cabin, pasted the dispatch barcode label in the dispatch book (9:06), returned the IP request slip to Mary who promptly put it in the IPD outbox (9:07). Ravi then went to pick up the next request for sample collection.

Ravi noticed several requests in the IPD inbox, and picked up the request at the top; the urgent request for Viral Patel in Medical ICU did not catch his attention. The request Ravi picked up carried an instruction to use a previous sample for the new tests ordered for an orthopedic patient Sanjay Doshi in the fourth floor. He generated a barcode, printed barcode labels, searched the previous samples of Sanjay Doshi kept in the laboratory, prepared samples for each section, pasted the barcode labels on each sample and gave them to the respective sections. He was then told by the Biochemist to draw fresh blood as the previous sample was 'too old' and hemolysed[iii] for sensitive tests. He was also advised to collect sufficient volume of blood, as several tests were to be performed. Ravi therefore took the IP request slip with the biochemistry worksheet, went up to the fourth floor, collected fresh blood sample from Sanjay Doshi, and pasted the barcode

---

[ii] The lab maintained a centralized dispatch book, where each phlebotomist pasted the dispatch label of the patient upon submission of the samples to the lab sections. This dispatch book was inspected by the supervisor every month to monitor the load handled by the phlebotomists.

[iii] Hemolysis is the breakage of RBC membrane causing the release of hemoglobin and other internal components into the surrounding fluid. It is usually visible as a pink/red tinge in serum or plasma. Hemolysis could be due to In-Vivo or In-Vitro.

label on the sample. Just when Ravi was about to return to his cabin, he was informed by the nursing station about another request for sample collection from Mr Mohan Solanki in the same floor. This was the usual practice followed in the Mahanagar Hospital laboratory to expedite sample collection. Ravi went to the nursing station, picked up Mohan's addressograph prepared by the nursing unit, as he did not have the barcode labels for Mohan Solanki. He then went to the patient's room, identified the patient, collected samples, pasted the addressograph on each sample, kept them in his red box, and returned to his cabin. There, he collected from Mary the computer printout of the IP request slip and the sectional worksheets for Mohan, generated barcode labels for Mohan, and pasted them on the samples already collected. After taking care of disposal of all used items, he gave the samples of Sanjay and Mohan to the respective lab sections, pasted the dispatch barcode labels (two labels, one for each patient) in the dispatch book, put the IP requests in the IPD outbox, and went to pick up the next request from the IPD inbox.

Ahmed Khan reached the emergency department with his red box within a few minutes (8:39) and took the written order for investigations from the Medical Officer (MO) in charge. He identified the patient and read the investigations ordered. It required collection of blood sample with EDTA for hematology tests. The patient was old, in severe pain and not cooperating with the phlebotomist for drawing blood. With a great deal of difficulty, Ahmed Khan managed to locate and detect an appropriate venous access for venipuncture to draw blood. The first blood sample became clotted before he left the patient's room and so another sample had to be drawn for hematology tests. Ahmed khan wrote the name of the patient over the collection tubes for identification, kept the samples in his red box, and disposed off all the used materials in the emergency room itself. He then gave to Mary the written investigation order slip given by the MO. Mary found out the inpatient ID from the list of recently admitted patients, entered all the details of investigation into the computer and generated a request slip, sectional worksheets, stapled the request slip with the written order slip, and put them in the IPD outbox. She handed over the worksheets to Ahmed who was waiting patiently by her side. Ahmed generated a unique barcode, pasted the barcode labels on the sample tubes, and took them to the respective sections in the laboratory. He then went back to his cabin, pasted the dispatch barcode label in the dispatch book (9:05).

Ahmed Khan then picked two request slips for sample collection from Abdul Malek and Purnima Trivedi from the same floor. With the barcode labels ready, he went to collect samples from Abdul Malek and realized that Abdul was taken for an X-ray. Ahmed khan therefore went to Purnima Trivedi, collected blood samples, and went back to his cabin as Abdul Malek was still away in the radiology wing. As soon as Abdul returned to his room, Ahmed collected his samples and returned to the cabin. Once in the cabin, he took out the samples collected from Abdul Malek and Purnima Trivedi, and gave them to the respective lab sections for analysis. Returning to his cabin, Ahmed pasted two dispatch barcode labels in the dispatch book, disposed off all used items, put both the request slips in the IPD outbox, and was ready for the next sample collection.

While Ravi and Ahmed were busy collecting samples from inpatients, another phlebotomist Maninder Singh called in two outpatients together who have paid their bills and were waiting with the requests for investigations and worksheets. Maninder entered the encounter numbers in his computer and generated unique barcode labels for both the outpatients. He then collected samples from both the patients wearing the same pair of gloves and pasted the barcode labels on respective samples, gave the samples to the lab sections, disposed off all used materials, pasted dispatch labels, returned to the receptionist cabin and put both the request slips in the OPD box. Mary requested him to take up the requests for two inpatients in the sixth floor.

Problems with night duty phlebotomists were of a different nature. Early morning sample collection load was usually very high, based on requests from the nursing stations overnight. The receptionist doing the night shift prepared all the worksheets for fifty to sixty IP request slips. The two phlebotomists on night duty (10:30 pm to 7 am) picked up all the IP requests for ICU cases (ten to twenty cases) around 5 am, generated barcode labels and were off for sample collection from ICU patients by 6 am. They were back by 7 am in their cabin, prepared slides, kept the samples and slides with correct barcode labels in the respective lab sections, disposed of all used materials, and pasted dispatch barcode labels in the dispatch book. They left behind the thirty to forty IP requests for sample collections (normal cases) to the phlebotomists who would report to work in the morning shift (7 am to 3:30 pm).

Sample Testing and Report Generation: The phlebotomists submitted the samples for testing to the appropriate analytical sections. The analytical sections did the necessary tests and sent the test result reports of inpatients to the physicians and to the nursing stations, while the reports of outpatients were sent to the lab receptionist for collection by the patients.

Questions

1. What are your observations on the pre-analytic practices followed by the physicians, phlebotomists, and the lab receptionist?
2. What are the likely pre-analytic lab errors resulting from their practices? A note on 'Pre Analytic Process' in a pathology laboratory is given in Annexure 1.

3. What are your recommendations to minimize pre-analytic lab errors at Mahanagar Hospital Lab?
4. How would you rate the performance of the pre-analytic phase in Mahanagar Hospital Lab?

Exhibit 10.5 Organogram of the Lab Department: Mahanagar Hospital Chief Pathologist and Laboratory Director (1)

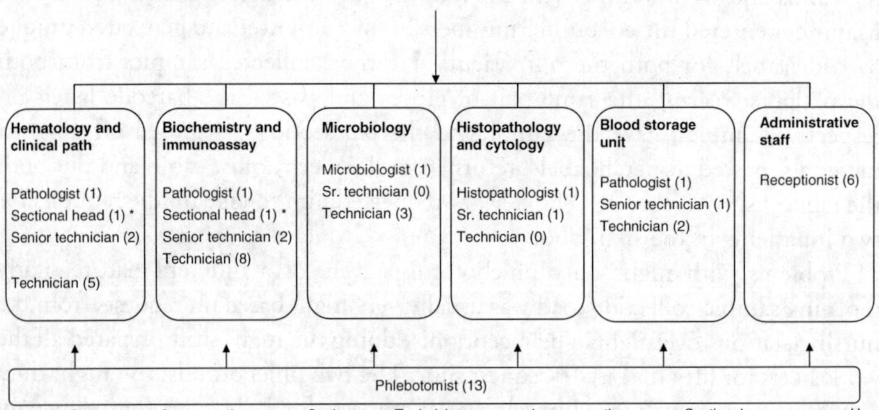

* One of the Senior Technicians is the Sectional Head

Exhibit 10.6 Load on Lab Department: Mahanagar Hospital

Section Name	From: 01/01/2007 to 31/12/2007	From: 01/01/2008 to 31/12/2008	From: 01/01/2009 to 31/12/2009
	Count	Count	Count
Biochemistry and immunoassay	117,194	132,871	137,133
Hematology	39,287	45,221	49,770
Blood storage centre (Test performed)	4,819	5,860	5,995
Blood storage centre (Product issued)	10,063	13,145	13,593
Clinical pathology	10,117	11,864	12,028
Histopathology and cytology	1,964	2,320	2,667
Microbiology	8,622	8,686	9,306
Outsourced test	1,915	1,720	1,517
Lab profiles (Department code: 30)	3,646	4,337	5,108
Lab profiles from health check up department	8,682	11,338	9,506
Total	**206,309**	**237,362**	**246,623**

Exhibit 10.7 IP Request Slip: Mahanagar Hospital

IP Request slip is a computer printout of tests ordered by a consultant for indoor patients. Each request slip has a unique ID number, known as Request Number, also called Encounter Number. Every time a consultant orders lab tests for an inpatient, a new request slip is generated and therefore a new encounter number by the HMS.

IP Request Slip

Request No. : 1022 RequestedOn :

Patient Name : IP No : 1072

Doctor's Name: Bed No. :

Ward No. :

Test Name

41- Blood Gases

299- GI PRE OP MAJOR-I

COMMENT:

Requested By : MO PrintedOn :

Collected Date/Time :
Collected By :
Received Date/Time :

Exhibit 10.8 IP Sectional Worksheet: Mahanagar Hospital

A Worksheet gives all the necessary information to the phlebotomist for drawing sample(s) from patients. If samples had to be sent to different sections in the lab for analysis (biochemistry section, hematology section and so on), the HMS automatically generated sectional worksheets for each.

IP - WORKSHEET SECTIONWISE

Lab Ref.No. : 4409 /1022 IP No : 1072
Date & Time of Posting : Ward :
Patient Name : Age/Sex :
Doctor's Name :
Credit Company Name :

SECTION : HEMATOLOGY/COAGULATION

299 GI PRE OP MAJOR-I

HB
TC
DC
PLT
BLOOD GROUP
ABO : " " Rh :
PT (Test) :
PT (Control) :
INR :
B T : C T :

Date of Worksheet Generation : Generated by : ps
Sample Run by: Inform to: Time: Informed by: Report printed by

Exhibit 10.8 (*Continued*)

```
                              IP - WORKSHEET SECTIONWISE
-------------------------------------------------------------------------------
Lab Ref.No. : 4409  /1022          IP No : 1072
Date & Time of Posting :                   Ward :
Patient Name :                             Age/Sex :
Doctor's Name :
Credit Company Name :
-------------------------------------------------------------------------------
              SECTION : BIOCHEMISTRY/IMMUNOASSAY/SEROLOGY
 41   Blood Gases

                pH :
                pCO2 :
                pO2 :
                TCO2 :
                HCO3 :
                Base Exe :
                O2 Satu :
                A-aDO2 :
                FIO2 :
                Sample ;  ARTERIAL / VENOUS             Time of Collection
 299   GI PRE OP MAJOR-I

                RBS:        (Urine R & M)
                TBIL:       BC:        BU:
```

Exhibit 10.9 OPD Requisition Slip: Mahanagar Hospital

REQUISITION SLIP Date: ____________

Dear Doctor,

Referring Mr./Mrs./Miss ______________________ Aged ____________

for the following investigations I.P. No. ____________

O.P. No. ____________

Lab Ref. No. ____________

HB
Protein
creatinine

Yours,

Short Clinical History

Provisional Diagnosis

Exhibit 10.10 OPD Cash Memo: Mahanagar Hospital

The cash memo for each outpatient is printed for the receptionist to collect the payment in cash for the investigations ordered.

```
                                    O P D   C A S H   M E M O
 no No.  : 3249                                        Date      :
 l Dept: PATH CASHIER
 : No.   : 5161
 ne      :                                             Age       :
 iss     : OP PAY                                      Visit/Case No :
 tor     :
-----------------------------------------------------------------------------------
 o  Charge Code    Service Description         Units        Amount        Lab N
o.
-----------------------------------------------------------------------------------
4   LAB. CHARGES   HEMOGLOBIN (HB)               1           48.00       376499
5   LAB. CHARGES   PROTEIN(SERUM)                1          216.00       376499
6   LAB. CHARGES   Creatinine (BLOOD)            1          108.00       376499

                                                            ==========
                                          Total Rs.:   372.00
                                                       ==========

unt In words : Three Hundred And Seventy Two  Only.
ayment Details :   Recd in Cash : 372
oncession    : 93
                                          Report Received By (Name  &  Sign)
                          Cashier
```

Exhibit 10.11 Materials Kept in the Phlebotomy Box (Red Box): Mahanagar Hospital

Sr. No.	Materials
1	Syringes
2	Needles (for vacuum and normal syringe): Mostly 22 G needle used
3	Tubes (for blood collection)
4	Spirit swab
5	Gloves
6	Scalp vein
7	Capillary
8	Heparin bulb
9	Belt/Strap
10	Bandage

ANNEXURE 1

Pre-analytic Phase in Pathology Lab Management

Pathology laboratories perform a number of clinical diagnostic procedures ordered by the physicians/consultants. Timely collection of samples and delivery of reliable accurate test results are therefore important quality indicators of performance of any laboratory.

Laboratory procedures are divided into three phases: Pre-Analytical, Analytical, and Post-Analytical phases.

1. **Pre-analytic phase** starts from the time the lab receives a request for investigations ordered by a consultant/physician and ends when the samples are handed over to the lab sections, such as biochemistry, hematology and so on for analysis.
2. **Analytic phase** involves testing, examination, analysis and interpretation of the investigations.
3. **Post-analytic phase** deals with reporting the results of investigations to the physicians and to their patients or patients' relatives. The physician's reaction to the report and interpretation of results would impact the future course of treatment and care.

Pre-analytic Phase

It is well known that more than 60 per cent of all lab errors occur at the pre-analytical phase, as sample collection calls for interaction with a number of people: physicians/consultants, nurses, lab receptionist, lab assistants, phlebotomists, patients and their relatives, lab analysts and so on.

This phase starts with the phlebotomists picking up their work orders from the lab receptionist, preparing bar-coded labels, collecting samples from patients, and submitting the samples to the analytic section of the lab for testing. This phase is known to account for almost 70 per cent of all lab errors, often leading to sample rejection. Hemolysed[iv] blood is the most common reason (as high

[iv] Hemolysis is the breakage of red blood cells causing the release of hemoglobin and other internal components into the blood serum or plasma. It can occur both in-vitro and in-vivo. In-vitro hemolysis happens mostly as a result of inappropriate blood collection practices, and is easily detected by the presence of pink or red color specimens in the serum/plasma after centrifugation. Causes for in-vivo hemolysis are many including hereditary, acquired and iatrogenic conditions such as autoimmune hemolytic anemia and other hemo globinopathies.Hemolysis is a very undesirable condition that influences the accuracy and reliability of lab tests.

as 55 per cent) for sample rejection. Other major reasons for sample rejection are insufficient sample quantity (20 per cent), incorrect samples (15 per cent), and lipemic[v], icteric[vi], and clotted blood samples [Bonini PA, et al 2002].

Sample collection requires strict adherence to safety procedures (safety to the phlebotomists and the patients), use of appropriate needles and well established procedures for drawing blood as well as correct identification of patient samples. Sample collection is followed by transportation of the samples to the lab for analysis. One of the major challenges in managing a pathology lab is to minimize the pre-analytic lab errors, so as to submit test worthy samples for analysis.

Table 10.1 Pre-analytic Phase

Phase	Sr. No.	Activity	
Pre-pre analytic	1	Physician/clinician orders tests for investigation	Orally
	2	Physician/clinician orders tests for investigation	Hand written
	3	Lab receptionist does not highlight 'URGENT' work orders	
Pre Analytic	4	Phlebotomist's habit of picking up work orders	
	5	Preparation of bar-coded labels for sample collection, identification	
	6	Patient identification	
	7	Use of gloves	
	8	Site selection for drawing blood	
	9	Site Preparation	
	10	Use of the tourniquet correctly	
	11	Identifying the order for sample collection	
	12	Vacutainers vs syringes, appropriate container for sample collection	
	13	Use of appropriate needle of gauge 21 or 22 if using a syringe	
	14	Sample collection	
	15	Proper mixing	
	16	Sample identification: Paste the bar-coded labels	
	17	Dispose off all used materials	
	18	Submit the samples to the lab for testing	

[v] Lipemia indicates the presence of fat in the blood serum, and is an inherent characteristic of the patient's blood. Lipemic sample can arise due to sample collection after heavy meals or the presence of some metabolic disorder. Lipemic samples become turbid making it difficult for investigation.

[vi] Icterus blood means jaundiced blood and cannot be used for testing.

RD CLINICAL LAB* CASE 10.3

Consumers are the reason for our existence. They are the reason for our growth. We are always looking at ways to improve our customer experience and their health through unsurpassed diagnostic insights.

– RD Lab mission statement

> Laboratory investigations help doctors make better judgments in providing patient care and treatment. Many physicians are therefore ordering a complete range of lab investigations which include routine and advanced tests. We serve about 500 hospitals and smaller labs for advanced investigations. Outstation samples account for more than fifty per cent of our total load. The growing demand from outstation clients over the years is an indication of the trust placed on our lab by the clients that tests would be done properly and the results reported speedily. As a stand- alone lab, we have to generate demand, unlike hospital based labs. With more labs coming up, how could we remain competitive in the market?

The CEO of RD lab welcomed us with the above comments on the working of his lab. He wanted our inputs to help him plan the future growth of RD lab.

RD Clinical Lab

RD Lab was set up in 1972 with a load of 25 walk-in patients per day. Over the years, RD lab has grown into a full range NABL accredited diagnostic testing laboratory, with eight technical departments: Biochemistry, Clinical Pathology, Cytology, Cytogenetics, Hematology, Histopathology, Microbiology and Radiology. The growth of RD labs over the years can be seen in Exhibit 10.12.

RD Lab employed about 80 technical and 90 administrative staff. Technical staff included pathologists, microbiologists, cardiologists, MOs, sonologists, 12–15 phlebotomists, and 55–60 technical analysts. Its administrative staffs looked after Front office, Back office, Logistics, Accounts, HR, Marketing, and House Keeping activities. All the employees were covered by Star Health Insurance or Employee State Insurance schemes.

---

* Reproduced with the permission of the copyright owner.

Prepared by Professor K.V. Ramani, Indian Institute of Management, Ahmedabad.

Cases of the Indian Institute of Management, Ahmedabad, are prepared as a basis for classroom discussion. They are not designed to present illustrations of either correct or incorrect handling of administrative problems.

© 2012 by the Indian Institute of Management, Ahmedabad, Revised 22 May 2012.

Many small hospitals relied on a full reference laboratory such as RD Lab to satisfy their customer needs. These hospitals carried out only routine biochemistry and hematology investigations, but not immunoassay investigations (hormone-based investigations such as Thyroid, Fertility, Vitamin D3, B12 and so on). This was mainly because their test volumes for such sophisticated tests did not justify the economics of investment in equipment, reagents, people, and training.

RD lab had a large number of outstation clients, who collected samples and sent them to the lab for advanced tests. Its outstation clients included physicians, hospitals, insurers, employers, clinical research foundations, and other laboratories (Exhibit 10.13). The lab served about 500 hospitals and smaller labs, with outstation samples accounting for more than 50 per cent of the total load on investigations.

RD Lab had four city centres for sample collection in addition to the main lab. It also accepted outstation samples, i.e., samples collected by other institutions. It was a one-stop shop for all diagnostic needs covering a wide portfolio of Lab tests, ECG, X-ray, Ultrasound, TMT, ECHO, PFT, and Color Doppler. A consultant physician was available for pre-employment medical assessment, insurance assessment, and for in-lab supervisory needs. Consumers were assured of high quality services and reliable results at affordable prices.

Pre-analytic Phase

RD Lab which accepted samples collected elsewhere by its outstation clients (non-RD staff) faced several additional challenges in controlling pre-analytic lab errors, not commonly encountered by institutions which tested their own samples only. It was well known that about 60 per cent of lab errors occurred in the pre-analytical phase of sample collection, transportation, and submission of test-worthy samples to the lab sections for analysis.

Sample Collection: Even though RD Lab gave clear instructions to its outstation clients for sample collection by trained phlebotomists/nurses; it had no direct control on sample collection procedures by its outstation clients. RD Lab received samples along with the request slips for investigation (Test Request Form) which was usually handwritten. Transcription errors could result in collecting wrong samples and/or conducting wrong tests[vii]. RD Lab could not be responsible

[vii] Transcription errors arise mainly from handwritten/ineligible Test Request Forms ordered by the physicians. In one case, testosterone was wrongly read by the lab receptionist as progesterone. In another case, a nephrologists asked for iron profile with ferritin. This was a verbal request to the staff nurse in – large hospital. The nurse in turn wrote the test request which did not include ferritin. The lab was not aware of the need for ferritin and so the test was done without ferritin.

for wrong identification of patients and/or samples, insufficient sample, use of non-standard containers, sample integrity[viii] and so on.

Sample Transportation: Certain tests were time sensitive and required such samples to be given to the lab on time; for example, samples for hematology investigations should reach the lab in less than 24 hours. Certain tests as Ammonia, Lactic Acid (for liver function), Free Beta HCG for pre-natal screening required the samples to be transported at 2–8° Centigrade. There were restrictions in transporting certain biopsy specimens; for example, biopsy specimens for immunofluorescence had be transported only in a special medium (Michel's Medium) and putting the biopsy in formalin had to be avoided as this would invalidate the immuno-fluorescence procedures. Also, there were tests which required sample integrity of a very high nature, for example Ammonia and Lactic Acid tests to ensure test worthiness of the samples.

RD Lab took full responsibility for transportation of samples at no burden to the institutions, financial or logistics. It had a tie-up with reputed courier agencies which followed strict guidelines prescribed by the Lab and was also in compliance with national, regional or local regulatory requirements.

Sample Receipt and Registration: Upon receipt of sample parcels from courier agencies, RD Lab carried out a number of activities before submitting the sample for testing.

The first step, called Courier Verification, involved verifying the courier contents by matching the parcel descriptions (number of parcels, place of dispatch, source of dispatch: Hospital/Lab details and so on) with the label which accompanied each parcel.

Courier verification was followed by Parcel Verification, which involved making a record of the sample details (number of samples, patient details, sample temperature, and so on) of each parcel. It was a common practice in RD Lab to make a scanned copy of the test request form signed by the outstation clinician and save a copy in its Lab Information System (LIS).

Parcel verification was followed by Test Registration where each sample was registered in the LIS with test details and patient's ID. Great care had to be taken to ensure that all tests requested by outstation clients were registered.

After test registration, the LIS generated a barcode for each sample, and these labels were pasted on the outstation sample containers. The RD staff entered the

[viii] Sample integrity means sample should not be hemolysed, lipemic, icteric or clotting. Hemolysed samples contain RBC breaks. Lipemia (lipid disorder) indicates presence of fat in blood serum. Icterus blood means jaundiced blood. It is well known that hemolysed, lipemic, and icteric samples interfere with analytical measurements of various parameters such as glucose, creatinine, and cholesterol.

details in a sample tracking system and dispatched the samples to the Lab for further processing.

Analytic Phase

Sample processing in the lab[ix] started with specimen preparation which involved centrifugation, aliquotting[x], pipetting, dilution, and so on and handing over the test-worthy samples to the respective departments. Specimen adequacy, a critical pre-analytic factor, affected test result accuracy and usefulness. Samples failing to meet acceptable criteria had to be rejected. Accepting specimen unsuitable for analysis could lead to erroneous information that could compromise patient care.

RD Lab had a number of machines that could run high volume of sample batches. Blood samples were analyzed (depending on the tests) in a machine called Blood Analyzer. These were also called Auto Analyzers. Depending on the nature of the tests, different machines were used for analyzing the sample. During the testing process, chemical reagents were used on the sample, depending on what test was being performed. Different machines were used for performing different types of tests on different types of samples. Most of the automated blood analyzers in use, automatically generated the results in electronic format, and many of them were interfaced to a computer. For some tests, analysis was done within hours, while some tests could take 48–72 hours or even longer to get the results. It depended upon the complexity of the test, processing frequency in the lab and other factors that were inherent to the test such as culture, histopathology and so on.

Post-analytic Phase

The post-analytic phase involved two sub processes: one within the lab and the other outside the lab. The one inside the lab consisted of technical and medical validation of results, production of a report, and its transmission to the requesting clinicians. The sub process occurring outside the lab was the clinician's reaction to the report and its interpretation for diagnosis and treatment.

[ix] Certain large hospitals and labs use conveyor belts for moving the sample to the processing departments. This avoids technicians walking back and forth with the sample and also improves the internal work flow, as samples could immediately leave the sample station to the processing station through the conveyor belt.

[x] Aliquotting is the process by which blood serum obtained from centrifugation is transferred into 2–3 tubes for different tests to be performed. Aliquotting makes it possible to perform different tests in parallel and thereby saves time in reporting the test findings.

At RD Lab, after the samples were processed in multiple analyzers and equipments, the results were verified and validated as part of the internal quality control process. Sometimes if the figures seemed too abnormal, which pre-empted some serious investigation, the lab would call the referring doctor directly, discuss the issues, and re-do the tests for reconfirmation. After verification they were consolidated and the results were fed into LIS. From here the reports were sent to a senior pathologist, who performed one more round of scrutiny before signing off. This was followed by report printing if requested.

Once the reports were signed, they were available for collection. At RD Lab, multiple report collection choices were provided for customer convenience. Reports could be collected in person from the front office, through courier, fax, email, SMS or through a secure internet-based result reporting system[xi]. It was a common practice in RD Lab to print test reports only when requested, so as to minimize the possibility of giving the wrong reports by the front office. Reports pertaining to the samples could be securely accessed online, much ahead of the physical reports. These reports were identical to the hard copy reports including header, footer, watermark, and signature. If report volumes were high, an off-line version of this tool was made available, so that these reports could be generated even without internet connectivity.

After report generation, the client institutions were billed as per the charges mentioned in the 'Price Booklet' made available to the clients. RD lab offered volume discount on investigation charges to all its client institutions, a conscious policy taken by RD lab to keep its outstation clients happy.

Managerial Challenges

In order to safeguard patients' interests and promote quality in laboratory testing, it was necessary to go beyond the traditional view of quality control activities in the analytic phase within the laboratory. Reliance of the pre and post analytical activities was very important to assure analytical accuracy of test results, since a large per centage of laboratory mistakes occurred in the pre and post analytical phases. It was imperative to strengthen the linkage between the analytic staff within the laboratory with the clinicians and personnel outside the laboratory.

With outstation samples contributing to more than 50 per cent of the total load, any failure in the logistics chain from sample collection at source to transportation to sample testing lab could lead to sample rejection.

[xi] Some labs also offer the option of report collection through report vending kiosk located outside the lab (the reports can be collected anytime from the kiosk).

Questions

1. What were the various reasons for sample rejection?
2. What were the managerial challenges facing RD Lab for serving its outstation customers for sample testing and communicating the test results?
3. What measures were needed to minimize lab errors?
4. Comment on the efforts of RD Lab to generate and sustain demand from its remote clients?

Exhibit 10.12 Growth of RD Lab

Year	Important Event (Milestone)	No. of Patients per Day (*)
1974	Started laboratory	25
1980	Started RIA analysis for hormones	100
1993	Auto analyzer for chemistry, Radiology services	200
1998	Upgraded LIS	300
2001	Acquired more space for lab	400
2003	Renovated lab to open hall concept, Started sample pick up from labs	400
2005	Started collection center	600
2006	Integrated system for Chemistry and Immunoassay, Pneumatic	700
2009	Started immunohistochemistry	800
2010	Started outstation laboratory	1,000

* *Note:* Each patient would give 2–3 samples and each sample would be subjected to 3–4 tests.

Exhibit 10.13 Number of Patients from Outstation clients

Outstation Clients	2005	2006	2007	2008	2009	2010
CRO	27	306	799	973	521	1,105
Hospital lab	13,648	43,812	58,033	74,217	82,922	88,215
Insurance	125	516	444	409	199	173
Company	4,861	8,088	6,827	5,595	4,748	7,201
Physician lab	6,554	16,675	13,820	16,463	20,467	21,720
Stand alone lab	22,381	55,019	59,950	66,328	72,119	94,095
TPA	101	2,606	5,997	9,160	7,730	6,763
Total Outstation Clients	**47,697**	**127,022**	**145,870**	**173,145**	**188,706**	**219,272**

part 4

A Framework for Case Analysis

CHAPTERS

OBJECTIVE

The main objective here is to outline a systematic methodology for case analysis.

We bring out the similarities between managing the case of a patient's health by a doctor and managing the case of a hospital's health—hospital management.

chapter 11

Hospital Management Cases: A Framework for Analysis

CHAPTER OUTLINE

CHAPTER OBJECTIVE

The main objective of this chapter is to show the similarities between the management of a patient's health by a doctor and the management of a hospital, and, thereby, evolve a framework for a case study approach to hospital management.

11.1 AN INTRODUCTION

Case study approach is not new to doctors. In managing the health of a patient, a doctor begins with preparing a case sheet of the patient, and then proceeds logically step by step to diagnose the health problems and recommends a line of treatment.

In the next section, we discuss the process taken by doctors for treating their patients' health.

11.2 PATIENT HEALTH MANAGEMENT

Step 1 (Case Sheet Preparation): The doctor (whom we refer to as patient manager) begins his consultation with the patient by taking some basic information of the patient such as name, age, occupation, and so on. The patient then describes his health concerns, such as 'high temperature', 'sore throat' and 'frequent coughs'. The patient manager may ask a few questions to get some more insight into the patient's health condition and then makes a case sheet of the patient with the inputs received thus far.

Step 2 (Physical Examination): Based on the symptoms of the patient (high temperature, sore throat, constant cough), the patient manager makes a physical examination of the patient to understand the magnitude of the patient's health concerns. The patient manager takes the temperature to know how high the temperature is, since the prescriptions would differ if the patient's 'high temperature' is 99° F or 102° F. He then examines the patient's 'sore throat' to check for possible throat infection, since he would prescribe antibiotic only if the throat is infected.

Step 3 (Preliminary Diagnosis and Prescriptions): The patient manager makes a preliminary assessment based on the case sheet information and the results of physical examinations and prescribes certain medications. The patient manager would like to confirm his preliminary diagnosis with additional data and, therefore, orders investigations.

Step 4 (Order Investigations): Additional information may come from the patient's complaint about frequent coughs. The patient manager may order certain clinical pathology tests and a chest X-ray to find out the reasons for constant cough. The patient manager is, thus, seeking additional information in order to provide the best treatment possible.

Step 5 (Final Diagnosis and Prescriptions): Based on the results of clinical lab test results and the X-ray observations, the patient manager makes a final diagnosis. There may be situations where the patient manager may order more investigations before making a final diagnosis; for example, a microbiology test of throat culture.

Based on the final diagnosis, the patient manager may prescribe new medications or continue with the old medications.

Step 6 (Monitor and Control): The patient manager continues to monitor the patient's health and, therefore, asks the patient to come back for repeat consultation after 2–3 days.

If the patient manager is not happy with the progress of his patient's health, a different line of treatment may be followed. There may be situations when the patient manager may refer the patient to a specialist or recommend that the patient be admitted for indoor care. In the case of referrals to specialists, the patient goes through the same cycle with the specialist doctor.

In the next section, we extend the logic of patient health management to managing a hospital's health.

11.3 HOSPITAL HEALTH MANAGEMENT

Managing an organization essentially means managing the health of the organization. Hospital management is, therefore, all about managing the health of the hospital departments[i] to address the health concerns of the hospital.

To a hospital manager, hospital departments which are not doing well are like his patients. Hence, the steps followed by the hospital manager would essentially be the same as those followed by a doctor to manage a patient.

Step 1 (Case Sheet Preparation): Managing a hospital, therefore, starts with preparing a case sheet of the hospital. This case sheet is prepared from the inputs to the hospital manager from the hospital departments which are not doing well. Large OPD load, shortage of staff, and so on are some of the symptoms of the departments not doing well. These departments are seeking some recommendations to improve their health status so that they can carry out their activities better.

Step 2 (Physical Examination): Based on the above symptoms, the hospital manager conducts a physical examination of his patient departments to understand (quantitatively) how serious the symptoms are. The hospital manager needs data on the OPD load and the staff strength of these departments in order to make a preliminary assessment of their health status. It is possible that the medicine department in a hospital is short of nursing staff for its OPD services (since the medicine department in any hospital attracts the largest number of outpatients), while its department of pediatrics faces shortage of skilled pediatricians

[i] A patient manager attends to many patients, possibly with different health complaints. Similarly, a hospital manager would need to attend to the health complaints of many hospital departments, each department with its own health concerns.

for neo-natal intensive care unit (NICU), the surgical department may be short of surgical materials and its radiology department may not have an MRI to estimate the size of tumours in cancer patients.

Step 3 (Preliminary Diagnosis and Prescriptions): Based on the physical examination measurements, the hospital manager develops an understanding of the magnitude, complexity and nature of the health concerns of his patient departments, and makes a preliminary assessment of the 'illness' of these departments and prescribes some actions. It is necessary that the hospital manager confirms his preliminary assessments with additional information.

Step 4 (Order Investigations): The hospital manager orders some investigations (calls for additional data collection) to get a better insight into the illness of the patient departments. For example, he may want to know the number of new and repeat patients for medicine OPD, since all new OPD patients usually follow-up their first visit with 2–3 follow up visits for repeat consultation. It is important to realize that new patients demand more hospital resources than repeat patients. For example, case sheets are prepared only for new patients, more investigations are ordered for new patients than repeat patients, and so on. Detailed investigation of OPD load would, therefore, provide additional inputs for decision making regarding the allocation of resources.

Step 5 (Final Diagnosis and Prescriptions): Based on additional data from the patient departments through detailed investigations, the hospital manager makes a final diagnosis of his patient departments. If necessary, the hospital manager could ask for additional investigations, such as the details of cross referrals in medicine OPD to assist in the final diagnosis.

With data from the case sheets and additional information from detailed investigations, the hospital manager makes a final diagnosis and either continues with the treatment based on preliminary diagnosis or changes the line of treatment based on additional data from investigations. The final prescriptions could be in the form of additional nurses to medicine OPD, posting a visiting pediatrician in the NICU, and so on.

Step 6 (Monitor and Control): It is the responsibility of the hospital manager to monitor the health of the patient departments to find out if his prescriptions do improve their health conditions. For example, are the additional resources helping the medicine and pediatrics departments to deliver their OPD and NICU services better? If not, the hospital manager has to intervene and do the needful (control) to ensure good quality service delivery.

In the next section, we bring out the similarities between managing a patient's health and managing a hospital's health.

11.4 PATIENT MANAGEMENT VS HOSPITAL MANAGEMENT

Table 11.1 shows the comparisons of management practices in managing a patient vs managing a hospital. It can be seen that activities are similar if we consider hospital as a patient for hospital management.

Table 11.1 Comparing Patient Management vs Hospital Management

Steps	Activities	Patient Management (for Illustration)	Hospital Management (for Illustration)
1	Case sheet	Record the symptoms of the patient: High temperature Sore throat Frequent coughs	Record the symptoms of the patient department: Large OPD load Shortage of staff Frequent machine breakdowns
2	Physical examination	Measure temperature Check for throat infection	Measure OP load Assess staff strength and workload Record machine breakdown times
3	Preliminary diagnosis and prescription	Prescription based on case sheet and physical examination	Recommends managerial interventions based on inputs thus far
4	Order investigations	Order chest X-ray and throat culture to aid final diagnosis and prescriptions	Get additional details on OPD workload, staff workload and machine utilization so as to give final recommendations for improved service delivery
5	Final diagnosis and prescriptions	Change the medications or continue with the on-going medicines	Change the managerial intervention or continue with the on-going interventions
6	Monitor and control	Monitor the health and intervene if progress is not satisfactory	Monitor the service delivery and intervene when required

It is clear from the above sections, that the hospital management can be more or less equated with patient management, if we consider hospital as our patient.

Based on these observations, we discuss in the next section, a framework for case analysis.

11.5 A FRAMEWORK FOR CASE ANALYSIS

Based on the discussions so far, we suggest the following framework for case analysis.

11.5.1 A Preliminary Analysis

Step 1 (Preliminary Diagnosis): Here the focus is on arriving at a basic understanding of the problem on hand. Any problem has four dimensions:

1. Magnitude of the problem
2. Nature of the problem
3. Complexity of the problem
4. Uncertainty, if any

For example, for a case study on 'OPD service management', magnitude of the problem would include:

- Total number of OPD patients
- Distribution of OPD patients into new patients and repeat patients
- Service time for each service
- Number of service providers for each service
- Time when each service is available

The nature of the problem would include:

- Sequentially interdependent queuing system

The complexity of the problem would include:

- Weekly schedule of doctors for OPD, especially in a teaching hospital
- Weekly schedule of OPD for each specialty (not all specialties have OPD every day)
- Assigning patients to doctors for consultation: patients assigned to the same doctor for new and repeat visits

The uncertainty of the problem would include:

- Arrival rate (new and repeat patients) for each service
- Service rate (new and repeat patients) for each service
- An element of uncertainty even in the diagnosis

Step 2 (Preliminary Recommendations): Based on the preliminary case analysis, it would be possible to suggest some preliminary recommendations or avenues for preliminary recommendations under certain element of uncertainty.

11.5.2 Final Recommendations

Step 3 (Final Diagnosis): The main focus here is to remove/minimize the element of uncertainty in the diagnosis arrived at in Step 1. This requires additional data collection and analysis. Based on the analysis, 3–4 feasible options would emerge as candidates for recommendations.

Step 4 (Recommendation): The final step is to evaluate the consequences of each option and select that option which is 'best for the hospital'. What is 'best for the hospital' would be decided by a number of factors such as implementation feasibility, cost vs revenue, service quality, and so on.

In the following sections, we demonstrate the usefulness of the above framework for analysing a case study in hospital management.

11.6 CASE ANALYSIS: AN ILLUSTRATION

CMC Hospital, Vellore (A)

Step 1 (Preliminary Analysis): Exhibits 1 and 2 of the case in Chapter 6 provide an overall picture of the growth of the CMC Hospital over the years, its active engagement in patient care, teaching and research, as well as the OPD load in the year 2010–11.

It can be seen that the medicine department alone handles the maximum OPD load, as is usually the case in any general hospital. Hence, our analysis would first focus on improving the OPD service quality by the medicine department. The experience gained from studying the med–OPD services can be later extended to OPD services by other departments at CMCH.

Managerial problems can be described across four components:

1. Magnitude of the problem
2. Nature of the problem
3. Complexity of the problem
4. Uncertainty, if any

Let us discuss the above four dimensions in the context of OPD services at CMCH.

1. Magnitude of the Problem: Med-OPD load at CMC at 122,028 cases per year works out to roughly 400 cases per day, assuming OPD is available for 300 days in a year (except Sundays and public holidays).

1.1 OPD Load on Consultants and Registrars (Staff Resources): The med department has 12 consultants (not including other related disciplines), 12 registrars (senior post graduate students), 13 interns and three nurses.

The med department is divided into three med units:

- Med Unit 1
- Med Unit 2
- Med Unit 3

Each med unit has four consultants, four registrars and one nurse.

As mentioned in the case, every outpatient makes three visits on an average; the first visit as a new patient and two repeat visits. Given the daily load of 400 med-OPD patients, the medicine department has about 130 new patients and 270 repeat patients every day.

Let us assume that private patients account for roughly 30 per cent of the total number of OPD cases. Table 11.2, therefore, provides a distribution of private and general patients into new and repeat cases:

Table 11.2 Distribution of Outpatients

Med Department	Private	General	Total
New	40	90	130
Repeat	90	180	270
Total	**130**	**270**	**400**

Time for consultation: It is important to realize that doctors spend more time on consultation with a new patient than a repeat patient, whether the patient is private or general. This is true because the first consultation requires preparation of a case sheet, detailed physical examination, decisions on the type of investigation and medication. Repeat visits rely on the case sheets already prepared and the reports on investigations already ordered. Also, the number of additional investigations ordered, if any, for a repeat patient would be much less than the number of investigations ordered in her/his first visit.

Let us, therefore, assume that the first consultation takes an average of about 20 minutes per private patient and 15 minutes per general patient. Repeat consultation takes, say, 10 minutes per private patient and 5 minutes for a general patient. Please note that consultants are also engaged in undergraduate teaching during OPD hours in their OPD clinic.

Let us do some simple arithmetic to estimate the total time required for consultation for a daily load of 400 outpatients.

OPD hours are from 8 am to 5 pm.

For the consultants, their consultation for private patients takes up 7 hours. Add at least another hour for lunch and tea/coffee breaks. That makes it a full working day of 8 hours. Where is the time for visiting their inpatients in wards? Is it not true that the private inpatients expect at least one visit by their consultants every day?

For the registrars, their consultation for general patients alone takes up all the 9 hours of OPD duty! When do they visit their inpatients?

The same observations can also be made on the nurse in each OPD clinic.

It is, therefore, very common to see consultants and registrars working beyond their working hours on their OPD days.

1.2 Outpatient Waiting Time for Consultation: Please note that registration window closes at 11 am. If doctors stay till 6 pm to complete all their appointments for OPD consultation, imagine the waiting time for the general patient who is seen last at 6 pm! A waiting time of at least 7 hours assuming he/she was the last patient to be registered at 11 am.

2. Nature of the Problem: The OPD process is a sequentially interdependent queuing system. Therefore, investigation services would start only after consultation is complete. Let us understand the impact of delayed OPD consultation services on investigation services.

2.1 Consequences of OPD Consultation Load on Investigations: Let us now analyse the consequence of OPD load on investigation which follows consultation. As mentioned in the case, sample collection service is available only till 1 pm. Many labs put this time limit on sample collection so as to ensure that test reports are available for *all samples* collected, before the lab closes at 6 pm for the day.

What are the implications on OPD service quality if the sample collection closes at 1 pm?

It is obvious that any outpatient seen after 1 pm cannot give samples for investigations the same day. Hence, all the outpatients seen after 1 pm have to make another visit to the hospital the next day for giving samples.

Private patients: How many such cases are likely to be there every day, on an average? Given that there are 4 consultants every day, it means about 12–16 new private patients and 20–30 repeat private patients cannot complete the OPD cycle of registration, consultation, investigation and medication on the same day. What is the service quality?

General patients: In the case of registrars, each registrar can see about 20–30 general patients (new and repeat cases combined) between 8 am and 1 pm. This leaves behind about 170 general patients who cannot give samples the same day! What is the quality of OPD services to general patients?

Delay in sample collection would also arise for those patients who are advised to fast overnight and come next day for blood sugar tests.

As a result, about 200–220 outpatients (private and general combined) have to return to CMCH the next day for giving samples for the tests ordered the previous day. In other words, only about 50 per cent of the total OPD load can complete the cycle of OPD services any given day. Is this acceptable service quality?

Please realize that about 40 per cent of OPD patients are from the far-east. For them, even a delay by one day in getting hospital services increases their cost of boarding and lodging (for patients and their attendants). While patients may get sick leave, their attendants end up losing salaries/wages. Hence, the cost to outstation OPD patients is very high.

3. Complexity of the Problem

3.1 Medical Council of India (MCI) Norms on Teaching Hospitals: The MCI norms put several demands on each department for offering teaching, research and patient care. The CMCH has scheduled all the activities of the doctors over a three day period, with each med unit assigned one full day for OPD. Therefore, each med unit has two days every week for OPD services. Hence, the OPD schedule for the med units given in the case is as follows:

- Med Unit 1 has Mondays, Thursdays for OPD services
- Unit 2 has Tuesdays and Fridays for OPD
- Unit 3 has Wednesdays and Saturdays for OPD

What are the implications of these OPD schedules on service quality?

3.2 Referred Cases: The OPD process gets very complex if a patient is referred to a specialist department for further consultation. For example, if a med-OPD patient is referred by the medicine consultant to diabetes department for specialist consultation, then the med patient has to repeat the same OPD process cycle in the diabetes department as well. The situation gets more complex if the OPD days for the diabetes department are different from the med department. Not all departments have OPD every day in many hospitals. After completing the OPD process in the diabetes department, the patient is required to report back to the med consultant.

4. Uncertainty: There is uncertainty regarding the turnaround time for OPD patients (time from registration till OPD treatment is complete: uncertainty on the number of repeat visits).

There is also uncertainty regarding delays in sample collection, mentioned above. If advanced tests are ordered (such as microbiology investigations), there could be delays in getting test reports. Uncertainty is more in the case of referred patients.

Summary of Our Preliminary Analysis: Some of the observations from our preliminary analysis are:

- **Load on Service Provider:** Are the consultants and registrars over worked? Does it have any impact on their (medical) service quality?
- **Customer Service Quality**: Long waiting time for consultation, only 50 per cent could complete the OPD cycle of services any day. The remaining 50 per cent of the outpatients come next day to give samples for the tests ordered the previous day.
- Uncertainty in total turnaround time.
- Total cost to outstation patients (hospital + board + lodge)

Please add to the above list of questions.

Step 2 (Preliminary Recommendations): Options for preliminary recommendations are:

- Increase staff resources in med department, say, one additional consultant and a registrar.
- Start an evening counter for med-OPD services. If yes, restrict the morning registration to say 300 OPD patients. The remaining outpatients can be given consultation in the evening OPD clinic.

Questions

1. What is an ideal OPD load which can be handled by a doctor in the medicine department?
2. What is the ideal number of doctors and registrars for medicine department for the proposed ideal load?
3. What is an ideal waiting time for consultation for general patients? Note that private patients come only as per their appointment.
4. Would you consider evening clinic as an option?
5. If answer to Question 4 is yes, what are its implications on service quality vs additional cost to CMCH?
6. Should we augment staff resources and not have any evening clinic? For example, employ one more consultant and one more registrar to each med unit, in order to bring down the OPD load per doctor?
7. If the answer to Question 6 is yes, what is its impact on service quality, such as
   7.1 How much load would be reduced on the doctors?
   7.2 What impact will it have on customer waiting time for consultation?
   7.3 How many patients could complete the OPD cycle of registration, consultation, investigation and medication the same day?
8. If the answer to Question 6 is yes, what is its impact on additional costs incurred by CMCH?
9. What is a good trade-off between a higher level of service quality and increased cost to CMCH?
10. What are the implications of augmenting staff resources on the total turnaround time for OPD service, given that almost 40 per cent of outpatients are from the north-east?
11. Uncertainty in turnaround time. Uncertainty in the number of repeat visits. How to address these?

Step 3 (Final Diagnosis): In order to get more clarity (to confirm your preliminary diagnosis), what additional data is required? What analysis you would undertake?

Step 4 (Final Recommendations): We now leave the rest of the case analysis to the readers and come up with final recommendations.

Please complete steps 3 and 4 for your hospital or a sample hospital.

11.7 SUMMARY

In this chapter, we have outlined a framework for addressing various problems faced by hospital managers. The above framework has been found to be very useful by the author in his various assignments on hospital management. We will follow this framework for analysing each study in this book.

Index